Cases on Multimorbidity and Its Impact on Elderly Patients

Adil Hamad Alharthi
King Fahad Armed Forces Hospital, Saudi Arabia

A volume in the Advances in
Medical Diagnosis, Treatment, and
Care (AMDTC) Book Series

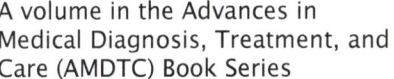 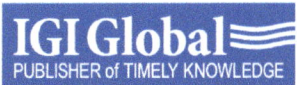

IGI Global
PUBLISHER of TIMELY KNOWLEDGE

Published in the United States of America by
    IGI Global
    Medical Information Science Reference (an imprint of IGI Global)
    701 E. Chocolate Avenue
    Hershey PA, USA 17033
    Tel: 717-533-8845
    Fax: 717-533-8661
    E-mail: cust@igi-global.com
    Web site: http://www.igi-global.com

Library of Congress Cataloging-in-Publication Data

Names: Alharthi, Adil, 1975- editor.
Title: Cases on multimorbidity and its impact on elderly patients / Adil
  Alharthi, editor.
Description: Hershey, PA : Medical Information Science Reference, [2023] |
  Includes bibliographical references and index. | Summary:
  "Multimorbidities is a common and important daily concept in Elderly
  patients and implies daily challenges to the treating internist. Our
  book is a practical case studies book aim for the internist on how to
  approach and manage different common aspect of Multimorbidities"--
  Provided by publisher.
Identifiers: LCCN 2022039347 (print) | LCCN 2022039348 (ebook) | ISBN
  9781668423547 (hardcover) | ISBN 9781668423554 (ebook)
Subjects: MESH: Multimorbidity | Geriatrics | Aged
Classification: LCC RC386.2 (print) | LCC RC386.2 (ebook) | NLM WT 100 |
  DDC 618.97/689--dc23/eng/20221025
LC record available at https://lccn.loc.gov/2022039347
LC ebook record available at https://lccn.loc.gov/2022039348

This book is published in the IGI Global book series Advances in Medical Diagnosis, Treatment, and Care (AMDTC) (ISSN: 2475-6628; eISSN: 2475-6636)

British Cataloguing in Publication Data
A Cataloguing in Publication record for this book is available from the British Library.

All work contributed to this book is new, previously-unpublished material.
The views expressed in this book are those of the authors, but not necessarily of the publisher.

For electronic access to this publication, please contact: eresources@igi-global.com.

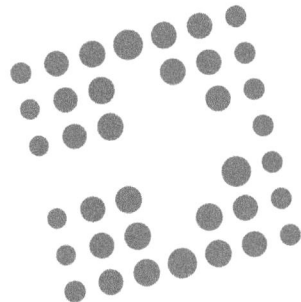

Advances in Medical Diagnosis, Treatment, and Care (AMDTC) Book Series

ISSN:2475-6628
EISSN:2475-6636

MISSION

Advancements in medicine have prolonged the life expectancy of individuals all over the world. Once life-threatening conditions have become significantly easier to treat and even cure in many cases. Continued research in the medical field will further improve the quality of life, longevity, and wellbeing of individuals.

The **Advances in Medical Diagnosis, Treatment, and Care (AMDTC)** book series seeks to highlight publications on innovative treatment methodologies, diagnosis tools and techniques, and best practices for patient care. Comprised of comprehensive resources aimed to assist professionals in the medical field apply the latest innovations in the identification and management of medical conditions as well as patient care and interaction, the books within the AMDTC series are relevant to the research and practical needs of medical practitioners, researchers, students, and hospital administrators.

COVERAGE

- Experimental Medicine
- Critical Care
- Diagnostic Medicine
- Emergency Medicine
- Chronic Conditions
- Medical Testing
- Internal Medicine
- Cancer Treatment
- Alternative Medicine
- Disease Management

IGI Global is currently accepting manuscripts for publication within this series. To submit a proposal for a volume in this series, please contact our Acquisition Editors at Acquisitions@igi-global.com or visit: http://www.igi-global.com/publish/.

Titles in this Series

For a list of additional titles in this series, please visit: http://www.igi-global.com/book-series/

Medical Cannabis and the Effects of Cannabinoids on Fighting Cancer, Multiple Sclerosis, Epilepsy, Parkinson's, and Other Neurodegenerative Diseases
Rana R. Zeine (Kean University, USA) and Brian W. Teasdale (Kean University, USA)
Medical Information Science Reference • © 2023 • 406pp • H/C (ISBN: 9781668456521) • US $345.00

Perspectives on Coping Strategies for Menstrual and Premenstrual Distress
B.S. Parimal (The Maharaja Sayajirao University of Baroda, India) and Kavita Gupta (The Maharaja Sayajirao University of Baroda, India)
Medical Information Science Reference • © 2023 • 344pp • H/C (ISBN: 9781668450888) • US $325.00

Pharmacological Benefits of Natural Agents
Narayanaswamy Radhakrishnan (St. Peter's Institute of Higher Education and Research (SPIHER), India) Srinivasan Vasantha (St. Peter's Institute of Higher Education and Research (SPIHER), India) and Ashok Kumar Pandurangan (B.S. Abdur Rahman Crescent Institute of Science and Technology, India)
Medical Information Science Reference • © 2023 • 335pp • H/C (ISBN: 9781668467374) • US $325.00

Cannabis sativa Cultivation, Production, and Applications in Pharmaceuticals and Cosmetics
Rafiq Lone (Central University of Kashmir, India) Aabid Hussain Mir (University of Kashmir, India) and Javid Manzoor (Jiwaji University, India)
Engineering Science Reference • © 2023 • 325pp • H/C (ISBN: 9781668457184) • US $250.00

Handbook of Research on Advanced Phytochemicals and Plant-Based Drug Discovery
Ajeet Singh (ICAR-Indian Institute of Wheat and Barley Research, India)
Medical Information Science Reference • © 2022 • 722pp • H/C (ISBN: 9781668451298) • US $545.00

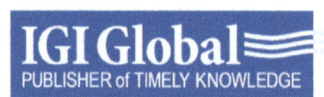

701 East Chocolate Avenue, Hershey, PA 17033, USA
Tel: 717-533-8845 x100 • Fax: 717-533-8661
E-Mail: cust@igi-global.com • www.igi-global.com

To my Family: my father and mother, my wife, my daughter Sarah and my son Hamad, for their continuous support.

Table of Contents

Detailed Table of Contents

Chapter 1
Multimorbidity, Ageing, and Frailty: Processes of Senescence and the
Pathologies of Progressive Functional Decline in Ambulation 1
  Catherine Hayes, University of Sunderland, UK

Being able to theoretically underpin the gerontology of ageing is a fundamental part of designing and constructing bespoke research and care interventions for the exploration of falls prevention in practice. Within the context of home care and community-based settings, being able to integrate falls prevention into the integrated care that older people receive, their ambulation, health, and wellbeing and subsequently their longevity in senior years can be extended and sustained in terms of quality and satisfaction. This chapter contextualises and frames falls and fall injuries as a societal challenge by deconstructing the characteristic physiological processes of senescence and identifying key areas for fundamental address in the prevention of falls 'in situ'. Chapter focus is predominantly aligned to those processes of natural senescence aligned with normal ageing processes, alongside those pathologies which constitute abnormal pathological processes, which occur more often in older adults as a consequence of these processes of senescence.

Chapter 2
Understanding Multimorbidity in the Elderly..27
  Adil Hamad Alharthi, King Fahad Armed Forces Hospital, Saudi Arabia
  Khalid Abdullah Almotari, King Fahad Armed Forces Hospital, Saudi Arabia
  Abdulaziz Ali Alghamdi, King Fahad Armed Forces Hospital, Saudi Arabia

Multimorbidity is the presence of two or more long-term conditions which are those that cannot be currently cured but can be controlled. Chronic conditions are the leading cause of death globally. The World Health Organization (WHO) predicted that 87% of deaths in high income countries were attributed to chronic conditions and the proportion of worldwide deaths caused by chronic conditions is expected to rise from 59% in 2002 to 69% in 2030. Fifty-five to ninety-eight percent of people 60 years or older are affected by two or more chronic diseases and patients with multimorbidity account for up to 80% of consultations with general practitioners and virtually all consultations with Geriatricians. Among the reasons are that Co-occurring diseases interact with each other increasing the risk of negative events beyond the sum of the risk of each disease alone.

Chapter 3

    Mahwash Iftikhar, Hayatabad Medical Complex, Pakistan
    Ayesha Jamal, Corydon Medical Clinic, Canada
    Mian Mufarih Shah, Hayatabad Medical Complex, Pakistan
    Sheraz Jamal Khan, Hayatabad Medical Complex, Pakistan

With obesity there is an increase in relative risk of type 2 diabetes, hypertension, and cardiovascular diseases. These can induce a vicious circle of a downward spiral of morbidity and mortality. Obesity is also associated with disability and health costs. In the US alone, it is $192.2 billion. This would be a formidable worldwide cost if interpolated globally. Obesity is also associated with sleep disturbance, respiratory difficulties, joint and mobility disorders, as well as social stigma. Treatments are varied and multifaceted and one shoe does not fit all. The different treatments are a low caloric diet (600 calories/day—this is quite debatable in the elderly); motivational and behavior approaches to sustain changes in eating and activity, these too need a lot of dedicated workforce; and drug treatment should be regarded as a therapeutic trial. Drugs should be stopped if there is no weight loss in two months' time. All drugs have side effects.

Chapter 4

    Adil Hamad Alharthi, King Fahad Armed Forces Hospital, Saudi Arabia
    Tabish Iqbal, Wadi Addawasir Military Hospital, Saudi Arabia
    Muhammad Adnan Haider, King Fahad Armed Forces Hospital, Saudi Arabia

Heart failure is a common disease worldwide. It is also an aging disease, being more common in the elder population; it is a multimorbidity disease as well, multimorbidity with heart failure became the norm; despite that, heart failure guidelines are still disease-specific, as well as multimorbidity and geriatric ignorant. To understand the unique, multimorbid, and geriatric characteristics of heart failure, one needs to understand the nature of the disease to shed light on the heart failure pathophysiological areas still in the shadows. Also needed is an understanding of symptom clusters in heart failure, their significance, and their unique relationship to each other.

Khawar Shabbir, University of Auckland, New Zealand
Adil Hamad Alharthi, King Fahad Armed Forces Hospital, Saudi Arabia
Aisha Alshehri, King Fahad Armed Forces Hospital, Saudi Arabia
Danyah Ahmed Katlan, King Fahad Armed Forces Hospital, Saudi Arabia
Alaa Shahbar, Umm Alqura University, Saudi Arabia

In many cases, the prescription medications are not taken as prescribed is because of failure to adhere to the medication regimen. The reason for not adhering to drug treatment include unpleasant or inconvenient side effects of the medications; dry mouth, change in taste, fatigue or frequent urination are various reasons of stopping a mediation. Older adults are at higher risk for medication nonadherence due to prevalence of multiple comorbidities, including cognitive deficit and polypharmacy. Medication adherence can be enhanced by considering geriatric's vision, hearing, swallowing, cognition, motor impairment, and health literacy while providing counselling and education. On the positive side, a study found that increased medication adherence was associated with fewer hospitalizations and decreased cost in patients with certain chronic medical conditions (e.g., diabetes, hypertension).

Aikaterini Christogianni, Loughborough University, UK
Suhaiza Hanim Suroya, Loughborough University, UK

Co-/multi-morbidities are prevalent in the elderly. Some noteworthy examples include the elderly with dementia, for example, elderly with Alzheimer's disease, Parkinson's disease dementia and vascular dementia diagnoses. Based on high prevalence rates, the elderly with dementia is likely to experience more than one disease. Usual co-/multi-morbidities in the elderly with dementia are epilepsy, diabetes, and cardiovascular diseases. For this reason, healthcare providers are tremendously challenged with demands for treatment and therapy plans to improve the quality of life and overall well-being of the elderly and their families. This Chapter discusses these co-/multi-morbidities and aims to inspire the translation of this knowledge into specialised services and therapy plans for the elderly.

Chapter 7

Karen Cordovil, Oswaldo Cruz Foundation, Brazil
Masato Hada, Independent Researcher, Japan
Zagami Francesco, Tabaka Mission Hospital, Kenya
Adil Al-Harthi, King Fahad Armed Forces Hospital, Saudi Arabia
Taha Hussein Musa, Southeast University, China

Sarcopenia is a generalized loss of muscle mass affecting muscle function and strength with age. The cause of sarcopenia is multifactorial and physiopathological mechanisms, including the decline of neuron numbers, changes in muscle metabolism, oxidative damage, reduced response to nutrients, and inflammation throughout proinflammatory cytokines that increase myofibrillar protein degradation and decrease protein synthesis. This chapter presents two case reports about sarcopenia and its associated multimorbidity impact on elderly patients. Sarcopenia in the elderly, when it advances to generalized muscle wasting, is mainly associated with multimorbidity which becomes a diagnostic, therapeutic, and palliative challenge to the physician; in these cases, a multidisciplinary approach is best for appropriate diagnosis and management results in a high-quality patient care setting.

Chapter 8

Ear, Nose, and Throat Complications and Challenges in the Elderly With

Samuel Oluyomi Ayodele, Obafemi Awolowo Teaching Hospital
        Complex, Nigeria

Elderly patients will not only present to specialists with specific ear, nose, and throat (ENT) complaints but will also seek treatment for comorbidities that have significant impacts on their quality of life; as well as the prognosis of the specific disease being managed the specialist with an increased demand on health care resources. While the principles of management of ENT disorders in the elderly are not so different from what is obtainable for other age groups, it is very important to take note of the specific differences and apply individualized treatment plan for better outcome. ENT diseases in the elderly may also present with unexpected or uncommon symptoms and this will mean that management must be carried out with caution. Medication dosage, performance scale, extent of surgical operations, and other treatment modalities are considerable in management of elderly ones. Subtle complaints from the elderly should not be over looked or managed by unqualified personnel. They should be referred early to specialists for proper management.

Stress is one of the main causes of various psychological and physiological changes. Those type of changes cause by excessive secretion of stress hormones like cortisol and adrenaline into the blood stream from adrenal gland in kidney. There is underline neuroendocrine pathways which carries signals from hypothalamus to pituitary gland than secretion of adrenocorticotropic hormone which ultimately stimulates the Adrenal cortex and release the Epinephrine and nor Epinephrine. When the cortisol and adrenaline level increase in blood stream. That causes the physiological changes like elevated level of blood pressure, glucose level, dilation of pupil and immunological response, as soon as, the threat is subsides this level down towards the normal. It is also a leading cause of hospitalization, especially in the elderly population. Elderly people who have comorbidities like Alzheimer's, cardiovascular disorders are more prone to wards minor stressors, it worsens their disease. It is essential to overcome the stress in elderly through various methods e.g., music therapy, social support.

This chapter will enlighten you to know about cognitive functions in the elderly and how these functions get affected and lead to downfall progression (neurodegeneration) with aging not only in terms of structural changes but also functional which cause age-associated illnesses. The evidence of cognitive deficit is obvious among the elderly population and needs to be tackled very effectively in keeping the view of maintaining functional independence in their routine activities. Throughout the chapter, different phenomena related to age-associated disorders and comorbidity have highlighted the high frequency of cognitive impairment and we will also be going to know about the role of the COVID-19 pandemic in worsening these symptoms. Neuropsychological assessment at an early stage plays a crucial role in pointing out cognitive deficits earlier which can further lead to decelerating of symptoms through pharmacological and psychosocial rehabilitation.

Chapter 11

An argument is made that multi-morbidity can be distinguished between three categories: male, female, and elderly. Another identifier linked to multi-morbidity is military service and veterans. Managed care and care planning are offered as common solutions when managing elder care. The topics of hypoxia, palliative care, abdominal distention, and pharmacology are examined to show their effects on elder care and multi-morbidity. For multi-morbidity, the role of chronic illnesses as a public health stressor must also be examined. Cases, solutions, and other outcomes in this chapter will discuss the overall diagnosis in some patients. Financial management in healthcare gains nominal attention because of its importance in our society, culture, and human behaviors.

Preface

The geriatric population is growing and it's expected to further grow in the future. One of the unique characteristics of this population is multimorbidity, which is having two or more chronic diseases. Any clinician treating elder people appreciates that multi morbidity in the elderly is now the norm rather than the exception, in spite of that we still lack clear, internationally agreed, multimorbidity management and prevention guidelines, compared to disease specific guidelines. We also need randomized controlled trials that contain a high multimorbidity sample contribution to give a fair representation of our elder patients with multimorbidity. We also need more longitudinal studies about multimorbidity, disease clustering, disease to disease interaction in the same cluster, its consequences, and its hazards and thus it's clinical translation. Due to multimorbidity in Elderly, elder people need multidisciplinary management teams. Healthcare providers managing elder people with multimorbidity need to understand and appreciate multimorbidity in its meaning, its risk factors, its significance on the patient's physical, mental, behavioral, cultural, and religious aspects, and the preventive strategies appropriate for it. We chose some topics that are of utmost importance in understanding multimorbidity and its impact on the elder population. Firstly, in order to understand multimorbidity, frailty and the effects of diseases on the elder patients, we need to understand the physiological changes of old age, it's reserve limitations and its physiotherapy and psychological empowerment and adaptation capabilities. Then we will talk about multimorbidity, its definition, its risk factors, its relation to frailty and the disease cluster concept, its relation to socio-economic status, and patient centered care, and its types most suitable to manage elders with multimorbidity. After that, we will talk about heart failure which is a fairly common disease worldwide and it is mostly related to the Elders with multimorbidity. We will review some of its underappreciated and under read pathophysiological mechanisms, the importance of the symptom cluster concept in heart failure, and we will review the guideline targeted management for heart failure patients. We will also talk about obesity in elderly and its relation with multimorbidity, its metabolic consequences, it's hazards and complications and the suggested therapeutic and preventive plans to manage it as well. After that we will talk about the important topic of medication non-adherence. We will review a practical day-to-day clinical case to draw out a couple of important topics related to medication nonadherence in Elders with multimorbidity and discuss them in details with the review of the literature for example, polypharmacy, depression, doctor-patient relationship, etc. Of the important topics in Elder with multimorbidity is dementia. We will discuss the prevalence, characteristics, complications of dementia associated with other chronic diseases like epilepsy and diabetes with the review of the recent medical literature. It is important to talk about sarcopenia in elder patients with multimorbidity as well, its definition, epidemiology, characteristic challenges. Then we will review two practical day-to-day cases as a doorway to talk about important concepts like sarcopenia in dementia, stroke related sarcopenia, sarcopenic obesity, and the review of artificial nutrition in older patients with advanced dementia. Followed by an interesting detailed review of the ENT manifestations and complications of the elderly with multimorbidity. Followed by an interesting literature review Of the manifestations and complications of stress in elder patients with Alzheimer's disease and it's relation to multimorbidity. Then we will talk about cognitive impairment in the elderly it's prevalence, importance, possible progression, different neurological types and its relation to multimorbidity. We will conclude with a literature review about the social, cultural and behavioral disparities in multimorbidity, the vulnerable populations with multimorbidity, the financial and cultural challenges and barriers in managing multimorbidity in elderly people around the world. Our reference studies are intentionally chosen from different countries in Europe, America, Asia, India, also involving both urban and rural populations as well in order to come up with an international, fair, practical and valid information about multimorbidity in the elderly, to attract the interest of the healthcare provider about its importance and possible complications and to promote them to activate multidisciplinary teams to better manage them. It's also a message to the researchers interested in trials related to elders with multimorbidity to further embark in the areas less investigated to upgrade our understanding of multimorbidity in the elderly, and thus improve our management and preventive strategies against it.

Adil Hamad Alharthi
King Fahad Armed Forces Hospital, Saudi Arabia

Chapter 1
Multimorbidity, Ageing, and Frailty:
Processes of Senescence and the Pathologies of Progressive Functional Decline in Ambulation

Catherine Hayes
University of Sunderland, UK

EXECUTIVE SUMMARY

Being able to theoretically underpin the gerontology of ageing is a fundamental part of designing and constructing bespoke research and care interventions for the exploration of falls prevention in practice. Within the context of home care and community-based settings, being able to integrate falls prevention into the integrated care that older people receive, their ambulation, health, and wellbeing and subsequently their longevity in senior years can be extended and sustained in terms of quality and satisfaction. This chapter contextualises and frames falls and fall injuries as a societal challenge by deconstructing the characteristic physiological processes of senescence and identifying key areas for fundamental address in the prevention of falls 'in situ'. Chapter focus is predominantly aligned to those processes of natural senescence aligned with normal ageing processes, alongside those pathologies which constitute abnormal pathological processes, which occur more often in older adults as a consequence of these processes of senescence.

DOI: 10.4018/978-1-6684-2354-7.ch001

INTRODUCTION

With increasing numbers of older adults living beyond the age of 65 years, so too is there a corresponding increasing number of falls in the home, which constitute the most significant number of injuries in adults of this specific age group (Moreland et al., 2020). Statistical analysis reveals that the risk of falls increases exponentially with age, which can lead to potentially long-term issues and challenges with the maintenance of ambulatory wellbeing as a consequence of resultant physical disability or impairment, and consequently contributes to poorer outcomes in quality and longevity of life (Tornero-Quiñones et al., 2020). Fatalities arising as a consequence of falls in those aged over 65 years and can be attributed to up to one third of all accidental deaths in this age group (Mielenz et al., 2020). These rates of mortality are largely preventable in relation to those necessitating long term care within nursing home and residential care settings (Drake et al., 2021). It is the normal processes of senescence, which impact on the physiological decline of ageing adults (Katsuumi, 2018; Faragher, 2017). Being able to accommodate and account for these within complex individual physical and social care provides a sound rationale for the integration of falls prevention strategies in the overall health continuum for older adults, where modifications can be made to prevent risk of future falls (Khong et al., 2017). Since once an older adult has fallen once, they are statistically two thirds more likely to fall again over the next 12 months, this can be a significant means of avoiding elevated rates of morbidity and mortality in this age group (Bartosch et al., 2020; Gazibara et al., 2017). This chapter constitutes a theoretical contribution to the gerontology of ageing, so that the target audience can potentially develop a comprehensive knowledge and understanding of the physiological processes of senescence. For those professionals seeking to align strategic interventions with what is practically achievable remains one of the greatest challenges in this field of gerontology (Schapmire et al., 2018; Skinner et al., 2017). Encouraging active and healthy processes of ageing not only benefits individual members of society, it has wider economic implications for health services, which deal with the implications of normal physiological senescence as greater numbers of older adults live into old age and, as a consequence of this, are more likely to live with morbidities which impact on their ambulatory health and wellbeing (Alcañiz & Solé-Auró, 2018).

Functional senescence is part of a normal process of physiological ageing. This encompasses the gradual deterioration of the organs and systems of the body alongside a progressively decreasing capacity for function by the body's processes of homeostasis (He & Sharpless, 2017). In terms of finality, the process of senescence leads to progressive dysfunction and eventual death. The fact that this is a normal trajectory for the ageing body also provides an insight into how disease and ageing synergistically contribute to the acceleration of death in older adults (Herranz & Gil,

2018). Providing an understanding of the basic physiological knowledge within the context of the process of senescence and disease, and their relevance to potential falls prevention initiatives is the overall aim of this chapter.

INTERRELATIONSHIPS OF MULTI-MORBIDITY AND SENESCENCE

As part of the trajectory of chronological ageing, statistical evidence provides an insight into the correlation between increasing age and increasing abnormal pathology. In this sense ageing is a natural process of physiological decline characterised by processes of physical change (Tieland et al., 2018). It is these processes of the ageing process which can be attributed to the often very serious consequences of illness, which amongst their younger counterparts, may be perceived and experienced as relatively minor. Comorbidities in ageing individuals are far more common in adults aged 65 years and older and these directly impact on the development, prognosis, and consequent management of illness (van Onna & Boonen, 2016). Those systems such as the neurological, vascular, respiratory and musculoskeletal systems demonstrate clear processes of degeneration with age, and as ageing progresses, pathology is statistically far more likely to present as being symptomatically atypical, meaning prompt assessment, diagnosis and management can be significantly delayed (Bisdorff et al., 2013). Depending on the nature of these presenting conditions, some of which may be progressive or even metastatic, in instances of cancer, this can have devastating consequences, which might otherwise have been far more treatable, if diagnosed at an earlier stage of the disease process. Similarly, many conditions arising in middle age or earlier may progress to conditions which in combination with natural processes of senescence can be potentially far more serious (Dodig et al., 2019).

Indicators of pathological processes, which might ultimately impact upon holistic processes of health and wellbeing are characterised by medical histories which for example may detail those conditions which were contracted or experienced in earlier life and which are now inactive but which may have a direct impact on an older person's capacity to cope with disease processes or indeed the degree of immune response they illicit in relation to infection (Rice et al., 2017). These medical histories may also provide an insight into current disease processes which are ultimately controlled by pharmacological and lifestyle changes, such as Diabetes mellitus or hypertension (Sciomer, 2019). In relation to this there can be an array of associated side effects of pharmacological interventions, which also mask signs and symptoms of pathologies which would benefit from early clinical diagnosis and management. The majority of these conditions can have a degree of relevance to the prevention of falls in ageing populations, since many develop slowly and can be termed progressive in terms of their degenerative impact. Typical example is atherosclerosis, which necessitates regular clinical monitoring so that medication can be appropriately modified to account for different stages of pathological change. Other conditions such as Multiple sclerosis or Rheumatoid arthritis can have relapsing and remitting stages, where preventative care in relation to the potential for temporary or progressive changes in ambulatory health and wellbeing can be successfully managed (Briggs et al., 2019; Mankia & Emery, 2019). This can have a direct impact on the overall longevity of these older adults where care interventions and preventative measures ought to be tailored to the individual needs of each (Stambler, 2017). The value of interprofessional and multi-disciplinary working arrangements between medical and allied healthcare practitioners cannot be underestimated here, and the capacity of these team members to accommodate functional change in ambulatory wellbeing is invaluable in the functional physiological avoidance of falls (Kenny et al., 2017).

COMPLEX MEDICAL HISTORIES AND FALLS IN AGEING POPULATIONS

Of those diseases, which more commonly manifest in ageing populations, many predispose older adults to falls, even those which may have started at an earlier stage in the life course trajectory (Brännström et al., 2019). In conjunction with this, the assessment, diagnosis and prompt management of conditions is made more complex by the fact that older people are far more likely to present with atypical or very non-specific signs, which are often overlooked and quite wrongly attributed to 'old age' (Buttigieg et al., 2018). What is worthy of note here, is that there is no one specific disease state that is particular to age, although the likelihood of occurrence may increase as part of normal processes of physiological senescence. Those disease states regarded as relatively minor in younger adults or children, can therefore lead to more serious outcomes for older people, especially in relation to falls when older adults are statistically far more likely to develop neurological, skeletal, or vascular pathologies, all of which have a potentially direct and negative impact on the quality and longevity of life (Cho et al., 2018). Given that these conditions rarely exist in abstraction from one another the higher numbers of pathologies evident in older adults can complicate diagnoses and predispose them to a greater likelihood of falling (Padrón-Monedero et al., 2020).

FUNCTIONAL DEFINITIONS OF 'OLD AGE'

Operationalising a functional definition of 'old age', is fraught with the danger of labelling someone on the basis of the chronology of their age, rather than their stage of functional senescence. Since ageing incorporates the age-related changes of functional decline (senescence) and those processes of pathological change which ought not to be normalised, since there is the potential for them to be identified as treatable and as a consequence curable or at least manageable. The associated decline in vitality and the reduction in physiological performance at a cellular level can lead to a reduced capacity to cope with environmental stressors and a correspondingly reduced capacity to cope either physically or psychologically with processes and outcomes of disease. Ageing is a slow and iterative process, which is largely variable impact at an individual level. The homogenisation that the term 'old age' brings to a whole generation is neither useful clinically or socially and often leads only to unintentional ageism, which directly impacts on the ability of older adults to access healthcare resources to the same extent as their younger counterparts (Covey, 1992). The need for accurate diagnosis and management of pathology ought not to be secondary to the recognition and value judgement attributable to changes in the visible appearance of people and biased assumptions of their physiological or anatomical status as a consequence. What cannot be denied is that the normal ageing process leads to death and that ageing impacts on all chronologically old people to a greater or lesser extent. The progressive and gradual deterioration of functionality and a lack of capacity for regulatory homeostasis in response to external stressors ensures a steady and progressive decline. Cytologically, there is a natural decline in the number of functional cells and in terms of medical assessment there is often a degree of ambiguity in relation to which cells are actually malfunctioning due to physiological change or whether these can, with any degree of confidence be attributed to the ageing process. Ultimately, there is no medical intervention that can halt this process and as a consequence the optimal quality of life for patients ought sometimes to be prioritised before the extension of their longevity. This systematic vulnerability to both disease and external stressors of human physiology are what actually characterise what is traditionally attributed to 'old age'. Disease and ageing in this sense, progressively and systematically cause the acceleration in a reciprocal and irreversible process.

FUNCTIONAL ANATOMICAL CHANGES IN AGEING

As an integral part of the ageing process, there are distinctive anatomical changes in organs and physiological alterations that primarily lead to:

- Compromised neurotransmission.
- Decrease in intellectual performance (e.g., leading to failing memory and confusion).
- Decreased renal perfusion.
- Deterioration of special senses (e.g., leading to poor vision and loss of hearing).
- Exacerbation of deformity (due to the rigidity of collagen).
- Poor breathing capacity.
- Poor oxygen uptake.
- Reduced cardiac output.
- Reduction in movement potential.
- Reduction in nerve conduction velocity.

PROGRESSIVE NERVOUS SYSTEM CHANGE IN AGEING

The sensitivity of the sympathetic receptors to circulating neurotransmitters is altered by the process of natural senescence in ageing. The greater intensity of response in the cardiac and vascular systems in older people have led to this being termed a hyperadrenergic state. In relation to a functional optimal nervous system in older years, no system demonstrates more clearly the need to remain active and to maintain a healthy lifestyle which engages capacity for ambulatory wellbeing and the prevention of falls in later life. The neurological system is dynamic in the sense that it changes throughout adulthood, but this trajectory of change increases exponentially after the age of sixty-five years. This manifests in a decreased awareness to the sensations of touch and vibration (Mahbub, 2020). Increasing numbers of neurofibrillary tangles which develop within nerve cell bodies as a consequence of ageing are evident in the hippocampus. This is seen across all older people but to an even greater extent in those patients living with dementia. Those who have dementia have an increased number of neurotic or senile plaques, which have come to characterise the anatomical and physiological changes of Alzheimer's disease (Sengoku, 2020). Senile plaques are thickened masses of degenerating neurites (constituted of small axons, some dendrites, astrocytes) with an amyloid (starchy glycoprotein) deposit in the centre. Plaques most commonly occur as a result of pathological ageing, as in Alzheimer's disease, although they have also been frequently observed in normal ageing, beginning in the fifth decade of life (Sharma et al., 2020).

From the perspective of biochemistry, the decrease in enzymes actively involved in processes of neurotransmitter synthesis has been recorded alongside a diminishing number of receptor sites or transmitters within the central nervous system and the peripheral nervous system. The reduction in motor system functionality is linked to the progressive decrease of dopamine uptake sites, which can be directly attributed to the loss of axons in basal ganglia pathways as part of age-related change. Higher order association areas lose a greater number of neurons than the primary motor or visual cortex during the process of ageing, which has led to theories of how forgetfulness develops in older adulthood. Even a minor degree of neuron loss and decline in the capacity of dendrites to produce new spines has an impact. Whilst structural losses can be attributed to age related decline, which is also associated with processes of synaptic remodelling. This is closely linked to an overall decrease in sensory perception, alongside the presence of arteriosclerosis.

The functional implications of these changes all impact on the reaction time of older people. These processes are often attributed to the overall slowing of reaction time and the process of voluntary motor movement. Linked to physiological changes in muscles, this is another clear indicator of the need for older people to maintain a degree of physical fitness, which contributes to the maintenance of optimal reaction time in old people (Toots et al., 2019). Exercise in itself is not proven to significantly improve reaction time though, since movement slowness is related to change in neural pathways rather than to the extent of muscle health alone. Reaction time can basically be defined as the length of time between stimulation and the motor response effected by it. It is also associated with nerve conduction velocity. In terms of growth and development at the other end of life's trajectory, reaction time progressively improves as a child develops more complex and developed motor skills. Scientific studies of complex reaction time detail that in research where there is a choice between two responses, that as the task becomes progressively more complex, then reaction time increases in line with the increasing age of the study participant. The complex neurological processes involved in maintaining balance, mean that the individual risk of falls is exponentially higher in relation to their age, and this is accompanied by a variable change in reaction times during progressive ageing, once people reach the age of 60 years.

In the prevention of falls, older patients typically may be living with a number of chronic disease states, for which they may be taking an equal number of medications. These systemic issues are predisposing factors to falling, which have a wider impact than just that of the individual who experiences them. Despite this, the chronologically aged ought never to be regarded as an indistinguishable category of personhood for whom there is minimal potential for the prevention of falls or systemic deterioration. The role of the health and social care multi-disciplinary team is invaluable in fulfilling this in the most optimal manner possible for the elderly.

FUNCTIONAL COGNITIVE ABILITIES

The synergistic relationship between the sensory and motor system is the basis for theories of intelligence, where cognition can be defined as the process of knowing and intelligence pertains to the application of knowledge (Sari et al., 2020). Cognitive processes specifically include:

- Attention.
- Decision making.
- Learning.
- Problem solving.
- Reasoning.

Without a degree of cognitive ability, negotiating the process of human ambulation is impossible and movement development is completely diminished. It is the nervous system which is responsible for cognition via the processing of thought and memory, where memories can be classified according to whether they are immediate, short, or long term in duration. Whereas declarative memory entails the immediacy of memory, which may only last seconds or at most minutes, longer term memories can be recalled years later as they result in structural changes to the synapses that have a long-lasting impact on signal conduction pathways. Ageing ensures an active decrease in capacity to undertake complex cognitive skills which involve memory. In those adults who are living with movement decline, it is also exceptionally important to consider their potential for change in memory ability.

Alongside these considerations, are considerations of what are termed either fluid or crystallised intelligence. Whereas fluid intelligence pertains to the logical capacity to form novel associations, and can be readily measured via tests of reaction time and memory, crystallised intelligence is linked to experience and the learning associated with it. Whereas fluid intelligence peaks early in the second decade and then diminishes, crystal intelligence forms the basis of wisdom and is deemed to increase with time. The reason why some adults remain alert and active mentally and others disengage or show signs of dementia still remains largely unknown and highlights the need for further research, which inevitably will impact on the field of falls prevention research.

Sensory Deficits

Motor activity in adulthood is guided by the sensory ability developed during adolescence. Decline in sensory function begins in adulthood and is progressive in nature. It is important that these may or may not link to a general decline in function and not necessarily all people experience them. From a somatic perspective, some ageing adults demonstrate a clearly diminished ability to effectively detect touch, vibration, temperature, and pain (Borzuola et al., 2020). The largest of the body's sense organs, the skin undergoes distinctive changes with ageing. From a structural perspective, the growth rate of the skin and its capacity to regulate temperature, injury response and to undertake growth diminish. Whilst extremes of temperature can be readily detected by older adults, their capacity to detect subtle temperature change is diminished. The sympathetic nervous system controls the degree of vasoconstriction and vasodilation to the skin, and this is also impaired. Pain perception is still not fully understood in relation to the ageing process. Whilst deep pain diminishes with age, as yet research reports both an increase and a decrease in superficial pain sensitivity. What is abundantly clear, however, is the degree of vibrationary sensation diminishment which occurs in older adults usually starting at around the age of 50 but mainly in the feet and legs. The decline in sense of where joint positions are in space declines more evidently in women, particularly in relation to static joint position sensation at the knee joint, which may or may not be attributable to the functional impact of a gynaecoid pelvic girdle and the position the knees relative to the hips, but this has not yet been proven (Maitre et al., 2013). This can impair balance and may contribute to the increased incidence of reported falls in elderly women, which is a significant aetiological factor in all-cause mortality and morbidity.

Motor Deficits

The incidence of vertigo and dizziness are very common presentations in general practice in patients aged over 50 years. The vestibular system and in particular hair cells are demonstrably degenerating with the consequent symptomology of dizziness. In relation to the vestibular nerve, by the time a person reaches the age of 75 years, the overall amount of myelinated nerve fibres has been reduced to just 60% (Liu et al., 2017). As a consequence of this, reliance on the vestibular system alone can result in falls, an important consideration in falls prevention strategies. Healthy older people with less of a degree of sensory deficit, have less of a degree of postural sway than those who do and as a consequence are far less likely to fall.

Ocular Changes

With a general increase in visual acuity increases in the twenties and thirties, which remains largely unaltered through to the forties and then declines, it is notable that by the age of 85 years there is an 80% less of visual acuity (Saftari & Kwon, 2018). It is the anatomical structural changes in the eye, which contribute to the apparent functional change. Accompanying processes of ageing, central vision may be impacted upon by the development of cataracts, which cause alteration of the lens. By the time people reach the age of 65, it is estimated that 60% of all people have a general reduction in their lens transparency (Donaldson et al., 2017). Cases of cataracts are more common in patients living with Diabetes mellitus.

VISUAL CHANGE IN RELATION TO THE POTENTIAL OF FALLS

Progressively the eye yellows due to the functional ageing process (Saftari & Kwon, 2018). The overall pupil size decreases and less light can enter the eye. By the time a person reaches the age of 60 years, the pupil has declined in size by at least 33%, with the resultant outcome that older people are far less likely to be able to detect low levels of light (Wolffsohn & Davies, 2019). If light becomes scattered over more of the retinal surface, then this results in glare. This glare then introduces external sources of light into the eye and because of retinal sensitivity loss, sudden flashes of light from headlights can transiently overstimulate the eyes. Alongside these manifestations, the contrast sensitivity, and processes of adaptation to the dark decline dramatically with age. The loss of contrast sensitivity causes a loss of perception of depth, a major cause of falls on dark staircases and consequently a major aetiological factor in the increased incidence and prevalence rate of falls in the elderly (Rubiño et al., 2020). Whereas an adolescent might have functional adjustment to the dark in less than seven minutes, an 80-year old's eyes may well take up to forty (Wang et al., 2020).

The gradual and progressive thickening of the lens and a consequent inability to focus is called presbyopia. With progressing age, from 40 onwards, there may be issues with adjustment from near sighted positions to long sighted perspectives. This can have important ramifications in being able to judge functional distance and can have an impact on falls and consequently falls prevention, where regular eye tests and the prescription of lenses for spectacles, where necessary, can be addressed. When there is a lack of functional capacity to adapt to change altogether, usually at the age of 60 or above, the person is said to have presbyopia (Mordi & Ciuffreda, 1998).

Whilst not especially relevant to the context of falls prevention, it is also important to remember the changes in hearing acuity, which occur as a consequence of the ageing process as an integral part of functional senescence. It is usually high frequency tones, which are first affected but the capacity for speech is less impacted upon, since speech is heard at a lower sound frequency, although in instances of presbycusis, there might also be issues with speech processing and discrimination. This lack of discriminatory ability has more of a functional impact than hearing loss alone. Over 75% of all adults aged over the age of 75 years will experience this to a certain extent (ibid, 1998). Other associated sensory losses are in relation to the perceptions of taste and smell. It is pressure detection on the tongue which progressively alters, rather than tastebud functional decline, which is widely reported. Odour intensity detection capacity also decreases with age. There may also be issues of memory distortion and changes in relation to the psychology of eating, which impact on the perception of flavour and consequently the appeal of food for older people (Locher et al., 2009).

ADJUSTMENT TO ENVIRONMENTAL CONTEXT AND SETTING

It is the modification of motor behaviour, which has the greatest impact in the consideration of the aetiological prevention of falls. This can impact directly, along with musculoskeletal change on the capacity of people to remain mobile on uneven terrain or in situations or environments with which they are unfamiliar (Lee & Ailshire, 2020). Sometimes older adults then need to use walking sticks or Zimmerframes, which can have an impact on self-image, as well as curtailing capacity for the individual movements they are capable of (Bertrand et al., 2017). Personality also impacts upon older peoples' perceptions of themselves in terms of their individuality and the homogenisation they sometimes feel as they are classified on the basis of their chronological age. This can also impact on their hesitancy to use aids to walking, which may be perceived as the preserve of the 'old aged' (Canada et al., 2020).

FUNCTIONAL ADAPTATIONS TO MOBILITY IN AGEING

Reaction time is commonly used to tangibly measure the capacity of an individual's central nervous system to pre-empt, initiate and sustain movement (Woo et al., 2020). It has been found that in people aged 50 to 90 there is a directly linear increase in the time needed to plan for precise movements of the distal extremities.

Whilst there is no universally accepted definition of fitness, and this is as individual as everyone alive, there are some very general definitions, which describe fitness as a state of optimal wellbeing and the capacity to successfully meet the present and potential physical challenges of life. This has obvious implications during the process of ageing and consequently senescence. To be fit, therefore, is to be adapted, adjusted, qualified, or suited to some purpose, function, or aim. 'Fit' also describes a person in good physical condition, or 'healthy'. Physical fitness allows one, regardless of their age, to carry out daily tasks with a degree of alertness, without any sense of undue fatigue and with remaining energy to enjoy leisurely activities as well as being deliberately productive (Gadelha, 2018).

FACTORS INFLUENCING HEALTH AND FITNESS IN AGEING

Various additional variables out with chronological age can impact on relative fitness levels, such as growth and gender (Rea, 2017). What is clear, however, is that the capacity to undertake physical tasks iteratively declines with increasing age. Whilst this decline is primarily attributable to physical changes of senescence it is also evident that social and environmental factors are also greatly influential. This may be due to the decreased level of physical activity that older adults partake exercise performance levels can also be unduly influenced by environmental factors such as levels of pollution and air quality.

SOCIAL FACTORS IMPACTING ON PROCESSES OF AGEING

As well as the concept of longevity, social determinants of health have a great impact on the overall quality of lives lived, in contemporary society, namely:

- **Educational Opportunity:** Which provides a mechanism which people can become upwardly socially mobile and in turn be empowered and inspired to maintain a standard of living associated with positive health and wellbeing choices (Breen & Müller, 2020).
- **Emergent Technologies:** Which have ensured an access to both knowledge and the capacity to communicate never experienced prior to now.
- **Public Safety:** Which ensures that societal protection is evident in relation to the overall health and wellbeing of citizens and which can positively impact on quality of life and wellbeing (Prince et al., 2015).
- **Social Norms and Attitudes, Such as Discrimination:** Being able to empower and provide a voice to what have been perceived as the most vulnerable members of society via democracy has enabled millions of people to live longer, more productive, and healthier lives, instead of the oppression caused by discrimination on the basis of gender, sexual orientation, race or religion (Burnes, 2019).
- **Social Order:** Which impacts on the capacity of all people to live in areas that have a tangibly lower degree of exposure to crime, violence, and social disorder, all of which can make a radical difference to perceived and actual health and wellbeing status (Baumann et al., 2020).
- **Social Support and Social Interactions Characterise Human Behaviour:** In instances where people do not have these, they are at an increasingly greater risk of the development of anxiety and depression, which can have

a cumulative and long-term impact on perceptions and lived experiences of health and wellbeing (Briggs et al., 2018).

- **Socio-Economics:** The impact of available finances obviously impacts on the ability of people to access a regular income and to sustain a level of living that is commensurate with positive health and wellbeing (Petrovic, 2018).
- **Transport Infrastructure:** Being able to have access to travel, being able to drive and having access to transport both enhance quality of life and achievable life experience. In some instances, this can also impact on the access to healthcare resources that people have, which can have a great impact on their capacity to regularly attend appointments or ensure their general health is optimal (Johnson et al., 2017).

PROGRESSIVE DEVELOPMENTAL CHANGE IN VASCULAR SYSTEM AGEING

Structural anatomical changes become evident in the heart, valves, and vasculature with natural processes of ageing and normal senescence (Laina et al., 2018). Within both the endocardium and the myocardium, elastic tissue, fat and collagen increase in the endocardium and myocardium of the heart, the outcome of which is a stiffer and far less compliant ventricular system (Laina et al., 2018). There is also an increased incidence of electrocardiographic abnormalities in the hears of older adults, with a demonstrable decrease beyond the age of 60years of cells in the sinoatrial node (Nishijima et al., 2018). Accompanying this, the valves become progressively more thick and calcified and this impacts on the closure and overall efficiency of the cardiac valves (Nishijima et al., 2018).

The proximal arteries have a tendency to dilate in parallel with increasing chronological age (Singam et al., 2020). The increased amount of connective tissue and lipid deposition leads to a progressive thickening of the blood vessels. The consequent outcomes of this are an increase in vascular rigidity and a reduction in vascular compliance.

Within the cardiovascular system there are also notable changes in relation to ageing, which are not immediately apparent during rest. The increases at rest of the systolic and diastolic blood pressure can be attributed to the increased stiffness of the vascular system and decreased size of the peripheral vascular bed.

The compliance and elastic recoil of the pulmonary system are impacted upon by processes of natural senescence too, making it harder for respiratory muscles to move air into the system (Romano & Romano, 2020). The most evident being:

- Increased anterior-posterior diameter of the thorax.

- Increased rigidity of the bronchioles.
- Increased stiffness of the chest wall.
- Structural changes in the elastic fibres of the lungs.
- Thickening of the mucous layer of the lungs.
- Thoracic ankylosis and kyphosis.

As a consequence of these changes, residual volume increases since more air is actively retained within the lungs. The amount of inspiratory reserve, expiratory reserve and vital capacity is reduced during both rest and active states. Alongside this, the surface area available for gas exchange also decreases due to changes in the function of the alveoli and substantial decrease in the number of pulmonary capillaries. Responses to ventilation in relation to increased levels of carbon dioxide or reduced levels of oxygen are also attributable to receptor, muscular or neuronal change. Ventilatory response in the elderly differs in older people can often be an indicator of exercise tolerance levels. There is evidence to suggest that training can effectively improve the changes in lung function which have been attributed to age (Seixas, 2020).

Older adults are generally happy with their level of fitness but underestimate their ability to exercise. Because of this, they are less inclined to engage in exercise that is challenging to them, which again can have an impact in terms of how they react to exercise (Heiestad et al., 2020). Consequently, this can place more physiological pressure on already vulnerable systems. where this develops to the worst extent older people may not be able to continue their daily activities of living with a functional state of dependency ensuing.

VISUAL INDICATORS OF AGEING

The gradual progression of grey and thinning hair, accompanied by skin wrinkling and decreased muscle tone and increasing fatty deposits, typically characterises old age. Physiologically comparable is the gradual deteriorating response to environmental stressors, with renal and digestive functionality progressively diminishing (Baker & Blakely, 2017). The functional response of the body to temperature regulation, dietary intake and oxygen supply means that the maintenance of a constant internal environment is more physiologically challenging. Alongside the progressive decline in the sheer number of cells older adults have, there is also a diminished functionality of those that remain. Beyond the context of the cells themselves, the extracellular fibres also change in terms of their quality, optimal strength, and overall number. The arterial walls harden and there is an increased incidence of arteriosclerosis. This is primarily attributable to the thickening of elastin and the uptake of calcium across the cell membrane, which causes the characteristic thickening and hardening of the condition. Processes of mitosis become progressively reduced and diminished leading to the production of fewer replacement cells in the heart, bones and muscles (Baker & Blakely, 2017).

In relation to the prevention of falls, these physiological changes are contributors to the physiological vulnerability of older people. Particularly where older adults develop more general issues in relation to their ambulatory health and wellbeing, where chronological age increases, the incidence of falls also exponentially increases. In relation to generalised pathological and age-related change in the feet and lower limbs. The likelihood of tissue breakdown in the foot and lower limb is increased by ischaemia and peripheral oedema (Muchna et al., 2018). Healing can be further impaired by poor dietary intake, avitaminosis and poor tissue perfusion. Elderly people are more prone to develop neoplastic disease, as the incidence of neoplasm increases with advancing age. The disease state in the elderly is predominantly one of multisystem pathologies, many of which will be chronic degenerative processes that impair healing and negatively impact on the individual's overall wellbeing.

Overall constitutional deterioration predisposes older adults to the development of pneumonia, particularly in those cases where they have been confined to bed for a prolonged period or in instances where there is a concomitant decreased cardiac or pulmonary function or respiratory infection (Focillo, 2020). As a clinical outcome, pneumonia is also a common and frequently fatal complication following the occurrence of cardiovascular accident (CVA) or hip fracture, where major orthopaedic intervention is required and prolonged periods of immobilisation occur. Since generalised arteriosclerosis is more common in elderly patients, there can be extensive pathological change to the renal, coronary and cerebral vessels, resulting in pulmonary and peripheral oedema (Ungvari, 2018).

FALLS IN THE ELDERLY: THE FUNCTIONAL PHYSIOLOGY

The physiological impact of falls in the elderly can also lead to what is commonly known as 'post-fall syndrome' (Meyer et al., 2020). This leads to a reluctance to resume normal activities, stunted progress in the restoration of occupational normality and potentially anxiety and depressive episodes. The origin of these falls is often systemic in nature but can sometimes also be attributed to extraneous variables such as the external environment or the introduction of new drug therapies (Musich et al., 2017). In addition to this, from an anatomical and physiological perspective the origins of falls in the elderly can emanate from dysfunction or impairment, most commonly in relation to:

- Connective tissue disorders.
- Dementia.
- Endocrine disorders.
- Myopathies.
- Neurological deficit.
- Vestibular function.
- Visual capacity.

THE FUNCTIONAL PHYSIOLOGICAL IMPACT OF POLYPHARMACY

As incidence and prevalence rates of multi-morbidity increase, so too do rates of polypharmacy (Kingston et al., 2018). Polypharmacy is defined as the concomitant use of five or more medications per 24-hour period by any individual, however many older patients use considerably higher numbers of medication (Delgado et al., 2020). Not only are prescribed medications used to treat the clinical symptomology of recognisable pathologies, they are often used to ensure that patients can live a more bearable life in relation to their potential to experience pain, as a consequence of natural processes of degeneration, so characterised by ageing and natural senescence (Veronese et al., 2017).

Since older adults can develop a pharmacokinetic and pharmacodynamics response to drugs as a consequence of increased physiological sensitivity, then they are also more likely to present with issues impacting upon their ambulatory health and wellbeing with symptoms such as dizziness (van den Anker, 2018). The need to reduce the amount of drugs taken due to the fact older people have decreased liver function and as such a correspondingly decreased capacity to optimally metabolise medication also places them at increased risk of adverse drug reaction (Drenth-van Maanen et al., 2020). Typical examples of these are local anaesthetics such as lignocaine or tricyclic anti-depressants, alongside stimulants such as caffeine. Systemic issues with renal clearance or renal dysfunction as part of the natural processes of senescence can also mean that drugs are not excreted effectively and remain in the system longer than they ought to – typical examples of these are those medications such as anti-hypertensive agents, which can directly result in postural hypotension and as a consequence of this, ambulatory unsteadiness and falls (Navaratnarajah & Jackson, 2017).

Added to the potential for complex dose regimen, for patients who might also have functional and/or untreated ocular decline, then the potential for drugs to be taken which are incompatible or even completely contradicted, is increased (Kim & Parish, 2017). Anti-hypertensive medications are not the alone as a significant drug group influencing the rate of falls in the elderly. Others include minor tranquillisers, hypnotics, and sedatives, all of which can instigate postural instability, another precursor to falls. Considering their potential to depress central nervous system, this is hardly surprising. Those medications prescribed to reduce pain and swelling for musculoskeletal pain and injury such as non-steroidal anti-inflammatory drugs can also have side effects of fluid retention or oedematous lower limbs accompanied by dizziness, postural instability, and a predisposition to fall. Postural hypotension can also be an unanticipated side effect of tricyclic antidepressants and diuretics, where blackouts, dizziness and fainting can be precursors to serious falls (Pan et al., 2018). Osteoporosis can be a side effect of the long-term use of systemic corticosteroids, which can also lower immunity to infection and predispose patients to an increased likelihood of falls and bone fractures (Rice et al., 2017).

CONCLUSION

The process of normal ageing is fraught with the potential for additional diseases which can run concurrently with abnormal pathologies, which may remain undiagnosed or undetected. All have the potential to impact on the general health and ambulatory wellbeing of older adults, which can accompany natural processes of senescence to the ultimate degenerative state of death. Being able to embed a working knowledge of the functional anatomy and physiology of old age, regardless of original academic discipline or professional identity is fundamental to being able to intervene with strategies to ensure optimal safeguarding against unintentional falls. This chapter has provided only a brief introductory overview to the most common physiological and anatomical changes, alongside considerations of polypharmacy and the wider implications of co-morbidities in older people. Whilst this chapter is relatively functional in approach to the annotation of anatomy and physiology, it ought also to be noted that beyond this underpinning knowledge, older people ought to be facilitated and empowered to share their own perceptions, needs and wants of how they wish to age and how they would prefer to live lives as fulfilling as they wish. As healthcare professionals, our privilege is to address and act on the seminally scientific facts, alongside their voices of lived experience in the co-construction of new knowledge.

REFERENCES

Alcañiz, M., & Solé-Auró, A. (2018). Feeling good in old age: Factors explaining health-related quality of life. *Health and Quality of Life Outcomes*, *16*(1), 48. doi:10.118612955-018-0877-z PMID:29534708

Baker, N. R., & Blakely, K. K. (2017). Gastrointestinal disturbances in the elderly. *Nursing Clinics*, *52*(3), 419–431. PMID:28779823

Bartosch, P. S., Kristensson, J., McGuigan, F. E., & Akesson, K. E. (2020). Frailty and prediction of recurrent falls over 10 years in a community cohort of 75-year-old women. *Aging Clinical and Experimental Research*, *32*(11), 1–10. doi:10.100740520-019-01467-1 PMID:31939201

Baumann, D., Ruch, W., Margelisch, K., Gander, F., & Wagner, L. (2020). Character strengths and life satisfaction in later life: An analysis of different living conditions. *Applied Research in Quality of Life*, *15*(2), 329–347. doi:10.100711482-018-9689-x

Bertrand, K., Raymond, M. H., Miller, W. C., Ginis, K. A. M., & Demers, L. (2017). Walking aids for enabling activity and participation: A systematic review. *American Journal of Physical Medicine & Rehabilitation*, *96*(12), 894–903. doi:10.1097/PHM.0000000000000836 PMID:29176406

Bisdorff, A., Bosser, G., Gueguen, R., & Perrin, P. (2013). The epidemiology of vertigo, dizziness, and unsteadiness and its links to co-morbidities. *Frontiers in Neurology*, *4*, 29. doi:10.3389/fneur.2013.00029 PMID:23526567

Borzuola, R., Giombini, A., Torre, G., Campi, S., Albo, E., Bravi, M., Borrione, P., Fossati, C., & Macaluso, A. (2020). Central and Peripheral Neuromuscular Adaptations to Ageing. *Journal of Clinical Medicine*, *9*(3), 741. doi:10.3390/jcm9030741 PMID:32182904

Brännström, J., Lövheim, H., Gustafson, Y., & Nordström, P. (2019). Association between antidepressant drug use and hip fracture in older people before and after treatment initiation. *JAMA Psychiatry*, *76*(2), 172–179. doi:10.1001/jamapsychiatry.2018.3679 PMID:30601883

Breen, R., & Müller, W. (2020). *Education and intergenerational social mobility in Europe and the United States*. Stanford University Press.

Briggs, R., Kennelly, S. P., & Kenny, R. A. (2018). Does baseline depression increase the risk of unexplained and accidental falls in a cohort of community-dwelling older people? Data from The Irish Longitudinal Study on Ageing (TILDA). *International Journal of Geriatric Psychiatry*, *33*(2), e205–e211. doi:10.1002/gps.4770 PMID:28766755

Burnes, D., Sheppard, C., Henderson, C. R. Jr, Wassel, M., Cope, R., Barber, C., & Pillemer, K. (2019). Interventions to reduce ageism against older adults: A systematic review and meta-analysis. *American Journal of Public Health*, *109*(8), e1–e9. doi:10.2105/AJPH.2019.305123 PMID:31219720

Buttigieg, S. C., Ilinca, S., de Sao Jose, J. M., & Larsson, A. T. (2018). Researching ageism in health-care and long term care. In *Contemporary perspectives on ageism* (pp. 493–515). Springer. doi:10.1007/978-3-319-73820-8_29

Canada, B., Stephan, Y., Sutin, A. R., & Terracciano, A. (2020). Personality and falls among older adults: Evidence from a longitudinal cohort. *The Journals of Gerontology: Series B*, *75*(9), 1905–1910. doi:10.1093/geronb/gbz040 PMID:30945733

Cho, B. Y., Seo, D. C., Lin, H. C., Lohrmann, D. K., & Chomistek, A. K. (2018). BMI and central obesity with falls among community-dwelling older adults. *American Journal of Preventive Medicine*, *54*(4), e59–e66. doi:10.1016/j.amepre.2017.12.020 PMID:29433954

Covey, H. C. (1992). The definitions of the beginning of old age in history. *International Journal of Aging & Human Development*, *34*(4), 325–337. doi:10.2190/GBXB-BE1F-1BU1-7FKK PMID:1607219

Delgado, J., Jones, L., Bradley, M. C., Allan, L. M., Ballard, C., Clare, L., ... Melzer, D. (2020). Potentially inappropriate prescribing in dementia, multi-morbidity and incidence of adverse health outcomes. *Age and Ageing*. PMID:32946561

Dodig, S., Čepelak, I., & Pavić, I. (2019). Hallmarks of senescence and aging. *Biochemia medica. Biochemia Medica*, *29*(3), 483–497. doi:10.11613/BM.2019.030501 PMID:31379458

Donaldson, P. J., Grey, A. C., Heilman, B. M., Lim, J. C., & Vaghefi, E. (2017). The physiological optics of the lens. *Progress in Retinal and Eye Research*, *56*, e1–e24. doi:10.1016/j.preteyeres.2016.09.002 PMID:27639549

Drake, S. A., Conway, S. H., Yang, Y., Cheatham, L. S., Wolf, D. A., Adams, S. D., Wade, C. E., & Holcomb, J. B. (2021). When falls become fatal—Clinical care sequence. *PLoS One*, *16*(1), e0244862. doi:10.1371/journal.pone.0244862 PMID:33406164

Drenth-van Maanen, A. C., Wilting, I., & Jansen, P. A. (2020). Prescribing medicines to older people—How to consider the impact of ageing on human organ and body functions. *British Journal of Clinical Pharmacology*, *86*(10), 1921–1930. doi:10.1111/bcp.14094 PMID:31425638

Faragher, R. G., McArdle, A., Willows, A., & Ostler, E. L. (2017). Senescence in the aging process. *F1000 Research*, 6. PMID:28781767

Foccillo, G. (2020). The Infections Causing Acute Respiratory Failure in Elderly Patients. In *Ventilatory Support and Oxygen Therapy in Elder, Palliative and End-of-Life Care Patients* (pp. 35–45). Springer. doi:10.1007/978-3-030-26664-6_5

Gadelha, A. B., Neri, S. G. R., Bottaro, M., & Lima, R. M. (2018). The relationship between muscle quality and incidence of falls in older community-dwelling women: An 18-month follow-up study. *Experimental Gerontology*, *110*, 241–246. doi:10.1016/j.exger.2018.06.018 PMID:29935953

Gazibara, T., Kurtagic, I., Kisic-Tepavcevic, D., Nurkovic, S., Kovacevic, N., Gazibara, T., & Pekmezovic, T. (2017). Falls, risk factors and fear of falling among persons older than 65 years of age. *Psychogeriatrics*, *17*(4), 215–223. doi:10.1111/psyg.12217 PMID:28130862

Heiestad, H., Gjestvang, C., & Haakstad, L. A. (2020). Investigating self-perceived health and quality of life: A longitudinal prospective study among beginner recreational exercisers in a fitness club setting. *BMJ Open*, *10*(6), e036250. doi:10.1136/bmjopen-2019-036250 PMID:32513890

Herranz, N., & Gil, J. (2018). Mechanisms and functions of cellular senescence. *The Journal of Clinical Investigation*, *128*(4), 1238–1246. doi:10.1172/JCI95148 PMID:29608137

Johnson, R., Shaw, J., Berding, J., Gather, M., & Rebstock, M. (2017). European national government approaches to older people's transport system needs. *Transport Policy*, *59*, 17–27. doi:10.1016/j.tranpol.2017.06.005

Katsuumi, G., Shimizu, I., Yoshida, Y., & Minamino, T. (2018). Vascular senescence in cardiovascular and metabolic diseases. *Frontiers in Cardiovascular Medicine*, *5*, 18. doi:10.3389/fcvm.2018.00018 PMID:29556500

Kenny, R. A., Romero-Ortuno, R., & Kumar, P. (2017). Falls in older adults. *Medicine*, *45*(1), 28–33. doi:10.1016/j.mpmed.2016.10.007 PMID:28298236

Kim, J., & Parish, A. L. (2017). Polypharmacy and medication management in older adults. *Nursing Clinics*, *52*(3), 457–468. doi:10.1016/j.cnur.2017.04.007 PMID:28779826

Kingston, A., Robinson, L., Booth, H., Knapp, M., & Jagger, C. (2018). Projections of multi-morbidity in the older population in England to 2035: Estimates from the Population Ageing and Care Simulation (PACSim) model. *Age and Ageing*, *47*(3), 374–380. doi:10.1093/ageing/afx201 PMID:29370339

Lee, H., & Ailshire, J. (2020). Neighborhood and Housing Conditions and Risk of Falls. *Innovation in Aging*, *4*(Suppl 1), 651–652. doi:10.1093/geroni/igaa057.2245

Liu, H., Yang, Y., Xia, Y., Zhu, W., Leak, R. K., Wei, Z., Wang, J., & Hu, X. (2017). Aging of cerebral white matter. *Ageing Research Reviews*, *34*, 64–76. doi:10.1016/j.arr.2016.11.006 PMID:27865980

Locher, J. L., Ritchie, C. S., Roth, D. L., Sen, B., Vickers, K. S., & Vailas, L. I. (2009). Food choice among homebound older adults: Motivations and perceived barriers. *JNHA-The Journal of Nutrition, Health and Aging*, *13*(8), 659–664. PMID:19657547

Mahbub, M. H., Hase, R., Yamaguchi, N., Hiroshige, K., Harada, N., Bhuiyan, A. N. M., & Tanabe, T. (2020). Acute Effects of Whole-Body Vibration on Peripheral Blood Flow, Vibrotactile Perception and Balance in Older Adults. *International Journal of Environmental Research and Public Health*, *17*(3), 1069. doi:10.3390/ijerph17031069 PMID:32046205

Maitre, J., Jully, J. L., Gasnier, Y., & Paillard, T. (2013). Chronic physical activity preserves efficiency of proprioception in postural control in older women. *Journal of Rehabilitation Research and Development*, *50*(6).

Mankia, K., & Emery, P. (2019). Palindromic rheumatism as part of the rheumatoid arthritis continuum. *Nature Reviews. Rheumatology*, *15*(11), 687–695. doi:10.103841584-019-0308-5 PMID:31595059

Meyer, M., Constancias, F., Vogel, T., Kaltenbach, G., & Schmitt, E. (2020). Gait Disorder among Elderly People, Psychomotor Disadaptation Syndrome: Post-Fall Syndrome, Risk Factors and Follow-Up–A Cohort Study of 70 Patients. *Gerontology*, 1–8. PMID:33254165

Mielenz, T. J., Kannoth, S., Jia, H., Pullyblank, K., Sorensen, J., Estabrooks, P., Stevens, J. A., & Strogatz, D. (2020). Evaluating a two-level vs. three-level fall risk screening algorithm for predicting falls among older adults. *Frontiers in Public Health*, *8*, 8. doi:10.3389/fpubh.2020.00373 PMID:32903603

Mordi, J. A., & Ciuffreda, K. J. (1998). Static aspects of accommodation: Age and presbyopia. *Vision Research*, *38*(11), 1643–1653. doi:10.1016/S0042-6989(97)00336-2 PMID:9747501

Moreland, B., Kakara, R., & Henry, A. (2020). Trends in nonfatal falls and fall-related injuries among adults aged[3] 65 years—United States, 2012–2018. *Morbidity and Mortality Weekly Report*, *69*(27), 875–881. doi:10.15585/mmwr.mm6927a5 PMID:32644982

Muchna, A., Najafi, B., Wendel, C. S., Schwenk, M., Armstrong, D. G., & Mohler, J. (2018). Foot problems in older adults: Associations with incident falls, frailty syndrome, and sensor-derived gait, balance, and physical activity measures. *Journal of the American Podiatric Medical Association*, *108*(2), 126–139. doi:10.7547/15-186 PMID:28853612

Navaratnarajah, A., & Jackson, S. H. (2017). The physiology of ageing. *Medicine*, *45*(1), 6–10. doi:10.1016/j.mpmed.2016.10.008 PMID:28065164

Nishijima, D. K., Lin, A. L., Weiss, R. E., Yagapen, A. N., Malveau, S. E., Adler, D. H., Bastani, A., Baugh, C. W., Caterino, J. M., Clark, C. L., Diercks, D. B., Hollander, J. E., Nicks, B. A., Shah, M. N., Stiffler, K. A., Storrow, A. B., Wilber, S. T., & Sun, B. C. (2018). ECG predictors of cardiac arrhythmias in older adults with syncope. *Annals of Emergency Medicine*, *71*(4), 452–461. doi:10.1016/j.annemergmed.2017.11.014 PMID:29275946

Padrón-Monedero, A., Pastor-Barriuso, R., García López, F. J., Martínez Martín, P., & Damián, J. (2020). Falls and long-term survival among older adults residing in care homes. *PLoS One*, *15*(5), e0231618.

Pan, Q., Zhang, Y., Long, T., He, W., Zhang, S., Fan, Y., & Zhou, J. (2018). Diagnosis of Vertigo and dizziness syndromes in a neurological outpatient clinic. *European Neurology*, *79*(5-6), 287–294.

Petrovic, D., de Mestral, C., Bochud, M., Bartley, M., Kivimäki, M., Vineis, P., & Stringhini, S. (2018). The contribution of health behaviors to socioeconomic inequalities in health: A systematic review. *Preventive Medicine*, *113*, 15–31.

Prince, M. J., Wu, F., Guo, Y., Robledo, L. M. G., O'Donnell, M., Sullivan, R., & Yusuf, S. (2015). The burden of disease in older people and implications for health policy and practice. *Lancet*, *385*(9967), 549–562.

Rea, I. M. (2017). Towards ageing well: Use it or lose it: Exercise, epigenetics and cognition. *Biogerontology*, *18*(4), 679–691.

Rice, J. B., White, A. G., Scarpati, L. M., Wan, G., & Nelson, W. W. (2017). Long-term systemic corticosteroid exposure: A systematic literature review. *Clinical Therapeutics*, *39*(11), 2216–2229.

Romano, A., & Romano, R. (2020). Gas Exchange and Control of Breathing in Elderly and End-of-Life Diseases. In *Ventilatory Support and Oxygen Therapy in Elder, Palliative and End-of-Life Care Patients* (pp. 15–20). Springer.

Rubiño, J. A., Gamundí, A., Akaarir, M., Canellas, F., Rial, R., & Nicolau, M. C. (2020). Bright Light Therapy and Circadian Cycles in Institutionalized Elders. *Frontiers in Neuroscience*, 14.

Saftari, L. N., & Kwon, O. S. (2018). Ageing vision and falls: A review. *Journal of Physiological Anthropology*, *37*(1), 1–14.

Sari, R. K., Sutiadiningsih, A., Zaini, H., Meisarah, F., & Hubur, A. A. (2020). Factors affecting cognitive intelligence theory. *Journal of Critical Reviews*, *7*(17), 402–410.

Schapmire, T. J., Head, B. A., Nash, W. A., Yankeelov, P. A., Furman, C. D., Wright, R. B., & Faul, A. C. (2018). Overcoming barriers to interprofessional education in gerontology: The interprofessional curriculum for the care of older adults. *Advances in Medical Education and Practice*, *9*, 109.

Sciomer, S., Moscucci, F., Maffei, S., Gallina, S., & Mattioli, A. V. (2019). Prevention of cardiovascular risk factors in women: The lifestyle paradox and stereotypes we need to defeat. *European Journal of Preventive Cardiology*, *26*(6), 609–610.

Seixas, M. B., Almeida, L. B., Trevizan, P. F., Martinez, D. G., Laterza, M. C., Vanderlei, L. C. M., & Silva, L. P. (2020). Effects of inspiratory muscle training in older adults. *Respiratory Care*, *65*(4), 535–544.

Sengoku, R. (2020). Aging and Alzheimer's disease pathology. *Neuropathology*, *40*(1), 22–29.

Sharma, P., Sharma, A., Fayaz, F., Wakode, S., & Pottoo, F. H. (2020). Biological Signatures of Alzheimer's Disease. *Current Topics in Medicinal Chemistry*, *20*(9), 770–781.

Singam, N. S. V., Fine, C., & Fleg, J. L. (2020). Cardiac changes associated with vascular aging. *Clinical Cardiology*, *43*(2), 92–98.

Skinner, M. W., Andrews, G. J., & Cutchin, M. P. (Eds.). (2017). *Geographical gerontology: Perspectives, concepts, approaches*. Routledge.

Stambler, I. (2017). Recognizing degenerative aging as a treatable medical condition: Methodology and policy. *Aging and Disease, 8*(5), 583.

Tieland, M., Trouwborst, I., & Clark, B. C. (2018). Skeletal muscle performance and ageing. *Journal of Cachexia, Sarcopenia and Muscle, 9*(1), 3–19.

Toots, A., Wiklund, R., Littbrand, H., Nordin, E., Nordström, P., Lundin-Olsson, L., & Rosendahl, E. (2019). The effects of exercise on falls in older people with dementia living in nursing homes: A randomized controlled trial. *Journal of the American Medical Directors Association, 20*(7), 835-842.

Tornero-Quiñones, I., Sáez-Padilla, J., Espina Díaz, A., Abad Robles, M. T., & Sierra Robles, Á. (2020). Functional ability, frailty and risk of falls in the elderly: Relations with autonomy in daily living. *International Journal of Environmental Research and Public Health, 17*(3), 1006.

Ungvari, Z., Tarantini, S., Donato, A. J., Galvan, V., & Csiszar, A. (2018). Mechanisms of vascular aging. *Circulation Research, 123*(7), 849–867.

van den Anker, J., Reed, M. D., Allegaert, K., & Kearns, G. L. (2018). Developmental changes in pharmacokinetics and pharmacodynamics. *Journal of Clinical Pharmacology, 58*, S10–S25.

van Onna, M., & Boonen, A. (2016). The challenging interplay between rheumatoid arthritis, ageing and comorbidities. *BMC Musculoskeletal Disorders, 17*(1), 184.

Veronese, N., Stubbs, B., Noale, M., Solmi, M., Pilotto, A., Vaona, A., & Maggi, S. (2017). Polypharmacy is associated with higher frailty risk in older people: An 8-year longitudinal cohort study. *Journal of the American Medical Directors Association, 18*(7), 624–628.

Wang, Y., Huang, H., & Chen, G. (2020). Effects of lighting on ECG, visual performance and psychology of the elderly. *Optik (Stuttgart), 203*, 164063.

Wolffsohn, J. S., & Davies, L. N. (2019). Presbyopia: Effectiveness of correction strategies. *Progress in Retinal and Eye Research, 68*, 124–143.

Woo, Y. S., Shin, G. I., & Park, H. Y. (2020). Comparative Analysis of Differences in Reaction Time and Divided Attention with Elderly Age: Using the Driving Ability Assessment Tool. *Therapeutic Science for Rehabilitation, 9*(3), 53–61.

ADDITIONAL READING

Ambrens, M., Tiedemann, A., Delbaere, K., Alley, S., & Vandelanotte, C. (2020). The effect of eHealth-based falls prevention programmes on balance in people aged 65 years and over living in the community: Protocol for a systematic review of randomised controlled trials. *BMJ Open*, *10*(1), e031200. doi:10.1136/bmjopen-2019-031200 PMID:31948985

Bjerk, M., Brovold, T., Skelton, D. A., & Bergland, A. (2017). A falls prevention programme to improve quality of life, physical function and falls efficacy in older people receiving home help services: Study protocol for a randomised controlled trial. *BMC Health Services Research*, *17*(1), 559. doi:10.118612913-017-2516-5 PMID:28806904

Davis, J. C., Bryan, S., Best, J. R., Li, L. C., Hsu, C. L., Gomez, C., Vertes, K. A., & Liu-Ambrose, T. (2015). Mobility predicts change in older adults' health-related quality of life: Evidence from a Vancouver falls prevention prospective cohort study. *Health and Quality of Life Outcomes*, *13*(1), 101. doi:10.118612955-015-0299-0 PMID:26168922

Dreinhöfer, K. E., Mitchell, P. J., Bégué, T., Cooper, C., Costa, M. L., Falaschi, P., Hertz, K., Marsh, D., Maggi, S., Nana, A., Palm, H., Speerin, R., & Magaziner, J. (2018). A global call to action to improve the care of people with fragility fractures. *Injury*, *49*(8), 1393–1397. doi:10.1016/j.injury.2018.06.032 PMID:29983172

Growdon, M. E., Shorr, R. I., & Inouye, S. K. (2017). The tension between promoting mobility and preventing falls in the hospital. *JAMA Internal Medicine*, *177*(6), 759–760. doi:10.1001/jamainternmed.2017.0840 PMID:28437517

Naseri, C., McPhail, S. M., Haines, T. P., Morris, M. E., Shorr, R., Etherton-Beer, C., Netto, J., Flicker, L., Bulsara, M., Lee, D.-C. A., Francis-Coad, J., Waldron, N., Boudville, A., & Hill, A. M. (2020). Perspectives of older adults regarding barriers and enablers to engaging in fall prevention activities after hospital discharge. *Health & Social Care in the Community*, *28*(5), 1710–1722. doi:10.1111/hsc.12996 PMID:32337796

Zanker, J., & Duque, G. (2020). Approaches for Falls Prevention in Hospitals and Nursing Home Settings. In *Falls and Cognition in Older Persons* (pp. 245–259). Springer. doi:10.1007/978-3-030-24233-6_14

KEY TERMS AND DEFINITIONS

Ageing: Ageing is the process of becoming older, which is characterised by a process of natural senescence in older adults.

Ambulation: Ambulation is the act, action, or an instance of moving about or walking.

Deterioration: Is the process of degenerating or becoming progressively worse.

Gerontology: Is the science and comprehensive multidisciplinary study of aging and older adults.

Morbidity: The term used to describe suffering from a disease or medical condition.

Mortality: Is the state of being subject to death.

Outcomes: The outcome of a phenomena is the way something turns out or the active consequence of something.

Physiology: The specific branch of biological sciences that deals with the normal functions of living organisms and their parts.

Polypharmacy: Polypharmacy can be defined as the concomitant use of five or more medications per 24-hour period by any individual person.

Psychology: Pertains to the mental factors governing a specific situation or process.

Chapter 2
Understanding Multimorbidity in the Elderly

Adil Hamad Alharthi
King Fahad Armed Forces Hospital, Saudi Arabia

Khalid Abdullah Almotari
King Fahad Armed Forces Hospital, Saudi Arabia

Abdulaziz Ali Alghamdi
King Fahad Armed Forces Hospital, Saudi Arabia

EXECUTIVE SUMMARY

Multimorbidity is the presence of two or more long-term conditions which are those that cannot be currently cured but can be controlled. Chronic conditions are the leading cause of death globally. The World Health Organization (WHO) predicted that 87% of deaths in high income countries were attributed to chronic conditions and the proportion of worldwide deaths caused by chronic conditions is expected to rise from 59% in 2002 to 69% in 2030. Fifty-five to ninety-eight percent of people 60 years or older are affected by two or more chronic diseases and patients with multimorbidity account for up to 80% of consultations with general practitioners and virtually all consultations with Geriatricians. Among the reasons are that Co-occurring diseases interact with each other increasing the risk of negative events beyond the sum of the risk of each disease alone.

DOI: 10.4018/978-1-6684-2354-7.ch002

INTRODUCTION

Multimorbidity is a phenomenon that is prevalent worldwide, it's common in the elderly and it's the norm rather than the exception, those healthcare providers who help the elderly need to understand and appreciate Multimorbidity to be able to deliver better care to their patient. currently multimorbidity is still suffering from lack of sufficient longitudinal studies to shed light on its risk factors, its disease clustering and its hazardous consequences. It's also suffering from lack of sufficient practical guidelines to orient healthcare providers, specifically primary care practitioners about its importance as well as its management requirements and prevention benefits. most of our knowledge about multimorbidity is prevalence and associated risk factors which are without an evidence base causation relationship. so, this important and relatively new concept is clearly with a knowledge gap, on the other hand new articles are enriching the literature about multimorbidity very rapidly.

PREVALENCE

Multiple comorbidities tend to appear as people age, the term multimorbidity identifies this condition (Calderón-Larrañaga et al., 2019). Beyond age 60 years, 55-90% gets affected by two or more chronic diseases, and those patients with multimorbidities account for up to 80% of consultations with practitioners and almost the majority of geriatrician consultations (Marengoni et al., 2011; Salisbury et al., 2011). In addition, co-occurring diseases tend to overlap, increasing the negative outcomes. The impact of multimorbidities is crucial as it triggers complex pharmacological regimes, increases the utilisation of health care resources and reduces the length and quality of life (Calderón-Larrañaga et al., 2019; Di Angelantonio et al., 2015; Dumbreck et al., 2015; Vetrano et al., 2018). Furthermore, this challenges physicians as they're practice are more toward considering only limited number of disease interactions, this eventually affects to offer elderly with multimorbidity comprehensive assessment, the most effective treatment and integrated paths. From another perspective, research conducted on the new horizons in multimorbidities in older patients reveals that the concept of multimorbidities is a growing interesting field over these years, especially with the publication of specific guidelines on multimorbidity by the National Institute for Health and Care Excellence (NICE) (NICE, 2016). Specifically, this is recognised as important to practitioners and relevant enough for elderly care, where the complexity of physical, mental health disorders, frailty, and polypharmacy overlaps (Yarnall et al., 2017). This overlap is in particular likely due to health deficit which leads to functional impairment in some cases. NICE guidelines outlines 'target groups' who may guarantee benefits from a tailored approach of care, thus increasing quality of life by reduction in unplanned or uncoordinated care, adverse events and treatment burden (Yarnall et al., 2017). Before the NICE guidelines, prioritising the multimorbidities was challenging, as percentages alone concludes a large number to target for intervention (Stott & Young, 2017). In addition, general multimorbidity measures of disease count and indices may not accurately reveal the characteristics of multimorbidity in elderly. NICE guidelines offer rather target groups with certain multimorbidities with high levels of complexity, so it allows for easier care and more focus. The majority of target groups are aligned with the population seen by geriatricians as those with a combination of functional impairment, falls and interactive mental and physical health conditions (Clegg et al., 2013). Large number of elderlies have two or more long term care, hence, consumes more primary and secondary care services, and requires more complex care compared to patients with only one or two comorbidities (Salisbury et al., 2011). Elder patients with multiple comorbidities are at a higher risk of being care dependent compared to those with single chronic condition, with around third and quarter requiring care home over a period of 5 years respectively (Koller et al., 2014). Geriatricians are more prone to aging syndromes like Parkinsonism, cerebrovascular disease and peripheral artery diseases, in relevance to the multimorbidities, this exposes them to experience other prone problems such as pain, falls and pressure ulcers (Vetrano et al., 2016). Research conducted on multimorbidity in older patients, they examined population bases-administrative claims indicating the health service delivery to about 31 million for 25 prevalent chronic conditions. 67% had multimorbidity, increased with age, for patients less than 65 was 50% to 62% for those aged 65-74 and for those ages more than 85 was 81.5%. Another systematic review included elder patients revealed a median prevalence of 63% (Salive, 2013). A study in India conducted showed that the proportion of elderly population is prone to increase from 5% in 2015 to 19% in 2050 and the older population was accounted for a third of the country's population. Multimorbidity is most common among elderly and its prevalence increases with age. Chronic conditions are present in clusters and the pattern of clustering needs to be explored for a better strategy plan directed by public health. In one of the cross-sectional studies conducted among 725 rural older adults above 60 of age in India, the multimorbidity was assessed using prior validated MAQ-PC tool. In conclusion, the prevalence of multimorbidity was 48.8%, the prevalence was higher in females 50.4% compared to males 47.4% (Kshatri et al., 2020). Multimorbidity refers to the presence of two or more chronic conditions, it has rapidly became common among elderly (Johnston et al., 2019). As multimorbidity is becoming a priority for health care due to the rapidly aging population, in addition it's also related to the increased risk of functional decline, higher burden on health care and mortality increase (Di Angelantonio et al., 2015). The outcomes associated with multimorbidity is not only restricted on the outcome measures like disability and mortality, but also subjectively like on quality of life, well-being and self-rated health (SRH) (Smith et al., 2018). SRH is a measure of psychosocial and physical status, which could be approached by a single question "how's your health now?". I'm addition SRH was also associated with well-being, physical functioning and mortality (Idler & Benyamini, 1997). A cohort study conducted that post midlife multimorbidity leads to reduction in subjective health (Mavaddat et al., 2014). In Japan, where the life expectancy is above 80 years, multimorbidity is a recognisable public health burden in Japan's society. The prevalence of multimorbidity is reported to have a jump with age, being 65% at 60s and nearly 100% at 85yrs (Barnett et al., 2012).

Definition

The coexisting of two or more chronic diseases within the same individual is termed as 'multimorbidity' (van den Akker et al., 1996). The term originated from 'comorbidity' (Salisbury, 2012) however it differed from comorbidity which signified a different additional clinical entity that occurs in the setting of indexed disease (Feinstein, 1970). Multimorbidity concept is human-centred and focuses more on exploration of the systemic methods of prevention and intervening on the common risk factors. Given that the world is witnessing a decrease in fertility rates and on the other hand an increase in life expectancy, aging population is growing worldwide (Divo et al., 2014). Globally, life expectancy increased 5.5 from the years 2000 to 2016 (Organization, 2018). As a result of aging, there are growing incidences of elderly with chronic multimorbidity which is found to be more in low and middle income countries (Garin et al., 2016). According the world health organisation definition of chronic multimorbidity, it's when two or more chronic diseases coexist at the same time (Mercer et al., 2016). The European General Practitioners Research Network (EGPRN) declares that the addition of another disease could be acute or chronic. The association of biopsychosocial either associated or not with previous disease or somatic factor (Le Reste et al., 2015) could lead to mismatch of multimorbidity mainly in terms of risk factors (Willadsen et al., 2016). Chronic multimorbidity leads to various adverse effects, including poor quality of life (Willadsen et al., 2016), poor physical function (Ryan et al., 2015), and an increase in demand toward healthcare (McPhail, 2016).Overall, multimorbidity increases the risk of all-cause mortality.

Risk Factors

In order to understand and study multimorbidity, we have to understand its risk factors. Multiple studies have addressed multimorbidity risk factors, its association, its importance and its harmful consequences. One of the important risk factors related to multimorbidity, is gender. Multiple studies have found that elder females have more multimorbidity compared to elder males (Sembiah et al., 2022). Studies done on middle aged and youth found there is no gender difference in multimorbidity (Everett, 2013), this could be explained by many factors first the protective role of the female hormones, second the socioeconomic difference between elder females and elder males. Elder females being deprived of retirement payrolls and deprived from financial support in cases of them being divorced, widowed or single in comparison to males. multimorbidity studies in rural and urban communities showed some controversial results (Romano et al., 2021). Most of them showed that elder females in urban communities have more multimorbidity then elder females in rural communities against what is logically expected, the explanation of this bias is that elder female in urban communities are more likely to be educated and aware about the importance of seeking healthcare and are less likely to have healthcare access challenges, compared to elder females in rural communities, who are more likely to be less educated, unaware about the importance to seek medical attention, and thus would be more difficult to identify the expected increase in multimorbidity among them (Sharma & Maurya, 2022).

Another important multimorbidity risk factor is obesity. One of the challenges is the way to measure obesity, which was mainly BMI. The problem is that taller men who have fat deposits restricted to their abdomen, may have normal or upper normal levels of BMI, that's why some studies have added measuring waist circumference to measuring BMI to avoid the bias. studies have showed that obese elders are more prone to multimorbidity not only that, but the level of obesity is related to higher levels of multimorbidity (Romano et al., 2021). Those elders with overweight are more prone to multimorbidity than those with healthy weights, but those elders with stage II or III obesity are prone to complicated multimorbidity (the coexistence of four or more chronic diseases). studies have also showed that middle aged individuals with obesity have a higher possibility of developing multimorbidity in their older ages. to complicate things not only obesity (Kivimäki et al., 2022), but also obesity related diseases was found to be associated with more prevalence of multimorbidity, those elder with obesity related diseases are more prone to have complicated multimorbidity (Kivimäki et al., 2022). Statistically obesity by itself without its obesity related diseases is associated with reduced disease-free survival but not with reduced overall survival, meaning that mortality in relation to obesity is only through its obesity related diseases.

Another multi morbidity risk factor is tobacco use. Multiple studies found that elders using tobacco are more porn to have multimorbidity, not only that but the type of tobacco use was also related to multimorbidity so studies showed that smoking tobacco is more related to multimorbidity then other types of tobacco use like chewing tobacco (Everett, 2013). One study found that Shisha smoking (water pipe smoking) is more related to multimorbidity then cigarette smoking (Bah et al.,

2022). Also, in keeping with the previous studies, it was shown that elder females using tobacco showed more relation to multimorbidity then elder men using tobacco, and this could be related to the socioeconomic differences between elder males and elder females that might cause them to smoke tobacco for longer times and use more cigarettes per week or even per day.

Another important risk factor for multimorbidity is reduced physical activity. Many studies show that elders with reduced physical activity, have a higher possibility of multimorbidity. Also, in keeping with the previous studies gender and generation difference exists as well, meaning that elder females with reduced physical activity are more prone to multimorbidity then elder men with reduced physical activity. Also, those middle-aged individuals with reduced physical activity and sedentary life, have a higher possibility of developing multimorbidity in older ages, not only that but studies showed that in elder females reduced physical activity is related to depression, whereas elder males reduce physical activity is related to diabetes (Gomes et al., 2020). depression related symptoms like apathy, blue mood and reduced physical activity are known to have a bidirectional relationship meaning that depressive symptoms can cause reduced physical activity, in the other hand increased physical activity can improve and prevent depression and depressive symptoms. Again, due to the known socioeconomic differences among older males and females, it is expected that older females are less likely to be involved in outside home activities and more restricted to indoors taking care of their home and family and are less likely to be involved in physical activity, thus more prone to reduced physical activity with its harmful consequences. It is clear from the previous review that most if not all of the risk factors are modifiable risk factors, reflecting on the importance of preventive strategies, not only that but gender specific preventive strategies need to be implemented community and population wise and further longitudinal studies need to follow these preventive measures both in urban and rural communities to study its benefits in reducing the harmful consequences of multimorbidity in Elderly (Bezerra de Souza et al., 2021).

Frailty

Multimorbidity in the elderly is also found to be related to Frailty. Frailty is defined as reduced Physiological reserve and reduced resistance to different stressors. This is called the phenotype definition of frailty. There is another definition called the accumulative deficit., in which Frailty is an accumulation of biological, psychological, culture and environmental injuries, causing sub clinical deficits, with further accumulation leading to dysfunction that leads to disability (Vassar et al., 2019). Deferent frailty screening indices are used in deferent studies, for example the Frailty index. Different frailty indices use different number of physiological deficits to assess the severity of frailty in elderly. The prevalence of frailty in multimorbidity depends on the definition considered, for those multimorbid with two diseases, and those considering frailty as having one physiological deficit the prevalence is around 18%, but for those considering multimorbidity having three diseases, and frailty as having two deficits, the prevalence increases to 24% and so on (Vassar et al., 2019).

It's also proven that frailty is a reversible condition in some elder patients. If we consider frailty as a pre-disability condition, then we have to consider these frail patients as at-risk patients and implement screening measures to discover them early and manage their frailty or at least prevent its deterioration into disability. Frailty has a multidisciplinary pathophysiology, one of its important hypotheses is energy imbalance in which there is a net catabolic outcome that can result in muscle loss and Sarcopina. Another important hypothesis is chronic Inflammation, in which increased inflammatory cytokines found in elder frail individuals proves that frailty is also a pro inflammatory condition (Wleklik et al., 2020). Of the important determinant of frailty is depression, actually frailty is considered an indicator for depression in elders and depression in the elderly is an indicator for Frailty, not only that, but due to symptoms overlap between Frailty and depression (Wleklik et al., 2020), it is mostly challenging to diagnose depression in elders with frailty, to add to this, most of the frail elders without depression can have isolated apathy, and those at risk multimorbid group could be targeted to prevent deterioration into depression with its harmful consequences. Another determinant of frailty is generalized muscle loss or Sarcopenia. Sarcopenia has multiple causes in frailty. One of them is malnutrition that occurs in frailty, the catabolic state network, and the protein catabolism that is common in elderly and especially in frailty and the pro inflammatory condition that is associated with it. This muscle mass loss will cause reduced energy, reduced activity, reduced gait speed, and thus more deterioration in elders with frailty. Another determinant of frailty is polypharmacy. The relationship between polypharmacy and multimorbidity is clear and polypharmacy is one of the important determinants in most elders with multimorbidity especially those elders with frailty, but the relation of polypharmacy and frailty is not only related to the number of medications but more importantly related to the drug to drug and drug to disease interaction (Wleklik et al., 2020), and thus the complication of drugs and the harmful outcome of the drug on the elder patients. This is one of the determinants that must be reviewed regularly being a preventable determinant in some if not most of the elder patients with frailty. Of the other examples of determinants of frailty syndrome are loneliness and social isolation, cognitive decline, malnutrition, weight loss, reduced gait speed, unintentional weight loss and others as well.

Many studies investigated the relationship between multimorbidity and Frailty in the elderly, these studies are cross-sectional and retrospective studies and they found that the number of diseases, the number of medications, the age of the patient and the level of fitness of the elders are all strong frailty risk factors in the elderly. It has been found also that having a low BMI in elders is a risk factor for Frailty meaning that overweight is a protective phenomenon in elderly, Physiological theories behind that mentioned that in elderly there is more protein catabolism and less fat burning, leading to significant weight loss that is more harmful than helpful (Lv et al., 2022). And that must be taken into consideration clinically when dealing with elder obese patients. Having frailty and multimorbidity in elder patients leads to further catastrophic consequence like higher risk of DVT for hospitalized patient, high risk of falls, fractures, high risk of institutionalization (Lv et al., 2022). Some studies have argued that elder diabetic patients with multimorbidity have a higher risk of frailty and frail elder diabetics have higher risk of multimorbidity (Sinclair & Abdelhafiz, 2022). Other studies went further than the disease count relationship between them, and went to study the dynamics of the Multimorbidity-frailty relationship, they found that Drug to drug, disease to disease, and drug to disease interaction all worsen the hazardous consequences of multimorbidity and frailty on each other, and on their outcome as well. One longitudinal study followed up a large number of elder patients with multimorbidity and Frailty. They found that between 65 and 85 years of Age the higher the number of diseases the more the severity of frailty, but after 85 the number of diseases becomes constant but the severity of frailty keeps rising i.e., Frailty severity is not affected by disease any more but affected by none disease related factors which are called symptoms, signs, lab and disability (SSLD) so after 85 years frailty is more related to SSLD factor than disease related factors (Carrasco-Ribelles et al., 2022). More longitudinal studies of multimorbidity and frailty will teach us more about their dynamics and more about their relationship and interactions with each other.

Multimorbidity Clusters

Most multimorbidity researches are limited to studying the prevalence and number of chronic diseases in the elderly, in order to understand the effects and consequences of multimorbidity on elder patients we have to understand its pathophysiology, it's disease to disease interaction, (Vetrano et al., 2020) it has been noticed in multimorbid patients that most chronic illnesses share the same risk factors. For example, cardiovascular diseases, chronic kidney diseases and peripheral vascular diseases, all share diabetes, hypertension, dyslipidaemia, and obesity as risk factors for their occurrence. In order to understand more in-depth relationship about chronic diseases clustering and grouping together in multimorbid patients and its consequence on the patient's health and prognosis, some studies underwent certain cross-sectional longitudinal studies, and used certain statistical analysis to understand the recurrent appearance of chronic diseases. Some frequently measured indices in these studies are the observed/expected ratios (O/E-ratios) that is obtained by dividing disease prevalence in the cluster by disease prevalence in the overall population. And the exclusivity (E), defined as the proportion of patients with the disease included in the cluster over the total number of patients with the disease (Guisado-Clavero et al., 2018; Vetrano et al., 2020; Violán et al., 2020). Chronic diseases which are highly prevalent and overrepresented in a specific cluster, are considered the nuclear chronic disease of the cluster, and the cluster is named according to them, by this statistical method we can form different Multimorbidity clusters with specific diseases sharing specific characteristics. Interestingly, a common finding in all Multimorbidity cluster researches, you will find one cluster that has high prevalence of chronic diseases but none over represented diseases, this cluster is called the nonspecific cluster, characterized by having younger patients with less chronic diseases, who retain their cognitive and performance capabilities, because these patients are common to have chronic diseases like hypertension, dyslipidaemia, obesity, pre-diabetes (Guisado-Clavero et al., 2018), this group is agreed to represent the high metabolic risk group which should be the focus of preventive strategies. in order to further understand the relationship and interactions of chronic diseases in the same group, some studies further investigated using different, statistical measures one of which is the lift analysis which is the ratio of the observed support to that expected if the two events were independent, by measuring the lift of two diseases in the same cluster we will know the possibility of these two diseases occurring in the same group, and the possibility of one condition occurring in the presence of another (Zemedikun et al., 2018). Some researchers took a further step in a more longitudinal cohort and followed up the same research sample over time to assess whether these patients remain in their same clusters or transition to other clusters. This phenomenon is called Multimorbidity trajectory. which is the transition of patients from one cluster to another overtime (Haug et al., 2020). Studying it allowed researchers, a plethora of information about Multimorbidity consequences, it's prognosis and mortality. Some studies followed patients over four years or even 12 years and these studies showed that the unspecific group described earlier is one of the large groups acquiring about 48% of the sample size (Vetrano et al., 2020). By labelling some clusters with cardiovascular diseases as high mortality clusters, researchers can study the significance of these Multimorbidity trajectories for example, those clusters that transition and step into the high mortality clusters are called high risk clusters, and those who less likely transition to them are called low or intermediate risk clusters. High risk clusters are the clusters who have high metabolic related diseases like dyslipidaemia, obesity and hypertension. These high-risk clusters are important clusters to understand as they should be the target of our elder preventive strategies (Carrasco-Ribelles et al., 2022; Vetrano et al., 2020). Unfortunately, Multimorbidity cluster studies, face multiple challenges, and it's difficult to compare one Multimorbidity research to another because of the wide variation in the methodology, data collection and patient characteristics involved. For example, some researches collect data by means of patient description and others collect data by means of medical record review, in order to be able to compare studies with each other and strengthen our understanding and progress in our crusade against multimorbidity, we have to overcome these challenges, and to overcome them, we have to appreciate them. So, among the challenges that we face:

- Most of Multimorbidity research are cross-sectional research and not longitudinal research, which cannot give any causation analysis.
- Some researches defer in the Multimorbidity definition for example some include infectious diseases as well, which gives over representation of Multimorbidity.
- The more diseases included in the Multimorbidity definition the higher the prevalence of multimorbidity.
- Some researches use patient self-description data while others use hospital records review for multimorbidity. The first type of data collection can result in under representation of multimorbidity, due to "the well- being paradox" in which patients may feel well with a good physical and cognitive capability, in spite of having multimorbidity.
- Most physicians are uncomfortable diagnosing and managing elder with Multimorbidity, due to the lack of experience and improper education about disease to disease and disease-to-drug interactions.
- Guidelines about diagnosis, management and follow-up of single diseases exist, but guidelines about proper management, follow up and prevention of Multimorbidity are still lacking
- Risk factors affect different multimorbidity clusters in different ways.
- Differences in elder population characteristics result in different multimorbidity clusters.
- Most multimorbidity studies search for disease Counts, rather than the impact of Multimorbidity on patient outcomes and prognosis.
- Contradicting Multimorbidity researches need to be explained by the research design, data collection and population characteristics.

Socioeconomic Status

Multi morbidity affect human well-being and quality of life and have a negative impact not only on the physical health but extends to include mental and psychological and social health. Being an old man with multi morbidity decrease functional and productive capacity, furthermore frequent visits to healthcare facilities, cut out valuable time and add extra loads on the weak shoulders of an old man or woman. The polypharmacy associated with multi morbidity Add extra financial and task to do burden on a retired old patient.

The current fragmented, single disease-oriented healthcare system (Fortin et al., 2007) forced the multimorbid patient to have frequent visits to healthcare facilities, at each visit the health staff obligate him with a different management plan, which may contradict another health staff plan or at least make the patient confused. Multimorbidity, is disabling and costly on healthcare system and patients.

The effect of socioeconomic status on multimorbidity, has been addressed in many studies. One of the retrospective cohort studies concluded that exposure to disadvantaged socioeconomic conditions in childhood or over the entire life course could predict the multimorbidity in older age (Jungo et al., 2022). Another family life survey, studied by determinants of multimorbidity among the elderly found that higher rates of multimorbidity in elderly is associated with low socioeconomic conditions and poor health behaviours (Mahwati, 2014).

Not only does socioeconomic status affects multimorbidity, but also multimorbidity affects the socioeconomic status of patients. In a systematic review (Larkin et al., 2021) which involved qualitative studies from six continents, the included 46 studies indicated that financial burden compromise patients health through non-adherence to medication, self-management practices, and non-attendance at healthcare appointment, which could create a negative cycles adding more stress, worries and frustration to patients life and negatively impacted their psychological well-being.

The effect of multimorbidity on the health system was elaborated on many studies. One systematic review, found that multimorbidity is associated with increased in hospitalization rate, and frequency of primary care and dental visits, hospital and total cost (Soley-Bori et al., 2021). In this systematic review studies demonstrated that depression is one of the important conditions associated with higher cost and hospital utilization. It was also found that those with four or more conditions have 14.38 times increased odds for unplanned potentially preventable hospitalization. Another systematic literature review emphasized the large effect of multimorbidities on hospital stays as well as total health coasts (Lehnert et al., 2011). The increase in frequency of ER and general practitioner visits is also supported by a population-based cohort study (Mbuya-Bienge et al., 2021). Patients with multimorbidity are shown to spend longer consultation time compared to those without multimorbidity (Tadeu et al., 2020).

The effect of educational level on multi morbidity has been investigated in different studies.

These studies range from systematic review to cross sectional types. All these studies found a high significant association between low educational level and increased odds of multimorbidity (Altonen et al., 2020; Bof de Andrade et al., 2022;

Frølich et al., 2019; Pathirana & Jackson, 2018). Diabetes, low back pain where notably independently associated with the lowest educational level (Frølich et al., 2019). Increasing educational attainment were found to be associated with the increase in the prevalence of multimorbidity (Bof de Andrade et al., 2022). Geographical distribution of multimorbidity varies from area to area, lower prevalence was found in areas with high educational level, and vice versa (Bof de Andrade et al., 2022). Contradicting all reviewed studies one meta-analysis found inconsistent relation between multi morbidity and the educational level in different countries, however these results could be related to different national contexts which are dependent on subjective self-reports rather than on objective data collection, such as physical examination which questions it's validity and reliability (Feng et al., 2021).

Other factors which affect multimorbidity include occupation, income, and higher deprivation.

Although occupation have been strongly associated with multimorbidity, dose response relationships were less marked (Altonen et al., 2020). Inconsistent studies were found for income in relation to multi morbidity risk, on the other hand, statistically significant association was found between higher deprivation levels and greater risk of morbidity (Pathirana & Jackson, 2018).

In conclusion, low socioeconomic status and educational levels are strongly associated with a higher rate of multimorbidity, these findings mandate hard work in improving the national and the individuals Socio economic status and offering mass Health education to its citizens.

PATIENT-CENTRED CARE

The complexity and heavy burden of multimorbidity on patient as well as healthcare system necessitates the transformation to an integrated patient cantered healthcare system which takes in account patients value.

More collaboration between patients and the healthcare team is needed. The patient must be considered a partner rather than a recipient of a list of tasks which concentrate mainly on healthcare system goals without paying attention to his own needs or feelings. If the patient understood the expected outcome and the odds of a successful caring plan its more likely that he will have a very positive experience and his engagement will more likely be insured.

In one systematic review it was shown that the more patient-centred organizations are, the more they are going to have positive outcomes in the form of improving patient quality of life,

Increasing professional job satisfaction and promoting safety and quality of the provided healthcare services (Rathert et al., 2013).

Patient-centred care can be defined as providing care that is respectful of and responsive to individual patients preferences, needs and values and ensuring that patient values guide all clinical decisions (Richardson et al., 2001).

The dimensions of patient centeredness are identified through a systematic review and include essential characteristics of clinician, clinician-patient relationship, clinician-patient communication, patient as a unique Person, biopsychosocial perspectives, patient information, patient involvement in care, involvement of family and friends, patient empowerment, physical support, emotional support, integration of medical and non-medical care, teamwork and teambuilding, access to care, coordination and continuity of care. It provides a foundation for healthcare provider and manager to establish patient-centred care (Scholl et al., 2014).

Every single patient with multimorbidity needs a care plan, which is tailored to his clinical conditions (Kuipers et al., 2020) meeting these needs based on the shared physician patient decision making contributes to the physical and social well-being of the patients (Kuipers et al., 2019). Poor health and cognitive impairment is considered as a barrier to shared decision making, while explicit invitation of an old patient to participate in decision making and good communication skills of healthcare professionals facilitate shared decision making (Pel-Littel et al., 2021).

General practitioners are frequently asked to manage patients with multimorbidity. They express their concerns about applying a single disease guideline to a multimorbid patient and the possibility of causing harm and subsequently failing to maintain a continuous positive trustful relationship with the patient. formulating multimorbidity management guidelines are highly requested by general practitioners (Damarell et al., 2020).

Multimorbidity Guidelines

Few Multimorbidity Guidelines were Published, all of which share patient-centred principles.

In 2016, The world health organization published multimorbidity technical series on safer primary Healthcare, it highlights the importance of safe practice. multimorbidity management guidelines need to be created and highly encouraged. Policymakers need to prioritize multi morbidity and train primary care physicians to understand it and adhere to it (Cohen, 2016).

In 2016, the UK national Institute for health and care excellence guidelines for multimorbidity explicitly recommend that patient's goals, values, and priorities should include establishment of disease and treatment burden and take in account improving coordination of care across services (UK, 2016).

The American Geriatrics Society has established guiding principles for the patient-centred care of older adults with multimorbidity. These include eliciting patient preferences and carefully weighing up individual burdens, risks, benefits, and prognosis (Stott & Young, 2012). In 2019 they translated these principles into a framework to assist clinicians decision making for specialties delivering the care to older people with multiple chronic conditions (Boyd et al., 2019).

In 2022, Italian scientific societies working in the field of aging, general and internal medicine, and pharmacology published Italian guidelines on the management of persons with multimorbidity and polypharmacy (Onder et al., 2022).

In 2022, a Germany Evidence-Based Decision Support on Polypharmacy in Multimorbidity guideline was published. It enabled 57% of GPs to identify problems, that lead to medication changes in 49% and self-assessed improvement in 56% of patients and recommended by 92% of GPs (Dinh et al., 2022).

Models for Care for Patients With Multimorbidity

During the last few years, several models for patients with multimorbidity were developed. However, few of them have been implemented and evaluated. The integrated multimorbidity care model was designed and called Chrodis-Plus, that was implemented in five European countries and found able to improve multimorbid patient care quality (Rodriguez-Blazquez et al., 2020).

The Ariadne principles was formulated by 19 experts from North America, Europe and Australia. Realistic treatment goals shared between physician and patient are at the core of these principles (Muth et al., 2014). The multi-pap intervention is a patient-centred intervention implementing the Ariadne principles, its effectiveness is studied by a systematic review and showed that it is effective in improving medication appropriateness however, the magnitude of the effect is small and cautious interpretation is advised (Prados-Torres et al., 2017).

The 3D (dimension of health, depression and drugs) is a patient-centred intervention, which wasn't found to be beneficial with regards to treatment burden or life quality in general practice sitting as reported by a systematic review (Salisbury et al., 2018). Minimally disruptive medicine (MDM) is defined as a patient-centred approach of care that focuses on achieving patient's goal for life and health, while imposing the smallest possible treatment burden on their lives (Leppin et al., 2015). Clinicians can assess the burden of treatment on patients using the instruments for patient capacity assessment (ICAN) (Trevena, 2018). In order to achieve minimally disruptive management, the clinical practitioner should use the principles of shared decision making guided by his own experience to provide optimal care. Minimally disruptive management had been applied on diabetic patient with multimorbidity, it was found to be beneficial in improving patient outcome through coordinating community and healthcare responses, lowering treatment burden and enhancing patient capacity to chase their dreams (Serrano et al., 2017).

Goal oriented care model is based on collaboration among professionals and patients to set goals, and identify strategies to achieve. Despite the sound rationale and the strong push towards dissemination, it is very difficult to find good quality 'unbiased homogeneous studies, more future studies are needed to give firm conclusions (Barbato et al., 2022).

Future Models of Multimorbidity Care

In order to advance multimorbidity management we need to develop strong accessible primary care, being a gate keeper and the most frequently visited medical staff by a multimorbid patient, primary care services must be given priority by policymakers and decisionmakers level, primary care physicians should be offered a focused multimorbidity management training program and equally importantly establishing a health system that enhances communication and coordination and service integration across different levels of a healthcare system (Aramrat et al., 2022).

Multimorbidity decision support systems enables healthcare professionals to get a tailored patient management plan and reduce costs, avoid unnecessary treatments, and reduce length of stay, one of the good example of decision support system for multimorbidity management is The Comorbidities Manger Launched recently by BMJ Best Practice (Rayman et al., 2022).

Future research should be directed at understanding the clustering and sequencing of diseases, with a view to determine key drivers and efficient preventive or curative interventions as needed (Whitty et al., 2020).

REFERENCES

Altonen, B. L., Arreglado, T. M., Leroux, O., Murray-Ramcharan, M., & Engdahl, R. (2020). Characteristics, comorbidities and survival analysis of young adults hospitalized with COVID-19 in New York City. *PLoS One*, *15*(12), e0243343. doi:10.1371/journal.pone.0243343 PMID:33315929

Aramrat, C., Choksomngam, Y., Jiraporncharoen, W., Wiwatkunupakarn, N., Pinyopornpanish, K., Mallinson, P. A. C., Kinra, S., & Angkurawaranon, C. (2022). Advancing multimorbidity management in primary care: A narrative review. *Primary Health Care Research and Development*, *23*, e36. doi:10.1017/S1463423622000238 PMID:35775363

Bah, S., Hussain, M., AlHotheyfa, R., AlNujaidi, H. Y., Al-Qahtani, M., AlAnsary, N., & Albagmi, F. M. (2022). *Multimorbidity Prevalence and Contributing Factors in Saudi Arabia*. Academic Press.

Barbato, A., D'Avanzo, B., Cinquini, M., Fittipaldo, A. V., Nobili, A., Amato, L., Vecchi, S., & Onder, G. (2022). Effects of goal-oriented care for adults with multimorbidity: A systematic review and meta-analysis. *Journal of Evaluation in Clinical Practice, 28*(3), 371–381. doi:10.1111/jep.13674 PMID:35355381

Barnett, K., Mercer, S. W., Norbury, M., Watt, G., Wyke, S., & Guthrie, B. (2012). Epidemiology of multimorbidity and implications for health care, research, and medical education: A cross-sectional study. *Lancet, 380*(9836), 37–43. doi:10.1016/S0140-6736(12)60240-2 PMID:22579043

Bezerra de Souza, D. L., Oliveras-Fabregas, A., Espelt, A., Bosque-Prous, M., de Camargo Cancela, M., Teixidó-Compañó, E., & Jerez-Roig, J. (2021). Multimorbidity and its associated factors among adults aged 50 and over: A cross-sectional study in 17 European countries. *PLoS One, 16*(2), e0246623. doi:10.1371/journal.pone.0246623 PMID:33571285

Bof de Andrade, F., Thumé, E., Facchini, L. A., Torres, J. L., & Nunes, B. P. (2022). Education and income-related inequalities in multimorbidity among older Brazilian adults. *PLoS One, 17*(10), e0275985. doi:10.1371/journal.pone.0275985 PMID:36227899

Boyd, C., Smith, C. D., Masoudi, F. A., Blaum, C. S., Dodson, J. A., Green, A. R., & Rich, M. W. (2019). Decision making for older adults with multiple chronic conditions: Executive summary for the American Geriatrics Society guiding principles on the care of older adults with multimorbidity. *Journal of the American Geriatrics Society, 67*(4), 665–673. doi:10.1111/jgs.15809 PMID:30663782

Calderón-Larrañaga, A., Vetrano, D. L., Ferrucci, L., Mercer, S., Marengoni, A., Onder, G., Eriksdotter, M., & Fratiglioni, L. (2019). Multimorbidity and functional impairment–bidirectional interplay, synergistic effects and common pathways. *Journal of Internal Medicine, 285*(3), 255–271. doi:10.1111/joim.12843 PMID:30357990

Carrasco-Ribelles, L. A., Roso-Llorach, A., Cabrera-Bean, M., Costa-Garrido, A., Zabaleta-del-Olmo, E., Toran-Monserrat, P., Orfila Pernas, F., & Violan, C. (2022). Dynamics of multimorbidity and frailty, and their contribution to mortality, nursing home and home care need: A primary care cohort of 1 456 052 ageing people. *EClinicalMedicine, 52*, 101610. doi:10.1016/j.eclinm.2022.101610 PMID:36034409

Clegg, A., Young, J., Iliffe, S., Rikkert, M. O., & Rockwood, K. (2013). Frailty in elderly people. *Lancet, 381*(9868), 752–762. doi:10.1016/S0140-6736(12)62167-9 PMID:23395245

Cohen, M. (2016). *Technical Series on Safer Primary Care: Multimorbidity.* World Health Organization.

Damarell, R. A., Morgan, D. D., & Tieman, J. J. (2020). General practitioner strategies for managing patients with multimorbidity: A systematic review and thematic synthesis of qualitative research. *BMC Family Practice*, *21*(1), 1–23. doi:10.118612875-020-01197-8 PMID:32611391

Di Angelantonio, E., Kaptoge, S., Wormser, D., Willeit, P., Butterworth, A. S., Bansal, N., & Burgess, S. (2015). Association of cardiometabolic multimorbidity with mortality. *Journal of the American Medical Association*, *314*(1), 52–60. doi:10.1001/jama.2015.7008 PMID:26151266

Dinh, T. S., Brueckle, M.-S., González-González, A. I., Fessler, J., Marschall, U., Schubert-Zsilavesz, M., & Schubert, I. (2022). Evidence-Based Decision Support for a Structured Care Program on Polypharmacy in Multimorbidity: A Guideline Upgrade Based on a Realist Synthesis. *Journal of Personalized Medicine*, *12*(1), 69. doi:10.3390/jpm12010069 PMID:35055383

Divo, M. J., Martinez, C. H., & Mannino, D. M. (2014). Ageing and the epidemiology of multimorbidity. *The European Respiratory Journal*, *44*(4), 1055–1068. doi:10.1183/09031936.00059814 PMID:25142482

Dumbreck, S., Flynn, A., Nairn, M., Wilson, M., Treweek, S., Mercer, S. W., & Guthrie, B. (2015). Drug-disease and drug-drug interactions: Systematic examination of recommendations in 12 UK national clinical guidelines. *BMJ, 350*.

Everett, J. A. (2013). The 12 item social and economic conservatism scale (SECS). *PLoS One*, *8*(12), e82131. doi:10.1371/journal.pone.0082131 PMID:24349200

Feinstein, A. R. (1970). The pre-therapeutic classification of co-morbidity in chronic disease. *Journal of Chronic Diseases*, *23*(7), 455–468. doi:10.1016/0021-9681(70)90054-8 PMID:26309916

Feng, X., Kelly, M., & Sarma, H. (2021). The association between educational level and multimorbidity among adults in Southeast Asia: A systematic review. *PLoS One*, *16*(12), e0261584. doi:10.1371/journal.pone.0261584 PMID:34929020

Fortin, M., Soubhi, H., Hudon, C., Bayliss, E. A., & Van den Akker, M. (2007). *Multimorbidity's many challenges* (Vol. 334). British Medical Journal Publishing Group.

Frølich, A., Ghith, N., Schiøtz, M., Jacobsen, R., & Stockmarr, A. (2019). Multimorbidity, healthcare utilization and socioeconomic status: A register-based study in Denmark. *PLoS One*, *14*(8), e0214183. doi:10.1371/journal.pone.0214183 PMID:31369580

Garin, N., Koyanagi, A., Chatterji, S., Tyrovolas, S., Olaya, B., Leonardi, M., & Ayuso-Mateos, J. L. (2016). Global multimorbidity patterns: A cross-sectional, population-based, multi-country study. *Journals of Gerontology Series A: Biomedical Sciences and Medical Sciences, 71*(2), 205–214. doi:10.1093/gerona/glv128 PMID:26419978

Gomes, R. S., Barbosa, A. R., Meneghini, V., Confortin, S. C., d'Orsi, E., & Rech, C. R. (2020). Association between chronic diseases, multimorbidity and insufficient physical activity among older adults in southern Brazil: A cross-sectional study. *Sao Paulo Medical Journal, 138*(6), 545–553. doi:10.1590/1516-3180.2020.0282.r1.15092020 PMID:33331604

Guisado-Clavero, M., Roso-Llorach, A., López-Jimenez, T., Pons-Vigués, M., Foguet-Boreu, Q., Muñoz, M. A., & Violán, C. (2018). Multimorbidity patterns in the elderly: A prospective cohort study with cluster analysis. *BMC Geriatrics, 18*(1), 1–11. doi:10.118612877-018-0705-7 PMID:29338690

Haug, N., Deischinger, C., Gyimesi, M., Kautzky-Willer, A., Thurner, S., & Klimek, P. (2020). High-risk multimorbidity patterns on the road to cardiovascular mortality. *BMC Medicine, 18*(1), 1–12. doi:10.118612916-020-1508-1 PMID:32151252

Idler, E. L., & Benyamini, Y. (1997). Self-rated health and mortality: A review of twenty-seven community studies. *Journal of Health and Social Behavior, 38*(1), 21–37. doi:10.2307/2955359 PMID:9097506

Johnston, M. C., Crilly, M., Black, C., Prescott, G. J., & Mercer, S. W. (2019). Defining and measuring multimorbidity: A systematic review of systematic reviews. *European Journal of Public Health, 29*(1), 182–189. doi:10.1093/eurpub/cky098 PMID:29878097

Jungo, K. T., Cheval, B., Sieber, S., Antonia van der Linden, B. W., Ihle, A., Carmeli, C., Chiolero, A., Streit, S., & Cullati, S. (2022). Life-course socioeconomic conditions, multimorbidity and polypharmacy in older adults: A retrospective cohort study. *PLoS One, 17*(8), e0271298. doi:10.1371/journal.pone.0271298 PMID:35917337

Kivimäki, M., Strandberg, T., Pentti, J., Nyberg, S. T., Frank, P., Jokela, M., & Sipilä, P. N. (2022). Body-mass index and risk of obesity-related complex multimorbidity: An observational multicohort study. *The Lancet. Diabetes & Endocrinology, 10*(4), 253–263. doi:10.1016/S2213-8587(22)00033-X PMID:35248171

Koller, D., Schön, G., Schäfer, I., Glaeske, G., van den Bussche, H., & Hansen, H. (2014). Multimorbidity and long-term care dependency—A five-year follow-up. *BMC Geriatrics, 14*(1), 1–9. doi:10.1186/1471-2318-14-70 PMID:24884813

Kshatri, J. S., Palo, S. K., Bhoi, T., Barik, S. R., & Pati, S. (2020). Prevalence and Patterns of Multimorbidity Among Rural Elderly: Findings of the AHSETS Study. *Frontiers in Public Health*, *8*, 582663. doi:10.3389/fpubh.2020.582663 PMID:33251177

Kuipers, S. J., Cramm, J. M., & Nieboer, A. P. (2019). The importance of patient-centered care and co-creation of care for satisfaction with care and physical and social well-being of patients with multi-morbidity in the primary care setting. *BMC Health Services Research*, *19*(1), 1–9. doi:10.118612913-018-3818-y PMID:30621688

Kuipers, S. J., Nieboer, A. P., & Cramm, J. M. (2020). Views of patients with multi-morbidity on what is important for patient-centered care in the primary care setting. *BMC Family Practice*, *21*(1), 1–12. doi:10.118612875-020-01144-7 PMID:32336277

Larkin, J., Foley, L., Smith, S. M., Harrington, P., & Clyne, B. (2021). The experience of financial burden for people with multimorbidity: A systematic review of qualitative research. *Health Expectations*, *24*(2), 282–295. doi:10.1111/hex.13166 PMID:33264478

Le Reste, J. Y., Nabbe, P., Rivet, C., Lygidakis, C., Doerr, C., Czachowski, S., & Assenova, R. (2015). The European general practice research network presents the translations of its comprehensive definition of multimorbidity in family medicine in ten European languages. *PLoS One*, *10*(1), e0115796. doi:10.1371/journal.pone.0115796 PMID:25607642

Lehnert, T., Heider, D., Leicht, H., Heinrich, S., Corrieri, S., Luppa, M., Riedel-Heller, S., & König, H.-H. (2011). Health care utilization and costs of elderly persons with multiple chronic conditions. *Medical Care Research and Review: MCRR*, *68*(4), 387–420. doi:10.1177/1077558711399580 PMID:21813576

Leppin, A. L., Montori, V. M., & Gionfriddo, M. R. (2015). Minimally disruptive medicine: A pragmatically comprehensive model for delivering care to patients with multiple chronic conditions. Healthcare.

Lv, J., Li, R., Yuan, L., Yang, X.-l., Wang, Y., Ye, Z.-W., & Huang, F.-M. (2022). Research on the frailty status and adverse outcomes of elderly patients with multimorbidity. *BMC Geriatrics*, *22*(1), 560.

Mahwati, Y. (2014). Determinants of multimorbidity among the elderly population in Indonesia. *Kesmas: Jurnal Kesehatan Masyarakat Nasional*, *9*(2), 187–193. doi:10.21109/kesmas.v9i2.516

Marengoni, A., Angleman, S., Melis, R., Mangialasche, F., Karp, A., Garmen, A., Meinow, B., & Fratiglioni, L. (2011). Aging with multimorbidity: A systematic review of the literature. *Ageing Research Reviews*, *10*(4), 430–439. doi:10.1016/j.arr.2011.03.003 PMID:21402176

Mavaddat, N., Valderas, J. M., Van Der Linde, R., Khaw, K. T., & Kinmonth, A. L. (2014). Association of self-rated health with multimorbidity, chronic disease and psychosocial factors in a large middle-aged and older cohort from general practice: A cross-sectional study. *BMC Family Practice*, *15*(1), 1–11. doi:10.118612875-014-0185-6 PMID:25421440

Mbuya-Bienge, C., Simard, M., Gaulin, M., Candas, B., & Sirois, C. (2021). Does socio-economic status influence the effect of multimorbidity on the frequent use of ambulatory care services in a universal healthcare system? A population-based cohort study. *BMC Health Services Research*, *21*(1), 1–11. doi:10.118612913-021-06194-w PMID:33676497

McPhail, S. M. (2016). Multimorbidity in chronic disease: Impact on health care resources and costs. *Risk Management and Healthcare Policy*, *9*, 143–156. doi:10.2147/RMHP.S97248 PMID:27462182

Mercer, S., Furler, J., Moffat, K., Fischbacher-Smith, D., & Sanci, L. (2016). *Multimorbidity: technical series on safer primary care*. World Health Organization.

Muth, C., van den Akker, M., Blom, J. W., Mallen, C. D., Rochon, J., Schellevis, F. G., & Kirchner, H. (2014). The Ariadne principles: How to handle multimorbidity in primary care consultations. *BMC Medicine*, *12*(1), 1–11. doi:10.118612916-014-0223-1 PMID:25484244

NICE. (2016). *Multimorbidity: Clinical assessment and management.* NICE guideline [NG56].

Onder, G., Vetrano, D. L., Palmer, K., Trevisan, C., Amato, L., Berti, F., & Kruger, P. (2022). Italian guidelines on management of persons with multimorbidity and polypharmacy. *Aging Clinical and Experimental Research*, *34*(5), 989–996. doi:10.100740520-022-02094-z PMID:35249211

Organization, W. H. (2018). *WHO methods and data sources for life tables 1990-2016*. Global Health Estimates Technical Paper WHO/HIS/IER/GHE.

Pathirana, T. I., & Jackson, C. A. (2018). Socioeconomic status and multimorbidity: A systematic review and meta-analysis. *Australian and New Zealand Journal of Public Health*, *42*(2), 186–194. doi:10.1111/1753-6405.12762 PMID:29442409

Pel-Littel, R. E., Snaterse, M., Teppich, N. M., Buurman, B. M., van Etten-Jamaludin, F. S., van Weert, J., Minkman, M. M., & Scholte op Reimer, W. J. M. (2021). Barriers and facilitators for shared decision making in older patients with multiple chronic conditions: A systematic review. *BMC Geriatrics*, *21*(1), 1–14. doi:10.118612877-021-02050-y PMID:33549059

Prados-Torres, A., del Cura-González, I., Prados-Torres, D., López-Rodríguez, J. A., Leiva-Fernández, F., Calderón-Larrañaga, A., & Pico-Soler, V. (2017). Effectiveness of an intervention for improving drug prescription in primary care patients with multimorbidity and polypharmacy: Study protocol of a cluster randomized clinical trial (Multi-PAP project). *Implementation Science; IS*, *12*(1), 1–10. doi:10.118613012-017-0584-x PMID:28449721

Rathert, C., Wyrwich, M. D., & Boren, S. A. (2013). Patient-centered care and outcomes: A systematic review of the literature. *Medical Care Research and Review: MCRR*, *70*(4), 351–379. doi:10.1177/1077558712465774 PMID:23169897

Rayman, G., Akpan, A., Cowie, M., Evans, R., Patel, M., Posporelis, S., & Walsh, K. (2022). Managing patients with comorbidities: Future models of care. *Future Healthcare Journal*, *9*(2), 101–105. doi:10.7861/fhj.2022-0029 PMID:35928198

Richardson, W. C., Berwick, D., Bisgard, J., Bristow, L., Buck, C., & Cassel, C. (2001). *Institute of medicine. Crossing the quality chasm: a new health system for the 21st century*. National Academy Press.

Rodriguez-Blazquez, C., João Forjaz, M., Gimeno-Miguel, A., Bliek-Bueno, K., Poblador-Plou, B., Pilar Luengo-Broto, S., & Rodríguez-Acuña, R. (2020). Assessing the pilot implementation of the integrated multimorbidity care model in five European settings: Results from the joint action CHRODIS-PLUS. *International Journal of Environmental Research and Public Health*, *17*(15), 5268. doi:10.3390/ijerph17155268 PMID:32707791

Romano, E., Ma, R., Vancampfort, D., Firth, J., Felez-Nobrega, M., Haro, J. M., Stubbs, B., & Koyanagi, A. (2021). Multimorbidity and obesity in older adults from six low-and middle-income countries. *Preventive Medicine*, *153*, 106816. doi:10.1016/j.ypmed.2021.106816 PMID:34599928

Ryan, A., Wallace, E., O'Hara, P., & Smith, S. M. (2015). Multimorbidity and functional decline in community-dwelling adults: A systematic review. *Health and Quality of Life Outcomes*, *13*(1), 1–13. doi:10.118612955-015-0355-9 PMID:26467295

Salisbury, C. (2012). Multimorbidity: Redesigning health care for people who use it. *Lancet*, *380*(9836), 7–9. doi:10.1016/S0140-6736(12)60482-6 PMID:22579042

Salisbury, C., Johnson, L., Purdy, S., Valderas, J. M., & Montgomery, A. A. (2011). Epidemiology and impact of multimorbidity in primary care: A retrospective cohort study. *The British Journal of General Practice*, *61*(582), e12–e21. doi:10.3399/bjgp11X548929 PMID:21401985

Salisbury, C., Man, M.-S., Bower, P., Guthrie, B., Chaplin, K., Gaunt, D. M., & Hollinghurst, S. (2018). Management of multimorbidity using a patient-centred care model: A pragmatic cluster-randomised trial of the 3D approach. *Lancet*, *392*(10141), 41–50. doi:10.1016/S0140-6736(18)31308-4 PMID:29961638

Salive, M. E. (2013). Multimorbidity in older adults. *Epidemiologic Reviews*, *35*(1), 75–83. doi:10.1093/epirev/mxs009 PMID:23372025

Scholl, I., Zill, J. M., Härter, M., & Dirmaier, J. (2014). An integrative model of patient-centeredness–a systematic review and concept analysis. *PLoS One*, *9*(9), e107828. doi:10.1371/journal.pone.0107828 PMID:25229640

Sembiah, S., Dasgupta, A., Taklikar, C. S., Paul, B., Bandyopadhyay, L., Burman, J., & Subbakrishna, N. (2022). Gender inequalities in prevalence, pattern and predictors of multimorbidity among geriatric population in rural West Bengal. *Journal of Family Medicine and Primary Care*, *11*(8), 4555–4561. doi:10.4103/jfmpc.jfmpc_565_21 PMID:36352948

Serrano, V., Spencer-Bonilla, G., Boehmer, K. R., & Montori, V. M. (2017). Minimally disruptive medicine for patients with diabetes. *Current Diabetes Reports*, *17*(11), 1–7. doi:10.100711892-017-0935-7 PMID:28942581

Sharma, P., & Maurya, P. (2022). Gender differences in the prevalence and pattern of disease combination of chronic multimorbidity among Indian elderly. *Ageing International*, *47*(2), 265–283. doi:10.100712126-021-09419-9

Sinclair, A. J., & Abdelhafiz, A. H. (2022). Multimorbidity, Frailty and Diabetes in Older People–Identifying Interrelationships and Outcomes. *Journal of Personalized Medicine*, *12*(11), 1911. doi:10.3390/jpm12111911 PMID:36422087

Smith, S. M., Wallace, E., Salisbury, C., Sasseville, M., Bayliss, E., & Fortin, M. (2018). A core outcome set for multimorbidity research (COSmm). *Annals of Family Medicine*, *16*(2), 132–138. doi:10.1370/afm.2178 PMID:29531104

Soley-Bori, M., Ashworth, M., Bisquera, A., Dodhia, H., Lynch, R., Wang, Y., & Fox-Rushby, J. (2021). Impact of multimorbidity on healthcare costs and utilisation: A systematic review of the UK literature. *The British Journal of General Practice*, *71*(702), e39–e46. doi:10.3399/bjgp20X713897 PMID:33257463

Stott, D. J., & Young, J. (2012). Across the pond'–a response to the NICE guidelines for management. *Lancet*, *380*, 37–43.

Stott, D. J., & Young, J. (2017). 'Across the pond'—A response to the NICE guidelines for management of multi-morbidity in older people. *Age and Ageing*, *46*(3), 343–345. doi:10.1093/ageing/afx031 PMID:28369219

Tadeu, A. C. R., de Figueiredo, I. J., & Santiago, L. M. (2020). Multimorbidity and consultation time: A systematic review. *BMC Family Practice*, *21*(1), 1–8. doi:10.118612875-020-01219-5 PMID:32723303

Trevena, L. (2018). Minimally disruptive medicine for patients with complex multimorbidity. *Australian Journal of General Practice*, *47*(4), 175–179. doi:10.31128/AFP-10-17-4374 PMID:29621856

UK, N. G. C. (2016). *Multimorbidity: assessment, prioritisation and management of care for people with commonly occurring multimorbidity*. UK.

van den Akker, M., Buntinx, F., & Knottnerus, J. A. (1996). Comorbidity or multimorbidity: What's in a name? A review of literature. *The European Journal of General Practice*, *2*(2), 65–70. doi:10.3109/13814789609162146

Vassar, M., Jellison, S., Wendelbo, H., Wayant, C., Gray, H., & Bibens, M. (2019). Using the CONSORT statement to evaluate the completeness of reporting of addiction randomised trials: A cross-sectional review. *BMJ Open*, *9*(9), e032024. doi:10.1136/bmjopen-2019-032024 PMID:31494625

Vetrano, D. L., Foebel, A. D., Marengoni, A., Brandi, V., Collamati, A., Heckman, G. A., Hirdes, J., Bernabei, R., & Onder, G. (2016). Chronic diseases and geriatric syndromes: The different weight of comorbidity. *European Journal of Internal Medicine*, *27*, 62–67. doi:10.1016/j.ejim.2015.10.025 PMID:26643938

Vetrano, D. L., Rizzuto, D., Calderón-Larrañaga, A., Onder, G., Welmer, A.-K., Bernabei, R., Marengoni, A., & Fratiglioni, L. (2018). Trajectories of functional decline in older adults with neuropsychiatric and cardiovascular multimorbidity: A Swedish cohort study. *PLoS Medicine*, *15*(3), e1002503. doi:10.1371/journal.pmed.1002503 PMID:29509768

Vetrano, D. L., Roso-Llorach, A., Fernández, S., Guisado-Clavero, M., Violán, C., Onder, G., Fratiglioni, L., Calderón-Larrañaga, A., & Marengoni, A. (2020). Twelve-year clinical trajectories of multimorbidity in a population of older adults. *Nature Communications*, *11*(1), 3223. doi:10.103841467-020-16780-x PMID:32591506

Violán, C., Fernández-Bertolín, S., Guisado-Clavero, M., Foguet-Boreu, Q., Valderas, J. M., Vidal Manzano, J., Roso-Llorach, A., & Cabrera-Bean, M. (2020). Five-year trajectories of multimorbidity patterns in an elderly Mediterranean population using Hidden Markov Models. *Scientific Reports*, *10*(1), 16879. doi:10.103841598-020-73231-9 PMID:33037233

Whitty, C. J., MacEwen, C., Goddard, A., Alderson, D., Marshall, M., Calderwood, C., & Stokes-Lampard, H. (2020). *Rising to the challenge of multimorbidity* (Vol. 368). British Medical Journal Publishing Group.

Willadsen, T. G., Bebe, A., Køster-Rasmussen, R., Jarbøl, D. E., Guassora, A. D., Waldorff, F. B., Reventlow, S., & Olivarius, N. F. (2016). The role of diseases, risk factors and symptoms in the definition of multimorbidity–a systematic review. *Scandinavian Journal of Primary Health Care*, *34*(2), 112–121. doi:10.3109/0281 3432.2016.1153242 PMID:26954365

Wleklik, M., Uchmanowicz, I., Jankowska, E. A., Vitale, C., Lisiak, M., Drozd, M., Pobrotyn, P., Tkaczyszyn, M., & Lee, C. (2020). Multidimensional approach to frailty. *Frontiers in Psychology*, *11*, 564. doi:10.3389/fpsyg.2020.00564 PMID:32273868

Yarnall, A. J., Sayer, A. A., Clegg, A., Rockwood, K., Parker, S., & Hindle, J. V. (2017). New horizons in multimorbidity in older adults. *Age and Ageing*, *46*(6), 882–888. doi:10.1093/ageing/afx150 PMID:28985248

Zemedikun, D. T., Gray, L. J., Khunti, K., Davies, M. J., & Dhalwani, N. N. (2018). Patterns of multimorbidity in middle-aged and older adults: An analysis of the UK biobank data. *Mayo Clinic Proceedings*, *93*(7), 857–866. doi:10.1016/j.mayocp.2018.02.012 PMID:29801777

Chapter 3
Obesity in the Elderly

Mahwash Iftikhar
Hayatabad Medical Complex, Pakistan

Ayesha Jamal
Corydon Medical Clinic, Canada

Mian Mufarih Shah
Hayatabad Medical Complex, Pakistan

Sheraz Jamal Khan
Hayatabad Medical Complex, Pakistan

EXECUTIVE SUMMARY

With obesity there is an increase in relative risk of type 2 diabetes, hypertension, and cardiovascular diseases. These can induce a vicious circle of a downward spiral of morbidity and mortality. Obesity is also associated with disability and health costs. In the US alone, it is $192.2 billion. This would be a formidable worldwide cost if interpolated globally. Obesity is also associated with sleep disturbance, respiratory difficulties, joint and mobility disorders, as well as social stigma. Treatments are varied and multifaceted and one shoe does not fit all. The different treatments are a low caloric diet (600 calories/day—this is quite debatable in the elderly); motivational and behavior approaches to sustain changes in eating and activity, these too need a lot of dedicated workforce; and drug treatment should be regarded as a therapeutic trial. Drugs should be stopped if there is no weight loss in two months' time. All drugs have side effects.

DOI: 10.4018/978-1-6684-2354-7.ch003

INTRODUCTION

Obesity is a global health issue (Centers for Disease Control and Prevention, 2010) and one of the most neglected too. It is mostly dealt with adequately in children who may be suffering from various genetic obesity syndromes. In the rapidly modernized and mostly urbanized world with varying unhealthy eating habits, sedentary lifestyle and lack of exercise and motivation to keep oneself healthy, it has evolved as a major health hazard (Bray et al., 2017; World Obesity Federation, 2021). There is relatively less research on obesity in the elderly, but it is more complicated in the geriatric population due to the comorbid conditions they frequently present with.

Statistics related to obesity are alarming. Globally, 13% of adults aged 18 years and older were obese in 2016. Obesity represents approximately 20% of the US population and 22% worldwide. The World Health Organization (WHO) estimates that approximately 40% of adults are overweight (BMI 25–29.9) and 30% of adults are obese (BMI over 30) (WHO, 2000) (Centers for Disease Control and Prevention, 2010; Bray et al., 2017; World Obesity Federation, 2021; World Obesity Federation, n.d.; Rimm, 2014). According to CDC by 2035 over one third of those over the age of 60 will be considered obese.

Interestingly but truly, they blame it on longevity, indiscriminate use of refined foods related to obesity, urbanization, lack of rural structure and many other factors that have become almost synonymous with the future life trends mankind is pursuing. This is not only a problem of the effluent societies, but this is fast growing into other less developed societies and countries. We are at the crossroads of famine and plenty. Obesity is considered like a saving account and it stays there till one gets old. To get rid of it, one has to spend it. Merely decreasing the amount putting into a saving account would still keep the bank fat and it would not do the job.

According to WHO: Basal Metabolic Index or BMI with certain caveats is considered the benchmark for obesity. A BMI of >30 is a marker of obesity. This concept has been challenged as it does not consider the central obesity (also called visceral or abdominal obesity). Currently, 7% of the world's population is over 65 years of age. This figure is projected to rise to 12% by 2030. Some 35% of world population is overweight or obese and so this is exponentially increasing with the baby boom. Simple statistics dictate that it is equally common across all age groups and elderly population is no exception.

Chronic conditions, such as arthritis, diabetes, hypertension, and heart disease, are among some of the most common, debilitating chronic conditions in older adults (Rubino et al., 2020; Brewis et al., 2018). These conditions are frequently accentuated by obesity and vice versa too (unfortunately).

Obesity is accumulation of excessive fat that presents an overall health risk (WHO). Fat accumulation however does not stay the only morbidity as it has close association with cardiovascular, metabolic, musculoskeletal, respiratory, and psychiatric conditions. Obesity begets obesity and once obese, always obese is a dreadful saying. Metabolic Obesity which leads to metabolic syndrome is characterized by abdominal or visceral obesity. This is measured by waist circumference. This is defined as a waist circumference of 40 inches in men and 35 inches in women. This measure has a strong association with metabolic syndrome and diabetes mellitus. It increases mortality and morbidity several folds.

An important determinant of body-fat mass is the relationship between energy intake and expenditure. Obesity occurs when a person consumes more calories than she/he burns. We need calories to sustain life and have the energy to be active and agile, yet to maintain a desirable weight. We need to balance the amount of energy we ingest in the form of food with the energy we use up during our activities of daily living and instrumental activities of daily living. The more sedentary and mechanized life would become, more would be its impact of the weight gain.

Weight gain occurs when the balance between intake and output is disturbed, and we take in more calories than we can consume. Most studies indicate that the amount of food we eat does not decline with advancing age. It stays steady state. Variation mostly occurs in consumption rather than intake. When consumption decrease due to decrease in activity with advancing age, the accumulated fat may further increase or at least it doesn't decrease. This positive balance or steady state both can be the cause of obesity.

"Thin people are beautiful, but fat people are adorable." – Jackie Gleason

Essentials

Obesity is more cumbersome in the elderly because:

1. With obesity, there is an increase in relative risk of type 2 diabetes, hypertension, and cardiovascular diseases. These can induce a vicious cycle of a downward spiral of mobility and mortality.
2. Obesity is also associated with disability and health costs. In the US alone, it is $192.2 billion. This would be a formidable worldwide cost if interpolated globally.
3. Obesity is also associated with sleep disturbance, respiratory difficulties, joint and mobility disorders, as well as social stigma.
4. Treatments are varied and multifaceted and one shoe does not fit all. The different treatments are:
    a. Low caloric diet (600 calories/day). This is quite debatable in the elderly.

b.   Motivational and behavior approaches to sustain changes in eating and activity. These too need a lot of dedicated workforces.

c.   Drug treatment should be regarded as a therapeutic trial. Drugs should be stopped if there is no weight loss in two months' time. All drugs have sides effects.

d.   Surgery is for people with morbid obesity or with associated complications. Surgery is usually marred with complications and contradictions due to other co-morbid conditions.

PATHOPHYSIOLOGY OF OBESITY IN THE ELDERLY

It is likely that a decrease in energy expenditure, particularly in the 50- 65-year-old age group, contributes to the increase in body fat as we age. In those 65 years of age and older, hormonal changes that occur during aging may contribute to the accumulation of fat. Hormonal changes are varied and protean and maybe there are different presentations in different individuals. Generally, aging is associated with a decrease in growth hormone secretions, reduced responsiveness to thyroid hormone, decline in serum testosterone, and resistance to leptin. Resistance to leptin could cause a decreased ability to regulate appetite downward. One thus stays hungry and gain more weight due to dysregulated satiety. Leptins should simply be considered as negative feedback to eat more, and its amount, or action is inversely related to hunger and putting on more weight. Leptins if decreased or its action stopped or inhibited would thus lead to obesity (World Health Organization, 2000; WHO, 1997; Ward et al., 2019; Amarya et al., 2014; Batsis & Dolkart, 2015; Do Cetin & Nasr, 2014; Coker & Wolfe, 2018; Dudeja et al., 2001; Zamboni & Mazzali, 2012; Zamboni et al., 2005; Stoever et al., 2015; Starr & Bales, 2015).

Genetic, environmental, and social, as well as several other factors can all contribute to obesity. Mostly this cause childhood obesity. Obese children however make obese adults. Though many of these syndromes do not have a normal life span but a proportion of them would grow into obese elderly and may make a small subset of obese elderly individuals. A detailed description would not be presented here as it is beyond the scope of this chapter. BMI may be complicated by some age-related anthropometric changes like height changes in women in the elderly. Women may lose 2-3 cm on average at the age of 65 and above from their male counterparts at similar age and may complicate the BMI calculation based on height and weight.

Sarcopenia defined as the loss of muscle mass with an increase in adipose tissue is common in the elderly and this may complicate the anthropometric measures further. Weight once a determinant of fats, muscles and bones is now constituted of more fat than muscles and bone. This interesting phenomenon may lead to steady or even decreased weight in the presence of accumulation of fats. Frailty syndrome is another caveat that is characterized by age-related loss and dysfunction of skeletal muscle as well as bone. This may have effects on weight. Sarcopenia and frailty both add to the complicated picture of obesity in the elderly.

To complicate things further, obesity is an independent risk factor for a number of cancers both in men and woman. It also leads to decreased healing and is usually associated with increased mortality due to varied conditions including infections. The recent COVID pandemic has confirmed that obesity was associated with a statistically significant mortality in all age groups and every geographical location.

Treatment modalities used in young people must be very carefully tailored while treating obesity in the elderly. One of the important treatment modalities to curtail obesity is caloric restriction and fasting. Calorie restricted diets can worsen sarcopenia, frailty syndrome and other nutritional deficiencies. This can be further hazardous than beneficial. Bariatric surgery has a limited role in selected older obese adults. This must not be offered as a routine to the elderly as it ultimately would lead to malnutrition.

Obesity has a great impact on rehabilitation from conditions like strokes, heart diseases and other illnesses peculiar to the geriatric population. These diseases may complicate each other and one cannot be complacent about any of these conditions. Geriatric units should have the services of exercise, physiotherapists, nutritionists, and endocrinologists and must have a close liaison with pulmonologist, respiratory therapist, and cardiologist to help these people (Misra & Khurana, 2008; Van Gaal et al., 2006).

HEALTH PROBLEMS ASSOCIATED WITH OBESITY

Health problems associated with obesity are classified as either nonfatal or life threatening by the World Health Organization:

1. Nonfatal Health Problems Related to Obesity

Conditions, such as those associated with respiratory, musculoskeletal, and skin problems are classified as nonfatal.

a. Respiratory Problems

The increased weight on the chest wall of obese patients and the difficulty they experience in lifting the heavy chest wall may contribute to difficulty in breathing. This is further complicated by abnormalities in gas exchange. The lung structure and function is also deteriorated and this is associated with normal aging. These changes in the lungs include decreased alveolar surface available for gas exchange, increased chest wall stiffness, and stiffening of the elastin and the collagen tissue supporting the lungs. Obese older patients often have a reduced respiratory efficiency that can reach the point of respiratory insufficiency in the presence of cardiovascular insufficiency of various degrees. Decreased respiratory functions further lead to sleep apnea syndrome, which, in these patients, is related to a greater risk of developing hallucinatory and cognitive disorders caused by hypoxia during sleep. This is further aggravated by the inner structures of throat including the tongue, palate and related structures and the shape of the neck. This would lead to a complicated phenomenon of both central and obstructive sleep apnea.

b.   Arthritis and Osteoarthritis

Arthritis, both axial and peripheral is the leading cause of disability in older adults. A high body mass index (BMI) is an independent risk factor for knee osteoarthritis (OA) in older persons. By 65 years of age the prevalence of osteoarthritis is 68% in women and 58% in men. This age-related increase in the prevalence of OA may reflect bodily changes as a result of a lifetime of being obesity that takes a toll on the weight bearing joints.

Cartilage damage is more prompt and the stress-pain-depression cycle is quite common. Obesity is the most important modifiable risk factor for osteoarthritis of the elderly.

c.   Skin Conditions

Itching, skin breakdown, redness, and rashes are very common in the obese elderly. This may lead to increased chances of pressure sores, infections, cellulitis, and septicemia. Incontinence to urine and feces is also common in the obese elderly and this may further complicate the skin conditions.

2.   Life-Threatening Illnesses Related to Obesity

The World Health Organization in 2005 has noted that life-threatening illnesses related to obesity include cardiovascular disease; conditions associated with insulin resistance, such as type 2 diabetes and certain types of cancers, especially hormonally related and large-bowel cancer (WHO, 2022).

a.   Cardiovascular Disease

Coronary heart disease is responsible for significant morbidity and mortality in older patients who are 65 years and older. It remains a leading cause of mortality in the US with 84% of persons 65 years or older dying from this disease. It is also a risk factor for type 2 diabetes.

b.   Diabetes

Type 2 diabetes, the most common type of diabetes in older adults, results from an interplay between genetic factors and environmental factors that contribute to obesity. There is an age-related increase in total body fat and visceral adiposity until age 65 that is often accompanied by diabetes or impaired glucose tolerance. In the Framingham Study 30-40% of people over 65 were found to have diabetes or glucose intolerance. Coronary disease is the most common and lethal sequel of type 2 diabetes. Lean-muscle mass begins to diminish after the age of 65. This decrease may be related to decrease in physical activity, disability, anabolic hormone production, or increased cytokine activity. If calorie intake continues at the same rate while the muscle mass decreases, the older person will most likely experience fat weight gain.

c.   Cancers

Obesity is also linked to higher rates of certain types of cancers. Breast cancer in older women is increasingly being linked to obesity. Twenty-five to 30% of several major cancers, including breast (postmenopausal), colon, kidney, and esophageal, have been linked to obesity and physical inactivity. Men who are obese are more likely to develop cancer of the colon, rectum, or prostate, than men who are not obese. Cancer of the gallbladder, uterus, cervix, or ovaries is more common in women who are obese compared with women who are not obese. Management of obesity is needed to decrease the incidence of these cancers.

Definitions

Who Is Elderly?

An older person is defined by the United Nations as a person who is over 60 years of age. However, families and communities often use other socio-cultural referents to define age, including family status (grandparents), physical appearance, or age-related health conditions. However, according to the United States Social Security Administration, anyone age 65 or older is elderly.

Who Is Obese?

Definition of Obesity

Obesity is the term used to indicate the high range of weight for an individual of given height that is associated with adverse health effects. WHO defines it as overweight and obesity are defined as abnormal or excessive fat accumulation that presents a risk to health. A body mass index (BMI) over 25 is considered overweight, and over 30 is obese. Cut off points proposed by WHO expert committee for the classification of overweight and obesity (World Obesity Federation, n.d.).

Table 1. BMI

BMI*	WHO Classification
<18.5	Underweight
18.5-24.9	Normal weight
25-29.9	Overweight
30.0-39.9	Obesity
40.0 or greater	Morbid obesity

BMI: BMI is calculated by dividing weight in kilograms by height in meters squared

Caveats

The definition of obesity based on BMI is not internationally universal. Individuals from India with a BMI over 25 are considered obese, whereas individuals from Asia are considered obese when their BMI is above 28. In order to prevent underdiagnosing obesity, clinicians caring for ethnic diverse populations must be aware of the variations in defining obesity based on BMI. Relying on BMI to define obesity can sometimes falsely under or overestimate an individual's obesity status. BMI does not differentiate between muscle, fat, and bone mass, and therefore cannot determine obesity status in all individuals.

What Is Abdominal Obesity?

BMI is not the only defining marker of obesity. The WHO defines obesity as the accumulation of excessive fat that presents an overall health risk. This accumulation of excess fat is often defined by using waist circumference. Waist circumference is a marker of intra-abdominal or visceral fat. Although the exact mechanism is not known, excessive adipose tissue is thought to increase inflammation and metabolic dysfunction of the organs within the abdominal region. Females with a waist circumference over 35 inches and males with a waist circumference over 40 inches are considered to be obese (World Health Organization, 2011; World Health Organization, 2000). These individuals display increased central obesity and have a statistically higher risk of developing insulin resistance, hypertension and dyslipidemia (Wormser et al., 2011).

What Are the Anatomic Consequences of Aging?

Anatomic consequences of aging are in part due to decreased bone density. They are mainly relating to decrease in bone density and muscle mass as well as an increase in adipose tissue. All of this is variable and unpredictable at times. The decrease in bone density results from a loss of vertebral height due to thinning of intervertebral discs typically seen in osteoporosis. Relying on BMI in the older population could underestimate the degree of adiposity due to the reduction of height. On average, women lose 2–3 cm more in height compared to their male counterparts which further decreases the validity of relying on BMI to determine obesity status.

Body composition of the obese older individual is different from their younger counterparts. With aging, individuals have redistribution of adipose tissue throughout their bodies. The older adult has an increased amount of intraabdominal fat with less subcutaneous fat. Intraabdominal fat accumulation is observed even in individuals with stable weight. Intrahepatic and intramuscular fat stores increase with age and are particularly prevalent in the thighs and calves. Ultimately the deposition of fat into the viscera and muscles result in increased insulin resistance that leads to a cycle of increased adipose tissue.

Sarcopenia and Frailty Syndrome in Aging

Aging is associated with a decline in muscle mass. Sarcopenia is defined as the loss of muscle mass with increases in adipose tissue. Sarcopenia is further defined as having decreased walking speed or grip strength. This condition is thought to affect up to 10% in individuals aged 50 and up to 35% of individuals over the age of 70. Decreased muscle mass results in a physiologic change that decreases the resting metabolic rate. This change is due to decreased mitochondrial volume and oxidative capacity resulting in a physiologic reduction in caloric metabolism (Barb et al., 2006; Alford et al., 2018; Andreyeva et al., 2004; Kjellberg et al., 2017; Upadhyay et al., 2018; Chooi et al., 2019). The physiologic changes leading to decreased muscle activity result in fat infiltration into the muscles leading to lipotoxicity, mitochondrial dysfunction, and inflammation. This further perpetuating underlying muscle dysfunction, insulin resistance, and increases in adipose tissue. These physiologic changes lead to difficulties with activities of daily living and overall increase in morbidity and mortality.

A lower BMI in the elderly population is associated with a higher risk of frailty syndrome in older adults. Frailty syndrome is characterized by age-related loss and dysfunction of skeletal muscle and bone. It is thought to affect multiple areas of human functioning in the geriatric population.

Sarcopenia and frailty syndrome can decrease the validity of current diagnostic measures of obesity in older adults. The clinician should evaluate patients' prior BMI trend, waist circumference, and muscle grip to determine the status of muscle loss and increased adiposity. Clinicians must first understand the complexity behind diagnosing elderly individuals with obesity prior to initiating treatment strategies.

What Is Morbid Obesity?

Morbid obesity is defined as a BMI above 35 with comorbidity (diabetes, hypertension, or obstructive sleep apnea) or over 40 without comorbidity.

Hormonal Changes With Aging

In those 65 years of age and older, hormonal changes that occur during aging may cause the accumulation of fat. Aging is associated with a decrease in growth hormone secretions, reduced responsiveness to thyroid hormone, decline in serum testosterone, and resistance to leptin. The body composition of an obese older individual is different from their younger counterparts.

Hormonal regulatory alterations predispose the old to increases in fat mass. There is redistribution of adipose tissue throughout the body with an increase in intra-abdominal fat with less subcutaneous fat. Aging results in decline in the growth hormone, insulin-like growth factor 1, testosterone in men and estrogen in woman. Testosterone is also reduced in obese men. Similar trends of lower levels of estrogens are known in obese women. The decrease in GH results in a decline in lean muscle mass. Sarcopenia may coexist with obesity and may cause frailty and associated complications. Obesity is a risk factor for type 2 DM, coronary artery disease, respiratory problems, dermatological problems, osteoarthritis, and above all many forms of cancer (pancreas, breast, colon, esophageal, endometrial, kidney, thyroid, liver, and gallbladder).

Obesity Paradox

In younger adults, obesity is known to increase the risk of developing diabetes, hypertension, and dyslipidemia. However, in older adults there is a phenomenon observed in which obesity may have a protective role. Obese older adults undergoing surgery or presenting with an acute critical illness, such as congestive heart failure exacerbation, had a lower mortality rate than overweight or underweight older adults (Cetin & Nasr, 2014). The belief is that obese older adults have increased energy stores that can withstand the demands of a critical illness. This phenomenon must be well respected while devising strategies for treatment of obesity in older populations. It may be prudent to leave alone the overweight or at least do fewer heroics to them and prevent them from complicated surgeries and starvation.

There are limitations to the obesity paradox. The mortality benefit applies to older adults with a BMI between 30 and 35, suggesting that older adults with a BMI categorized as morbidly obese no longer have this benefit.

Ways to Lose Obesity

The elderly should exercise daily for at least 30 minutes. By being engaged in physical exercise regularly, elders can easily prevent the risk of obesity. Physical exercise will not only help them to avoid obesity but also lead them towards a healthy and fit body.

Older people do not lose weight easily. It is much harder to lose weight as one gets older. Muscle loss is more significant than adipose tissue in old age. This has a bigger impact than the fact of simply losing muscle definition and tone. Muscle actually burns more calories than fat, so having less muscle means it's harder to use the calories one eats. Fats would accumulate these calories rather than burning them. The weight usually remains stable in such situations or there may be some gain, but weight loss must be taken seriously (WHO, 1997; Ward et al., 2019; Amarya et al., 2014; Batsis & Dolkart, 2015).

When the elderly lose weight rapidly one should look for comorbidities that may be playing in the background like heart diseases, gastrointestinal disorders, and cancers. These are the leading causes of weight loss in the elderly. Poor circulation causes a decrease in body mass because of the heart's inability to effectively pump and deliver nutrients to the various parts of the body. Excess weight in older people can have negative effects on their daily functioning, their social lives, and their mental health. High BMI is associated with a greater risk of functional limitation, especially mobility, among older people.

The giants of geriatrics are immobility, instability, incontinence, and intellectual impairment. They also have in common: a chronic course, deprivation of independence, depression and lack of self-esteem and no simple cure. One of the most significant complications of obesity in the elderly is the metabolic syndrome. This clustering of risk factors including increased waist circumference, hypertension, dyslipidemia, and glucose intolerance. Metabolic syndrome increases the likelihood of diabetes and cardiovascular disease.

Obesity puts people at risk for heart disease, type 2 diabetes, high blood pressure, stroke, and some types of cancer. In patients over 65, the increase in chronic diseases associated with aging reduces physical activity and exercise capacity, making it more difficult for elderly persons to lose weight. In the elderly population, weight loss is recommended in those with obesity (body mass index [BMI] 30 or higher) by a combination of diet and when possible exercise. There is an emphasis on resistance training with a gradual weight reduction diet to protect lean muscle mass and bone mineral density during weight loss.

APPROACHES TO WEIGHT LOSS AND TREATMENT IN THE ELDERLY

Approach should be individually tailored taking into account the individual circumstances and disease states in the elderly.

Goals of Weight Loss

Ideal body weight is not achievable and should not even be the goal especially in the elderly population. There is evidence that modest weight loss of the order of 5-10% from the initial weight is associated with significant reduction in comorbidities like hypertension, diabetes mellitus and dyslipidemia. All-cause mortality is reduced by 20-25% only with a 10 kg weight loss from the initial body weight.

Dietary Management

Caloric restriction is often the first modification that individuals implement to lose weight. Caution should be exercised in promoting caloric restriction in the old, as this can lead to increased risk for developing sarcopenia (Mathus-Vliegen et al., 2012; Hamerman, 1999; Ahmed et al., 2007). Weight loss can be achieved alone by a moderate caloric deficit of 500-1000 kcal/day which leads to 1-2 pounds lost per week and 8-10% over 6 months. The program must always be supervised. The low-calorie diet plan is usually to reduce the caloric intake up to 600kcal/day from the baseline caloric intake and over 6-12 months, it may reduce the weight by 8%.

A very low caloric diet where the minimum of calories in the range of 500 kcal/ day for men and 400 kcal/ day for women is used is neither beneficial nor safe in the elderly. The low caloric diet is equally effective as the very low caloric diet. The caloric restriction however must always be supervised by a physician and a nutritionist who should take into account the vitamin intake and micronutrients, lack of which can have very detrimental effects upon the elderly (Bray et al., 2016; Villareal et al., 2011; Aminian et al., 2015).

In order to avoid sarcopenia, the PROT-Age study provides guidelines with regard to daily protein requirements in the older adult (Bauer et al., 2013). Younger adults can maintain lean body mass when consuming 0.8 g/kg/day (Bauer et al., 2013; Jankovic et al., 2015). Older adults require a higher amount of daily protein; they require 1.2–1.5 g/kg/day of protein to compensate for age-related metabolic dysregulation, immune status, and hormonal fluctuations (Coker & Wolfe, 2018; Petroni et al., 2019).

In order to prevent muscle catabolism, elderly individuals with obesity with or at risk for sarcopenic obesity should be counseled on a less restrictive caloric deficit of 200-500 kcal/day combined with a recommended protein intake of 1.0-1.5 gm/ kg assuming normal renal function.

Behavioral Therapy and Exercise

Behavioral approaches would help the elderly to implement the eating patterns and activity (Bouchard et al., 2009). Only implementation should not suffice. They should sustain these activities for a long term as well. Daily exercise is necessary and a cumulative exercise of 150 minutes per week activity would help lose weight in the range of 4-6% of initial body weight. Type of physical activity (aerobic vs resistance) has no bearing on weight loss though resistance exercise may be more beneficial in the elderly to reduce sarcopenia and build muscle bulk.

Exercise is a reliable form of weight loss in obese older adults. The American College of Sports Medicine has issued an updated position on the benefits of exercise and physical activity for older adults. The updated guidelines recommend that older adults engage in 150 min of moderate intensity exercise (Shah et al., 2008; Shea et al., 2010; Witham & Avenell, 2010; Jensen & Hsiao, 2010; Rejeski et al., 2010; Jackson Leach et al., 2020). However, these recommendations are unlikely to elicit the amount of weight loss needed to improve metabolic and cardiovascular health (Jackson Leach et al., 2020; Simmonds et al., 2016; Angelidi et al., 2022). There is an emerging consensus that older adults should be encouraged to perform resistance training as it improves the muscle quality of older adults and is useful in combating sarcopenia and frailty syndrome (Sundell, 2011; Martínez et al., 2014).

Drug Therapy

The FDA has approved five medications for chronic weight management: Semaglutide, Liraglutide, Naltrexone/Bupropion, Phentermine/Topiramate, and Orlistat. Additionally, there is a trial on Empagliflozin undergoing in Japan since 2021 and Metformin has been used in obese nondiabetic elderly since long.

Previous anti-obesity drugs targeted central signaling like targeting cannabinoid signals (Rimonabant), noradrenergic (Phentermine) serotoninergic signaling (Fenfluramine), serotonergic reuptake (Sibutramine). These were moderately effective but were off target and had many central side effects (Pilitsi et al., 2019; Vosoughi et al., 2021).

Orlistat inhibits pancreatic and gastric lipases and would decrease triglyceride hydrolysis. It would maximally inhibit fat absorption at a dose of 120 mg / day at the expense of fatty stools and malabsorption of fat-soluble vitamins. This may not be very likeable for the elderly. The loose or liquid stool and urgency complicated with incontinence may be a menace for the elderly though it has the potential of behavior change that the user would avoid fats while in this drug.

Sibutramine promotes and prolong satiety by inhibiting the reuptake of serotonin and noradrenaline. The adverse effects of nausea, dry mouth and constipation may not be to the personal liking of the geriatric population. Recent concerns about cardiovascular mortality preclude its use in the elderly especially with established cardiovascular diseases.

Newer drugs like Lorcaserin, a selective 5HT receptor agonist has potential valvulopathy and cancer risk. Bupropion and naltrexone-bupropion due can be moderately effective too with anorexigenic effects. Synthetic GLP-1 Leraglutide effective in type 2 diabetes is approved by FDA for obesity and maybe useful for the elderly diabetic. It may not be tolerated however due to this nauseating potential. Many of the currently approved medications for weight loss are contraindicated in patients with hypertension, mood disorders, or glaucoma. These contraindications are clearly more prevalent in the geriatric population.

Liraglutide, a daily injectable GLP-1 receptor agonist was approved at doses of 3mg daily for weight loss by the FDA in 2014 for chronic weight management. This incretin-based therapy appears to have a short-term effect on decreasing gastric emptying but a long lasting central anorectic effect leading to a mean weight loss of 5.8kg in clinical studies.

Contrave, the combination of naltrexone, an opioid antagonist, and bupropion, an aminoketone antidepressant, was FDA approved in 2014 for chronic weight management. Only 2% (62 of 3,239 subjects) in the Contrave clinical trials were over age 65 years and none older than 75 years.

Surgery in Elderly Obese

It is usually reserved for selected patients with certain cut offs like BMI of more than 40 or BMI of more than 35 with comorbid conditions. Most of these are done laparoscopically. Almost all surgical procedures have the potential for malabsorption. These patients must return to see their doctor for readjustments like balloon and band readjustments that maybe hectic and time consuming.

Bariatric surgical interventions are increasingly common (Elbahrawy et al., 2018; Dorman et al., 2012; Contreras et al., 2013) to treat the morbidly obese and obese individuals with multiple comorbid conditions after those individuals who failed behavioral and medical interventions. The indications for bariatric surgery in the older adult are same as those in younger individuals. Selection for surgery has to be made based on comorbid conditions, surgical risk, and life expectancy. The older literature from the 2000s reported significantly worse outcomes in those older adults undergoing bariatric surgery compared with younger patients. Presently, there is a changing trend with the outcomes of bariatric surgery in the older adult (WHO, 2000; Maggard et al., 2005; Batsis & Dolkart, 2015).

Most procedures have operative mortalities around 0.2% and are not considered very safe in the elderly. Current surgical options include Roux-en-Y gastric bypass, sleeve gastrectomy, biliopancreatic diversion with duodenal switch, adjustable gastric banding, and intermittent vagal blockade. There are newer endoscopic approaches that include an expandable gastric balloon and gastric suturing. Despite the numerous options for surgical and endoscopic therapies for weight loss, there are a small number of studies that focus on the outcome of bariatric surgical procedures in the elderly population. The consensus thus is towards a very careful planning keeping in mind the age, life expectancy, comorbid conditions, and benefit vs. risk in all individuals.

Cryolipolysis is a newest procedure that is FDA approved for treatment of focal fat deposits in the flanks, abdomen, and thighs. In this procedure, fat cells are destroyed through a process of thermal reduction by which temperatures below normal but above freezing induce apoptosis-mediated cell death. Damaged adipocytes are then removed via an inflammatory response (Derrick et al., 2015).

REFERENCES

Ahmed, N., Mandel, R., & Fain, M. J. (2007). Frailty: An emerging geriatric syndrome. *The American Journal of Medicine*, *120*(9), 748–753. doi:10.1016/j. amjmed.2006.10.018 PMID:17765039

Alford, S., Patel, D., Perakakis, N., & Mantzoros, C. S. (2018). Obesity as a risk factor for Alzheimer's disease: Weighing the evidence. *Obesity Reviews*, *19*(2), 269–280. doi:10.1111/obr.12629 PMID:29024348

Amarya, S., Singh, K., & Sabharwal, M. (2014). Health consequences of obesity in the elderly. *Journal of Clinical Gerontology and Geriatrics*, *5*(3), 63–67. doi:10.1016/j. jcgg.2014.01.004

Aminian, A., Brethauer, S. A., Kirwan, J. P., Kashyap, S. R., Burguera, B., & Schauer, P. R. (2015). How safe is metabolic/diabetes surgery? *Diabetes, Obesity & Metabolism*, *17*(2), 198–201. doi:10.1111/dom.12405 PMID:25352176

Andreyeva, T., Sturm, R., & Ringel, J. S. (2004). Moderate and severe obesity have large differences in health care costs. *Obesity Research*, *12*(12), 1936–1943. doi:10.1038/oby.2004.243 PMID:15687394

Angelidi, A. M., Belanger, M. J., Kokkinos, A., Koliaki, C. C., & Mantzoros, C. S. (2022). Novel noninvasive approaches to the treatment of obesity: From pharmacotherapy to gene therapy. *Endocrine Reviews*, *43*(3), 507–557. doi:10.1210/endrev/bnab034 PMID:35552683

Barb, D., Pazaitou-Panayiotou, K., & Mantzoros, C. S. (2006). Adiponectin: A link between obesity and cancer. *Expert Opinion on Investigational Drugs*, *15*(8), 917–931. doi:10.1517/13543784.15.8.917 PMID:16859394

Batsis, J. A., & Dolkart, K. M. (2015). Evaluation of older adults with obesity for bariatric surgery: Geriatricians' perspective. *Journal of Clinical Gerontology and Geriatrics*, *6*(2), 45–53. doi:10.1016/j.jcgg.2015.01.001

Bouchard, D. R., Soucy, L., Sénéchal, M., Dionne, I. J., & Brochu, M. (2009). Impact of resistance training with or without caloric restriction on physical capacity in obese older women. *Menopause (New York, N.Y.)*, *16*(1), 66–72. doi:10.1097/gme.0b013e31817dacf7 PMID:18779759

Bray, G. A., Frühbeck, G., Ryan, D. H., & Wilding, J. P. (2016). Management of obesity. *Lancet*, *387*(10031), 1947–1956. doi:10.1016/S0140-6736(16)00271-3 PMID:26868660

Bray, G. A., Kim, K. K., & Wilding, J. P. H. (2017). Obesity: A chronic relapsing progressive disease process. A position statement of the World Obesity Federation. *Obesity Reviews*, *18*(7), 715–723. doi:10.1111/obr.12551 PMID:28489290

Brewis, A., SturtzSreetharan, C., & Wutich, A. (2018). Obesity stigma as a globalizing health challenge. *Globalization and Health*, *14*(1), 1–6. doi:10.118612992-018-0337-x PMID:29439728

Centers for Disease Control and Prevention. (2010). *Defining Childhood Overweight and Obesity*. CDC. https://www.cdc.gov/obesity/childhood/defining.html

Chooi, Y. C., Ding, C., & Magkos, F. (2019). The epidemiology of obesity. *Metabolism: Clinical and Experimental*, *92*, 6–10. doi:10.1016/j.metabol.2018.09.005 PMID:30253139

Coker, R. H., & Wolfe, R. R. (2018). Weight loss strategies in the elderly: A clinical conundrum. *Obesity (Silver Spring, Md.)*, *26*(1), 22–28. doi:10.1002/oby.21961 PMID:29265771

Contreras, J. E., Santander, C., Court, I., & Bravo, J. (2013). Correlation between age and weight loss after bariatric surgery. *Obesity Surgery*, *23*(8), 1286–1289. doi:10.100711695-013-0905-3 PMID:23462862

Derrick, C. D., Shridharani, S. M., & Broyles, J. M. (2015). The safety and efficacy of cryolipolysis: A systematic review of available literature. *Aesthetic Surgery Journal*, *35*(7), 830–836. doi:10.1093/asjjv039 PMID:26038367

Do Cetin, D. C., & Nasr, G. (2014). Obesity in the elderly: More complicated than you think. *Cleveland Clinic Journal of Medicine*, *81*(1), 51–61. doi:10.3949/ccjm.81a.12165 PMID:24391107

Dorman, R. B., Abraham, A. A., Al-Refaie, W. B., Parsons, H. M., Ikramuddin, S., & Habermann, E. B. (2012). Bariatric surgery outcomes in the elderly: An ACS NSQIP study. *Journal of Gastrointestinal Surgery*, *16*(1), 35–44. doi:10.100711605-011-1749-6 PMID:22038414

Dudeja, V., Misra, A., Pandey, R. M., Devina, G., Kumar, G., & Vikram, N. K. (2001). BMI does not accurately predict overweight in Asian Indians in northern India. *British Journal of Nutrition*, *86*(1), 105–112. doi:10.1079/BJN2001382 PMID:11432771

Elbahrawy, A., Bougie, A., Loiselle, S. E., Demyttenaere, S., Court, O., & Andalib, A. (2018). Medium to long-term outcomes of bariatric surgery in older adults with super obesity. *Surgery for Obesity and Related Diseases*, *14*(4), 470–476. doi:10.1016/j.soard.2017.11.008 PMID:29249586

Hamerman, D. (1999). Toward an understanding of frailty. *Annals of Internal Medicine*, *130*(11), 945–950. doi:10.7326/0003-4819-130-11-199906010-00022 PMID:10375351

Jackson Leach, R., Powis, J., Baur, L. A., Caterson, I. D., Dietz, W., Logue, J., & Lobstein, T. (2020). Clinical care for obesity: A preliminary survey of sixty-eight countries. *Clinical Obesity*, *10*(2), e12357. doi:10.1111/cob.12357 PMID:32128994

Jensen, G. L., & Hsiao, P. Y. (2010). Obesity in older adults: Relationship to functional limitation. *Current Opinion in Clinical Nutrition and Metabolic Care*, *13*(1), 46–51. doi:10.1097/MCO.0b013e32833309cf PMID:19841579

Kjellberg, J., Larsen, A. T., Ibsen, R., & Højgaard, B. (2017). The socioeconomic burden of obesity. *Obesity Facts*, *10*(5), 493–502. doi:10.1159/000480404 PMID:29020681

Mathus-Vliegen, E. M., Basdevant, A., Finer, N., Hainer, V., Hauner, H., Micic, D., Maislos, M., Roman, G., Schutz, Y., Tsigos, C., Toplak, H., Yumuk, V., & Zahorska-Markiewicz, B. (2012). Prevalence, pathophysiology, health consequences and treatment options of obesity in the elderly: A guideline. *Obesity Facts*, *5*(3), 460–483. doi:10.1159/000341193 PMID:22797374

Misra, A., & Khurana, L. (2008). Obesity and the metabolic syndrome in developing countries. *The Journal of Clinical Endocrinology and Metabolism*, *93*(11, supplement_1), s9–s30. doi:10.1210/jc.2008-1595 PMID:18987276

Pilitsi, E., Farr, O. M., Polyzos, S. A., Perakakis, N., Nolen-Doerr, E., Papathanasiou, A. E., & Mantzoros, C. S. (2019). Pharmacotherapy of obesity: Available medications and drugs under investigation. *Metabolism: Clinical and Experimental*, *92*, 170–192. doi:10.1016/j.metabol.2018.10.010 PMID:30391259

Powis, J., Jackson Leach, R., Barata Cavalcanti, O., & Lobstein, T. (2021). *Clinical care for obesity*. Available at: data.worldobesity.org/publications/wof-health-systems-final.pdf

Rejeski, W. J., Marsh, A. P., Chmelo, E., & Rejeski, J. J. (2010). Obesity, intentional weight loss and physical disability in older adults. *Obesity Reviews*, *11*(9), 671–685. doi:10.1111/j.1467-789X.2009.00679.x PMID:19922431

Rimm, A. (2014). Prevalence of obesity in the United States. *Journal of the American Medical Association*, *312*(2), 189–189. doi:10.1001/jama.2014.6219 PMID:25005660

Rubino, F., Puhl, R. M., Cummings, D. E., Eckel, R. H., Ryan, D. H., Mechanick, J. I., Nadglowski, J., Ramos Salas, X., Schauer, P. R., Twenefour, D., Apovian, C. M., Aronne, L. J., Batterham, R. L., Berthoud, H.-R., Boza, C., Busetto, L., Dicker, D., De Groot, M., Eisenberg, D, & Dixon, J. B. (2020). Joint international consensus statement for ending stigma of obesity. *Nature Medicine, 26*(4), 485–497. doi:10.103841591-020-0803-x PMID:32127716

Shah, K., Wingkun, N. J. G., Lambert, C. P., & Villareal, D. T. (2008). Weight loss Therapy Improves Endurance Capacity in Obese Older Adults. *Journal of the American Geriatrics Society, 56*(6), 1157–1159. doi:10.1111/j.1532-5415.2008.01699.x PMID:18554372

Shea, M. K., Houston, D. K., Nicklas, B. J., Messier, S. P., Davis, C. C., Miller, M. E., Harris, T. B., Kitzman, D. W., Kennedy, K., & Kritchevsky, S. B. (2010). The effect of randomization to weight loss on total mortality in older overweight and obese adults: The ADAPT Study. *Journals of Gerontology Series A: Biomedical Sciences and Medical Sciences, 65*(5), 519–525. doi:10.1093/gerona/glp217 PMID:20080875

Simmonds, M., Llewellyn, A., Owen, C. G., & Woolacott, N. (2016). Predicting adult obesity from childhood obesity: A systematic review and meta-analysis. *Obesity Reviews, 17*(2), 95–107. doi:10.1111/obr.12334 PMID:26696565

Starr, K. N. P., & Bales, C. W. (2015). Excessive body weight in older adults. *Clinics in Geriatric Medicine, 31*(3), 311–326. doi:10.1016/j.cger.2015.04.001 PMID:26195092

Stoever, K., Heber, A., Eichberg, S., Zijlstra, W., & Brixius, K. (2015). Changes of Body Composition, Muscular Strength and Physical Performance Due to Resistance Training in Older Persons with Sarcopenic Obesity. *The Journal of Frailty & Aging, 4*(4), 216–222. PMID:27031021

Upadhyay, J., Farr, O., Perakakis, N., Ghaly, W., & Mantzoros, C. (2018). Obesity as a disease. *Medicina Clínica, 102*(1), 13–33. PMID:29156181

Van Gaal, L. F., Mertens, I. L., & De Block, C. E. (2006). Mechanisms linking obesity with cardiovascular disease. *Nature, 444*(7121), 875–880. doi:10.1038/nature05487 PMID:17167476

Villareal, D. T., Chode, S., Parimi, N., Sinacore, D. R., Hilton, T., Armamento-Villareal, R., Napoli, N., Qualls, C., & Shah, K. (2011). Weight loss, exercise, or both and physical function in obese older adults. *The New England Journal of Medicine, 364*(13), 1218–1229. doi:10.1056/NEJMoa1008234 PMID:21449785

Vosoughi, K., Atieh, J., Khanna, L., Khoshbin, K., Prokop, L. J., Davitkov, P., Murad, M. H., & Camilleri, M. (2021). Association of glucagon-like peptide 1 analogs and agonists administered for obesity with weight loss and adverse events: A systematic review and network meta-analysis. *EClinicalMedicine*, *42*, 101213. doi:10.1016/j.eclinm.2021.101213 PMID:34877513

Ward, Z. J., Bleich, S. N., Cradock, A. L., Barrett, J. L., Giles, C. M., Flax, C., Long, M. W., & Gortmaker, S. L. (2019). Projected US state-level prevalence of adult obesity and severe obesity. *The New England Journal of Medicine*, *381*(25), 2440–2450. doi:10.1056/NEJMsa1909301 PMID:31851800

WHO. (1997). *Obesity: preventing and managing the global epidemic. Report of a WHO consultation on obesity*. WHO.

WHO. (2000). Obesity: Preventing and managing the global epidemic. *World Health Organization Technical Report Series*, *894*, 1–253. PMID:11234459

WHO. (2022). *Draft recommendations for the prevention and management of obesity over the life course, including potential targets*. WHO. www.who.int/teams/noncommunicable-diseases/governance/obesityrecommendations

Witham, M. D., & Avenell, A. (2010). Interventions to achieve long-term weight loss in obese older people: A systematic review and meta-analysis. *Age and Ageing*, *39*(2), 176–184. doi:10.1093/ageing/afp251 PMID:20083615

World Health Organization. (2011). *Waist circumference and waist-hip ratio: report of a WHO expert consultation*. WHO.

World Obesity Federation. (2021). *Obesity is a disease*. WOF. www.worldobesityday.org/assets/downloads/Obesity_Is_a_Disease.pdf

Wormser, D., Di Angelantonio, E., Sattar, N., Collins, R., Thompson, S., & Danesh, J. (2011). Body-mass index, abdominal adiposity, and cardiovascular risk–Authors' reply. *Lancet*, *378*(9787), 228. doi:10.1016/S0140-6736(11)61122-7

Zamboni, M., & Mazzali, G. (2012). Obesity in the elderly: An emerging health issue. *International Journal of Obesity*, *36*(9), 1151–1152. doi:10.1038/ijo.2012.120 PMID:22964828

Zamboni, M., Mazzali, G., Zoico, E., Harris, T. B., Meigs, J. B., Di Francesco, V., Fantin, F., Bissoli, L., & Bosello, O. (2005). Health consequences of obesity in the elderly: A review of four unresolved questions. *International Journal of Obesity*, *29*(9), 1011–1029. doi:10.1038j.ijo.0803005 PMID:15925957

Chapter 4
Multimorbidity and Heart Failure

Adil Hamad Alharthi
King Fahad Armed Forces Hospital, Saudi Arabia

Tabish Iqbal
Wadi Addawasir Military Hospital, Saudi Arabia

Muhammad Adnan Haider
King Fahad Armed Forces Hospital, Saudi Arabia

EXECUTIVE SUMMARY

Heart failure is a common disease worldwide. It is also an aging disease, being more common in the elder population; it is a multimorbidity disease as well, multimorbidity with heart failure became the norm; despite that, heart failure guidelines are still disease-specific, as well as multimorbidity and geriatric ignorant. To understand the unique, multimorbid, and geriatric characteristics of heart failure, one needs to understand the nature of the disease to shed light on the heart failure pathophysiological areas still in the shadows. Also needed is an understanding of symptom clusters in heart failure, their significance, and their unique relationship to each other.

INTRODUCTION

Heart failure is a common disease worldwide. It is also an aging disease being more common in the elder population, it is a multimorbidity disease as well, multimorbidity with heart failure became the norm, in spite of that heart failure guidelines are still disease specific, as well as multimorbidity and geriatric ignorant. To understand the

DOI: 10.4018/978-1-6684-2354-7.ch004

unique, multimorbid and geriatric characteristics of heart failure, we need to understand the nature of the disease to shed light on the heart failure pathophysiological areas still in the shadows, we also need to understand symptom clusters in heart failure, their significance, and their unique relationship to each other.

LITERATURE REVIEW

In spite of the high prevalence of multimorbidity in heart failure, studies about it are relatively small. One Spanish study considered the different clustering of Multimorbidities in heart failure patients, their large retrospective study found that there are different cluster patterns in heart failure patients, of those are the cardiovascular pattern which includes ischemic heart disease, HTN, arrhythmia, coronary kidney disease and anticoagulation, preceded by the respiratory pattern, which is includes mainly COPD. Followed by the neuro-vascular pattern that includes mainly dementia, cardio embolic diseases, cerebral hypoperfusion and end organ pathologies like lower limbs and eyes. The authors argue that each cluster has relatively common risk factors and mechanisms making it unique from the others. In spite of the difficulty to make hard lines between each cluster still you can notice their differences. They also argued that each cluster is expected to have a range of different prognosis and complications, and they concluded that future studies should be directed to further investigate the comorbidity clusters in heart failure to more understand not only it's prevalence but how much each comorbidity in the same cluster affect each other i.e., the level of pathogenic synchronicity and specific health hazard consequences that is caused by each cluster to better understand its tailored approach and preventive strategies (Gimeno-Miguel et al., 2019). An American study was interested on the ethnic disparities in heart failure Multimorbidity patients. They investigated certain common morbidities in elder heart failure patients to unlock the disparities and struggles unique to ethnic groups. They found that in spite of hypertension being common in US heart failure patients, about 50%, in spite of that Elder African American heart failure patients with hypertension have a more difficult hypertension to manage, that ultimately needs multiple antihypertensive medications. In regard to dyslipidemia, they found that African Americans have a 20% higher prevalence of dyslipidemia than non-Hispanic whites, and when they have dyslipidemia their chances of having an atherosclerotic event is higher than the non-Hispanic whites, the authors concluded that these findings could be related to the poor health care services directed to the African-Americans compared to the non-Hispanic whites, the healthcare access is more difficult to them. They are more likely to be health illiterate then their non-Hispanic white counterparts, and they concluded that ethnic disparities in heart failure with multimorbidity is less investigated and they recommend that future heart failure studies have to ensure an appropriate representation of different ethnic populations to insure a fair research result and a fair ethnic management spectrum (Blach et al., 2022). Another study investigated an important topic which was noticed by a group of Japanese authors, they noticed that multimorbidity is under-represented in guideline directed medical therapy trials in which the representation of multimorbidity is between 5-10% in spite of multimorbidity being a common phenomenon in the real world. In their Japanese study having two comorbidities was around 90% whereas having five Multimorbidities was around 30%. The study discussed the possible effects of multimorbidity on guideline directed medical therapy that was not properly represented in the trials. For example, ACE inhibitors are also important for chronic kidney disease, but in cases of advanced chronic kidney diseases ACE inhibitors have hazardous consequences and they are withheld. They found that in elders with multimorbidity guideline directed medical therapy tends to be associated with more adverse events. They recommend that guideline directed medical therapy trails should have higher representation of multimorbidity. They also concluded that physicians should approach the patient individually and understand all his comorbidities including polypharmacy, drug to drug and drug to disease possible associations (Takeuchi et al., 2022). Another Australian cross-sectional study about Multimorbidities in elder Australians with heart failure found similar results in which heart failure with multimorbidity is fairly common. They also found that GPs manage patients in a guideline directed management approach rather than an individual approach, which can affect the patient's health and lead to the under appreciation of possible disease to disease or disease to drug interaction. They came with a conclusion that heart failure related guidelines need to change heart failure approach to one that understands and respects multimorbidity. They also encourage GPs to adapt an individualized management approach rather than a disease specific one (Taylor et al., 2017).

PATHOPHYSIOLOGY

When talking about heart failure pathophysiology, we need to talk about adaptive mechanisms. Some of the cardiovascular adaptive mechanisms are well-known due to the many randomized controlled trial's that investigated them like the Renin-angiotensin-aldosterone system, others do not have strong evidence base and thus are less read nor understood by the front line clinician, of those we will be talking about cardiorespiratory reflex arcs, the inflammatory role in heart failure, and the lymphatic system role in congestive heart failure.

Firstly, the cardiorespiratory reflex arcs, in normal physiology in order to maintain a healthy cardio-vascular function in a delicate beat by beat monitoring during rest and exercise and to prevent any sudden changes in Blood pressure we will need a couple of highly sensitive mechanisms mainly the Cardiorespiratory reflexes (Boyes et al., 2022). and like any other cardiovascular mechanism, they are adaptive cardiovascular mechanisms aiming to improve cardiac function in early heart failure, but with advanced heart failure, they become maladaptive, and they contribute to the harm and complications of heart failure.

1. The carotid baroreceptors are physiologically important in regulating heart rate, blood pressure and vascular resistance, when a sudden gush of blood flow cause stretch to the carotids that stimulates its baroreceptors to send sympatho-inhibitory feedback and prevents cardiac overload in cases of exercise. In healthy individuals its aim is to prevent sudden changes in blood pressure after sudden changes from exercise to rest by preventing the sudden change from sympathetic to parasympathetic flow that leads to blood pressure and heart rate pathological shifting (Pachen et al., 2021).

In congestive heart failure patients, the carotid baroreceptor is altered, and it becomes hypersensitive causing an exaggerated sympatho-excitatory tone, increasing the heart rate, blood pressure and vascular resistance contributing to physical intolerance during congestive heart failure. The BeAT-HF Trial, in which an electrical stimulation of the efferent arm of the baroreflex arch was used in Heart failure patients. Initial results showed that individuals with high NT proBNP levels might not benefit from this form of treatment (Biegus et al., 2021).

2. The Chemoreceptor reflex. These are mainly positioned in the carotid body and are strongly sensitive to changes in oxygen, CO2 and acid levels that are physiologically important in the autonomic regulation of ventilation during exercise and movement. applying its effect through positive feedback on the sympathetic, autonomic tone not only that but also by stimulating the carotid baroreceptors as well, so that they are responsible for the sympatho-excitatory tone, directly and indirectly by stimulating the carotid baroreceptor (Ponikowski et al., 2001). In congestive heart failure peripheral and central chemoreceptors are altered causing increased sensitivity which results in an exaggerated sympatho-excitation that results in the increased sympathetic tone during rest and exercise, and the ventilation intolerance i.e., dyspnea and tachypnea during exercise and rest.

In a first human clinical trial, on a small group of moderate to advanced heart failure and enhanced sensitivity of peripheral chemoreceptors, in which surgical carotid body resection resulted in decreased sympathetic tone measured by microneurography. The procedure improved the exercise tolerance in all post-surgical patients, nonetheless the improvement was not accompanied by improvements in LVEF (Left Ventricular Ejection Fraction) nor NT proBNP this improvement also has some important drawbacks showed in the form of a decreased acute hypoxic sensing.

Periodic breathing in advanced heart failure including its severe form the Cheyne-stokes respiration is mainly due to oversensitive peripheral and central chemoreceptors (Biegus et al., 2021). According to the BREATH study, which showed that central sleep apnea in heart failure can be improved using buspiron which is a 5HT1A receptor agonist that decreases chemosensitivity to CO_2 (Biegus et al., 2021).

3. The muscle pressor receptors. These are important receptors found in the skeletal muscles, which are divided into mechano-receptors stimulated by voluntary muscle contraction and metabo-receptors stimulated by byproducts of metabolism e.g., ATP. Physiologically in the healthy person, these muscle pressors exert their effect through exacerbating the sympathetic system, and thus preventing peripheral blood flow from surpassing cardiac output during exercise (Boyes et al., 2022). During heart failure, this mechanism is exaggerated, contributing to the sympatho-excitatory tone seen in heart failure patients. It has been shown repeatedly in small studies that physiotherapy and supervised aerobic exercise decreases the oversensitivity of these muscle pressure receptors and improves the physical intolerance that is known with congestive heart failure. One study showed that selective lumbar area fentanyl induced intrathecal blockage of the afferent neurons lead to improved cardiac output in heart failure (Biegus et al., 2021).

Another study showed that physical training led to autonomic resetting by improving skeletal muscle metabolism as proven by magnetic resonance spectroscopy (Biegus et al., 2021).

Many studies were done on heart failure patients investigating the cardiorespiratory reflexes, trying to reduce their devastating consequence but most of these studies are small studies, and they showed controversial results indicating that we need to understand the pathophysiology of these cardiorespiratory reflexes better in order to know their unclear connections and their hidden autonomic branches to be able to suppress their effect in a therapeutic manner needed in congestive heart failure.

Second, the lymphatic system which is strongly related to fluid accumulation in heart failure, but underappreciated due to improper imaging techniques of lymphatic drainage. Compared to the cardiovascular system, which is a closed high-pressure circulatory system with the heart being a central pump, the lymphatic system is an open low pressure circulatory system without a central pump that has a pivotal role in fluid hemostasis as well as an immune system and a cellular catabolism role (Fudim, Hernandez, & Felker, 2017). Lymphatic system collects fluid from the vascular system at the level of the interstitial space which circulates in lymphatic vessels in the form of lymph and returns it to the vascular system again. Lymph formation occurs at the level of the interstitial space and is governed by starling law through differences in hydrostatic and oncotic pressures in which hydrostatic interstitial pressure is always sub atmospheric ensuring a flow of fluid from the capillary to the interstitium in a process called filtration, fluid then moves from the interstitial space to the lymphatic capillaries due to its unique histological characteristics lacking a basement membrane and with larger inter-endothelial bores this process called interstitial drainage is organ specific depending on the capillary's hydrostatic and histological properties of the organs, soft tissue capillary hydrostatic pressure being around 35 mm Hg where's hepatic sinusoidal hydrostatic pressure is around 5 mmHg because the hepatic sinusoids have different histological characters in the form of larger enter-endothelial bores to allow large proteins to enter the lymphatic space of disse to ensure more filtration that aids in its conjugative and fat absorption functions (Itkin & Itkin, 2021). After fluid is removed from lymphatic capillaries they move to lymphatic collectors and lymphatic vessels, the later properties change, developing smooth muscle lining its wall that resembles cardiac and blood vessel muscle capabilities in the form of contractions that respect the starling law forces. It also possesses lymphatic valves to ensure a Uni directional flow of lymph. The space between two lymphatic successive valves is called the lymphangiom, which is the functional unit of the lymphatic system that is responsible for its contraction and represents the main factor for lymph propulsion through the lymphatic vessel Network. Ultimately delivering the Lymph to the thoracic duct and draining it back into the systemic venous circulation. Lymphatic histopathological and anatomical properties are highly organ specific, for example Serosal lymphatic system are different from muscular lymphatic system in which the lymphatic system of the pleura and diaphragm have unique characteristics that would ensure its full benefit from the respiratory cycle ensuring a pressure supporting fluid filtration in the entire Respiratory cycle. fluoroscopic imaging of the lymph flow in the pleura and diaphragm showed different perpendicular and longitudinal lymph vessel patterns in respect to the to the deferent superficial and deep muscles surrounding the diaphragm allowing the muscles external pressure to help propulsion of lymph through the lymphatic system (Solari et al., 2022). Another example is the kidney, due to its unique histological and anatomical properties in which the tight renal capsule causes increased intrarenal pressure seen in cases of renal vein congestion resulting in renal dysfunction. Renal lymphatics are found to be a safeguard against increased intrarenal pressure. It was found that in cases of obstructive uropathy and renal vein congestion, renal lymphatic flow increases to prevent building up intra renal pressure (Itkin et al., 2021). It also has been shown that therapeutic thoracic duct drainage in congestive heart Failure patients causes an increase in urine flow, that results in improving renal lymphatic function to ensure fluid hemostasis as well as increasing its lymphatic flow to prevent interstitial fluid accumulation, in spite of this during states of congestive heart failure in which central venous pressure increases and excessive fluid filtration causes excessive interstitial fluid accumulation that exceeds the capability of the lymphatic systems clearance which leads to fluid accumulation, congestion and edema. Most of experimental studies are small and done on animals, few only are done on human samples. These studies showed that the therapeutic drainage of the thoracic duct in congestive heart failure causes a reduction in the central venous pressure that results in improvement of heart failure symptoms, reduction in pulmonary congestion, reduction in plural effusion and increase in urine flow. Patients with congestion secondary to congenital heart diseases can acquire certain complications due to an overwhelmed lymphatic system. for example some patients with congenital heart diseases may develop anasarca and hypoalbuminemia secondary to protein losing entropy, new imaging techniques like contrast dynamic magnetic resonance lymphangiography (CDMRL) has shown that this condition is due to spilling of the albumin rich hepatic lymph through abnormal, hepato-duodenal Lymphatic connections in the G.I. system, as the contrast media (gadolinium) injected in the livers interstitium was found in the duodenal interstitium and the duodena's lumen indicating the phenomena (Itkin et al., 2021). An invasive treatment was performed in the form of thoracic duct to atrial anastomosis to these patients that resulted in improvement of fluid accumulation and resolution of their protein losing condition. In spite of the common prevalence of congestive heart failure, which is one of the commonest reasons of admission worldwide, its treatment still depends on frusemide loop diuretic which ultimately causes intravenous collapse, hypotension and renal impairment. A decongestive therapy that is directed towards the interstitium or its fluid drainage (the lymphatic system) is theoretically a more suitable alternative. Multiple small animal studies showed that thoracic duct drainage or more invasively lympho-venous anastomosis showed improvement in the form of reduced central venous pressure, reduced pulmonary congestion, increased urine flow, and generalized symptom improvement as mentioned earlier. To conclude the Lymphatic system has a pivotal role in fluid accumulation in congestive heart failure, more understanding of the lymphatic systems pathophysiology by new imaging techniques, and the therapeutic effect by thoracic duct drainage techniques will improve our understanding of congestive heart failures dynamics, and lead to newer therapeutic modalities.

Third, the role of inflammation in heart failure is well known and well documented but remains with unclear clinical translation, many human and experimental studies proved that many pro-inflammatory cytokines, are increased in heart failure patients in relation to comparable healthy subjects. Although both types of heart failure, i.e., systolic, and diastolic, have a pro-inflammatory role, the Pathophysiology of both roles are different. It is hypothesized to be organ-specific inflammation in systolic heart failure and metabolic driven low-grade systemic inflammation in diastolic heart failure (Ho et al., 2020). Due to the heterogenicity and different phenotypes of diastolic heart failure, managing heart failure through controlling its inflammatory rule is still a challenge. The role of some cytokines is extensively studied in heart failure, and they are shown to have higher levels in heart failure patients, for example the tumor necrosis factor alfa (TNF), Interleukin one (IL-1) and Interleukin six (IL-6). TNF which is one of the oldest and most extensively studied cytokines is found to have high circulating levels in heart failure patients, as well as increasing levels in specific cells like the cardiomyocytes, fibrocytes and vascular cells. Importantly, TNF exerts its effect through two different receptors TNFR1 and TNFR2, it is hypothesized that stimulating these two receptors may cause different contradicting effects on the inflammation as one of them exerts a protective inflammatory effect, the other may exert a harmful effect (Hanna & Frangogiannis, 2020). Randomized controlled studies trying to stop the harmful role of TNF using a monoclonal antibody against TNF has unfortunately showed contradicting results and did not clearly show a benefit (Rolski & Błyszczuk, 2020). Another important cytokine involved in the local and systemic inflammatory consequence of heart failure is IL-6 which is part of a family of cytokines who exert their effect through a specific type of cell membrane called Glycoprotein 130 (gp 130) its effect is initiated by binding to the interlukine six receptor (IL-6R) on the cell wall creating an IL-6/IL-6R complex that activates the gp 130/STAT3 axis. Molecular and genetic studies found that IL-6 is able to stimulate cells that lack IL-6R by a process called Trans signaling of interleukin 6 (Ho et al., 2020) which complicates the pathophysiology and thus determines more studying and understanding of these cytokines and their complicated contradicting roles in heart failure. Most of these well studied cytokines stimulate specific molecules in target cells, one of them is a transcription factor called nuclear factor kaba beta (NFKB), and this molecule binds to specific binding areas in the DNA resulting in different molecular and cell functions that promote inflammation (Hanna & Frangogiannis, 2020). Another way that cytokines exert their effect is by stimulating specific pattern recognition receptors on some cells, in which the most famous are the toll like receptors 4 (TLR4) and the toll like receptor 9 (TLR9), these family of receptors are stimulated by either pathogen recognition protein stimulation or damage recognition pattern stimulation (Hanna & Frangogiannis, 2020). The above brief explanation of the inflammatory role in heart failure reflects the heterogeneous and complicated inflammation effect that requires a more in-depth understanding of the pathophysiology of each related Cytokine and its different connections, more cytokine receptor specific blocking may be needed or more damage recognition pattern receptor specific blocking may be needed in order to reach a beneficial clinical result from this complicated inflammatory role.

Symptom Clusters

A cluster is a combination of more than two symptoms which manifest simultaneously and are connected, which are essential to investigate in heart failure since individuals who have HF typically suffer several symptoms, many of which appear simultaneously in groups or clusters rather than alone. In patients with heart failure, our perception of the function that heart failure clusters play and the characteristics of these clusters are limited. Uncertainty about the illness can make it more difficult to evaluate symptoms and begin treatment appropriately.

Patients diagnosed with heart failure (HF) may complain of various symptoms, the most prevalent of which are dyspnea on exercise, tiredness, and peripheral edema. Because HF is a chronic condition that worsens over time, these symptoms might appear even in patients who appear to be doing well clinically. Nevertheless, a significant early predictor of decompensation is a change in the intensity of these signs or a rise in the frequency with which they occur. Patients who suffer from heart failure frequently have difficulties recognizing their symptoms, isolating the root cause of those symptoms, and differentiating the symptoms of heart failure from those of associated illnesses or the consequences of normal ageing (Miller et al., 2012).

Clusters of symptoms have been investigated in different diseases, most frequently cancer. Cancer symptom clusters have been discovered to help determine the impact that many symptoms simultaneously have on the patients, including their standards of living and their health abilities. If groups of symptoms associated with HF could be isolated, it could be possible to assist people with HF in recognizing the early symptoms of decompensation in their condition. In other words, patients may have an easier time attributing their symptoms to their heart condition if they are better aware of the links between symptoms that occur simultaneously with heart failure. Accurately attributing symptoms makes it easier to provide prompt self-care and makes it possible to avoid admission to a hospital for acute symptom management (Miller et al., 2012).

The significance of taking this viewpoint comes from the fact that when symptoms are complex, it may be difficult to separate and thus appropriately diagnose underlying diseases, since cognitive, affective, and environmental inputs can play a role in doing so. Patients may have trouble differentiating their shortness of breath from other social, sentimental, and situational factors that contribute to symptom recognition and thus better react to signs when there is an interaction between symptoms. Patients may also have difficulty distinguishing between their shortness of breath and other symptoms. This can make it difficult for patients to get an accurate diagnosis. Patients' views of their symptoms can be influenced by circumstances such as depression or previous experiences with the disease. A patient who is depressed may be less attentive to the Aspects of new-onset edema including its duration, strength, and character, as well as its stress contributions (Salyer et al., 2019).

Although the difficulty associated with particular symptoms may vary between men and women, both sexes reported experiencing the same clusters of symptoms. The only cluster that correctly predicted an increased risk for a cardiac event was the emotional/cognitive one. Based on these findings, it is recommended that management decisions should be made according to symptom clusters. Targeting patients experiencing significant levels of discomfort due to emotional or cognitive symptoms may be of utmost importance because these individuals may be the most susceptible to negative results (Song et al., 2010).

Two significant symptom clusters were found to be present in every country. These findings show that the disease pathogenesis of HF symptom clusters is the same across all ethnicities and that society does not influence the formation of these clusters in any manner. Cultures do not play any role in the emergence of these clusters. Many researchers have looked into the connection between specific symptoms and outcomes. Some of the manifestation, particularly breathlessness and depressive symptoms, are linked to an increased chance of hospital readmission and an increased risk of death. These statistics are essential for drawing attention to the significance of investigating the symptoms patients with heart failure report experiencing. A study found that supporting individuals or medical practitioners in appropriately detecting signs of deteriorating heart failure may not be adequately addressed by focusing on specific symptoms alone (Ahmad et al., 2014).

The segmentation of symptomatology adjacent to each other means putting patients at a higher risk for poor outcomes, together with adverse health outcomes; however, this risk does not become instantly obvious when symptoms are taken individually. The data comes from a wide variety of patient populations and shows that clinical signs frequently occur together. For instance, the presence of both anxiety at the same time in individuals who have coronary artery disease is connected to a greater mortality risk than the prevalence of either stress or depression alone. Cardiovascular disease is the leading cause of death in the United States. Patients with cancer who exhibit more symptoms are more likely to pass away from the disease. One study found that individuals who presented with four symptoms had a ninefold increased risk of death compared to patients with only one symptom. One research suggests that symptom appearance is universal, in addition to symptom clustering, which would be beneficial to physicians as they try to determine the significance of symptomatology in their patient populations who have HF, as well as when they try to start educating their patients on how to react adequately to illnesses. It is likely that clinicians could benefit from knowing symptom clusters to better risk stratify their patients (Horiuchi et al., 2018).

After conducting an analysis on a large sample of hospitalized HF patients, researchers discovered that these patients had three separate clusters of signs: acute fluid overload, psychosocial, and chronic volume overload. Comorbid illnesses did not serve as a reliable assessment of symptom clusters; hyperglycemia was the only ailment that was related with the emotional symptom cluster. Elders 75 or older have more frequent clusters, although they had a less negative influence on their ability to live as they wished. All three symptoms that made up the cluster happened more frequently in older patients, but the symptoms had less impact on their quality of life. Others have observed that the severity of the symptoms decreases with age, but relatively little literature explains why older adults are substantially less sensitive to symptoms. Variations in the adrenergic function associated with ageing, changes in individual body and fitness levels, and symptom proneness, also known as the inclination, to be conscious of and report symptoms, can all affect cardiac symptoms (Miller et al., 2012).

A study found that more pain from the breathlessness symptom cluster didn't appear to anticipate cardiac rehospitalization free survival; even so, it predicted impartial cardiac death-free survival after adjusting for age, sex, causative agents of HF, and Mass index. This was the case even though higher anguish from the shortness of breath symptom cluster was not really shown to anticipate cardiac rehospitalization free survival. It was found that there was an increase of one unit in the probability of cardiac mortality for every one unit rise in the average distress score of the dyspneic symptom cluster. On the other hand, increased discomfort from the Weary symptom cluster was found to significantly predict cardiac rehospitalization free survival despite adjusting for the same clinical factors. This was discovered even though cardiac rehospitalization free survival was the primary outcome of interest. There was a proportional increase in the likelihood of cardiac rehospitalization proportional to the amount by which the average distress score in the Weary symptom cluster rose by one unit. The anguish that was brought on by the Weary symptom cluster was unable to provide an appropriate prediction of survival independent of cardiac death (Araiza-Garaygordobil et al., 2020).

Patients with heart failure who had increased distress due to the Weary symptom cluster had a 50% higher probability of being readmitted to the hospital within one year of being discharged from the hospital for aggravation of their heart failure. Patients with greater discomfort due to the dyspneic symptom cluster had roughly twice the risk of passing away from cardiac causes within one year of being discharged from the hospital. The evidence currently available from prior studies indicating the detrimental effect physical symptoms have on clinical outcomes focuses on quality of life and functional status as outcomes. The bulk of these researchers investigated the impact of the influence of physical symptoms on the results of individuals with heart failure (HF). Just one previous study looked at how heart failure symptoms relate to hospitalization and death, and that study found conclusions that were consistent with these results (Yu et al., 2018).

The chronic volume overload cluster was only responsible for a minor portion of the observed variation in the severity of the symptoms. This discovery may have one possible explanation: the early signs of HF decompensation, such as these, typically worsen subtly over the course of several weeks while having no effect either physically or emotionally. Consequently, patients might not even be aware of the symptoms that belong to this cluster until they are in a very impaired state. Patients can also alleviate their symptoms by engaging in less activity throughout the day. This can help make the patient's symptoms appear less severe. According to a well-known study, patients hospitalized with decompensated heart failure frequently failed to recognize edema detected during a physical exam. The patient's level of concern is not necessarily proportional to the intensity of the patient's physical symptoms. Finally, changes in the status of heart failure that can be neglected without particular instructions from healthcare experts include increased shortness of breath with physical activity, as well as a concurrently increased urge to rest (Jurgens et al., 2009).

It is common knowledge that heart failure patients who frequently use acute care facilities have poor prognosis. As a result, people who are suffering from heart failure who have to return to the hospital on a regular basis because of their heart failure have become a primary focus of quality improvement initiatives. Patients dealing with heart failure in the real world are plagued by various comorbidities, many of which are not related to the heart but affect their outcomes. Although it is common knowledge that patients with HF who present to the emergency room have a significant risk of short-term death after discharge, it is not common knowledge what happens to patients with HF who make several visits to the emergency room in short time span. Research discovered that individuals with HF who presented to the emergency room more than three times in six months had a heavier cardiac and non-cardiac comorbidities threshold. Additionally, a markedly greater mortality rate than patient populations with non-clustered visits for HF, even when adjusting for chronic patient conditions. In addition, patients with non-clustered visits for HF had a significantly higher burden of both cardiac and non-cardiac comorbidities (Moser et al., 2014).

MANAGEMENT

Treatment of Advanced HF May Be Divided Into Conventional and Advanced

Conventional Treatment

General Measures

The treatment of underlying causes should be eradicated if possible (e.g., revascularization in ischemic heart disease or aortic valve replacement in severe aortic stenosis) and comorbidities treated (e.g., supplemental intravenous iron in iron deficiency with or without iron deficiency anemia) when feasible (Silverberg et al., 2002). Sleep related breathing disorders are common in heart failure (Bradley & Floras, 2003). Forty percent of patients have central sleep apnea (CSA) and 10% have obstructive sleep apnea (OSA). Sleep apnea causes nocturnal catecholamine surge, hypertension and cardiac arrhythmias and may represent an independent risk factor for increased mortality in heart failure. CSA improves with intensification of heart failure therapy and nocturnal oxygen may be helpful in some cases (Bradley & Floras, 2003).

Medical Treatment

It starts with the treatment of the Syndrome of Clinical HF in patients with Pre-HF (with LVEF £40%), ACEi should be used to prevent symptomatic HF and reduce mortality (Heidenreich et al., 2022). In patients with heart failure with Reduced Ejection Fraction (HFrEF) and NYHA class II to III symptoms, the use of Angiotensin Receptor-Neprilysin Inhibitors (ARNi) is recommended to reduce morbidity and mortality (Heidenreich et al., 2022). However, in patients with previous or current symptoms of chronic HFrEF, the use of ACEi is beneficial to reduce morbidity and mortality when the use of ARNi is not possible. In patients with previous or current symptoms of chronic HFrEF who are intolerant to ACEi because of cough or angioedema and when the use of ARNi is not feasible, the use of ARB is recommended. It must be clarified that ARNi should not be administered concomitantly with ACEi or within 36 hours of the last dose of an ACEi. It is also reminded that either ACEi or ARNi should not be administered to patients with any history of angioedema (Heidenreich et al., 2022).

Treatment of congestion is of the upmost importance but is frequently challenging as diuretic resistance is a characteristic feature of advanced HF. Diuretic resistance implies a failure to increase fluid and sodium (Na+) output sufficiently to relieve volume overload, oedema, or congestion, despite escalating doses of a loop diuretic to a ceiling level (80 mg of furosemide once or twice daily or greater in those with reduced glomerular filtration rate) (Wilcox et al., 2020). The mechanisms implicated are reduced renal perfusion, the activation of the renin-angiotensin-aldosterone system and the escape mechanisms in the kidney such as the "braking phenomenon" (Vargo et al., 1995; Ellison & Felker, 2017). Other mechanisms such as the impaired intestinal absorption of oral diuretics due to the intestinal wall oedema or hypoalbuminemia may be involved (Vargo et al., 1995). Various strategies have been successfully used to alleviate diuretic resistance, including dose escalation and continuous loop-diuretic infusion as well as diuretic combinations like loop and thiazide diuretics (Vargo et al., 1995; Charokopos et al., 2019). When ascites and oedema persist in the setting of rising creatinine and hyponatremia, ultra-filtration may be utilized (Blázquez-Bermejo et al., 2020).

In patients with HFrEF, with current or previous symptoms, use of 1 of the 3 beta blockers have proven to reduce mortality (e.g., bisoprolol, carvedilol, and sustained-release metoprolol succinate) is recommended to reduce mortality and hospitalizations. The beta blockers should be started with lowest possible dose and gradually titrated up to achieve full benefit (Heidenreich et al., 2022).

In patients with HFrEF (LVEF £40%) and NYHA class II-IV symptoms, an MRA (spironolactone or eplerenone) is used to reduce morbidity and mortality, if eGFR is >30 mL/min/1.73 m2 and serum potassium is <5.0 mEq/L. Careful monitoring of potassium, renal function, and diuretic dosing should be performed at initiation and closely monitored thereafter to minimize risk of hyperkalemia. In patients with HF who experience hyperkalemia (serum potassium level [3]5.5 mEq/L) while taking a renin-angiotensin-aldosterone system inhibitor (RAASi), the effectiveness of potassium binders (patiromer, sodium zirconium cyclosilicate) to improve outcomes by facilitating continuation of RAASi therapy is uncertain (Bradley, & Floras, 2003; Heidenreich et al., 2022).

Sodium-Glucose Cotransporter 2 Inhibitors (SGLT2i) are recommended to reduce hospitalization for HF and cardiovascular mortality, irrespective of the presence of type 2 diabetes (Bradley & Floras, 2003; Heidenreich et al., 2022).

In patients with current or previous symptomatic HFrEF who cannot be given first-line agents, such as ARNi, ACEi, or ARB, because of drug intolerance or renal insufficiency, a combination of hydralazine and isosorbide dinitrate might be considered to reduce the symptoms (Bradley & Floras, 2003).

Drugs of unproven value or drugs that may worsen HF like vitamins, nutritional supplements, hormonal therapy and dihydropyridine calcium channel-blocking drugs should be avoided (Silverberg et al., 2002; Bradley & Floras, 2003).

Antiarrhythmic medications and dronedarone, the dipeptidyl peptidase-4 (DPP-4) inhibitors saxagliptin and alogliptin, NSAIDs worsen HF symptoms and should be avoided or withdrawn whenever possible (Silverberg et al., 2002).

Device Treatment

Cardiac resynchronization therapy (CRT) is indicated in HF patients in NYHA class II or III that remain symptomatic despite optimal medical treatment and have a LVEF £ 35% and a QRS width > 130 ms or [3]150 ms depending on the presence or absence of left bundle branch block (LBBB), respectively (McMurray et al., 2014). The potential additional placement of an implantable cardioverter-defibrillator (ICD) on CRT (CRT-D) depends on factors unrelated to LVEF such as age, extent of myocardial fibrosis, the presence or absence of coronary artery disease, life expectancy, comorbidity burden, and patients' preference (Packer & Metra, 2020). Echocardiography data shows that CRT-D is associated with decrease in LV size, reduced mitral regurgitation and improvement in LVEF (St John Sutton et al., 2003).

Advanced Treatment

Patients with advanced HF and hemodynamic instability are candidates for temporary mechanical circulatory support (MCS) (37), chronic MCS including myocardial recovery, or heart transplantation. Currently MCS is indicated for: 1) Post cardiotomy-pump failure,2) AMI with cardiogenic shock, and 3) as a bridge to transplantation (Jaski et al., 2003; Combes et al., 2020).

Long-term (durable) MCS. Left Ventricular Assist Device (LVAD) are indicated in inotrope-dependent heart failure (HF) patients with pure or predominant LV dysfunction (Jiritano et al., 2020). The phenomenon of recovery during the support was noticed early in the LVAD bridge to transplant experience. Some worked so well that the pump was removed, and transplant avoided (Hetzer et al., 2000).

Multimorbidity and Guideline-Directed Medical Treatment: Therapeutic Challenges and Opportunity in Advanced Heart Failure

Heart failure (HF) is a major cause of mortality, hospitalizations, and reduced quality of life and a major burden for the healthcare system. The number of patients that progress to an advanced stage of HF is growing. Only a limited proportion of these patients can undergo heart transplantation or mechanical circulatory support (Truby & Rogers, 2020). HF guidelines recommend the use of these drugs at maximally tolerated target doses to reduce mortality and/or re-hospitalizations due to HF (Esposito et al., 2017; Jiritano et al., 2020). Guideline-directed medical therapy (GDMT) remains effective in patients with advanced HF. However, patients with advanced HF are less likely to tolerate it because of hypotension, low cardiac output, and severe kidney dysfunction. Physicians should be aware that the proper use of

GDMT is associated with a better prognosis and its implementation is of central importance (Truby & Rogers, 2020).

Definition and Epidemiology

In the most recently published ESC guidelines, advanced HF has been defined as the presence of all the following criteria: (1) severe and persistent symptoms of HF [NYHA class III (advanced) or IV]; (2) severe cardiac dysfunction [left ventricular ejection fraction (LVEF) £ 30% in the setting of HFrEF]; (3) episodes of pulmonary or systemic congestion requiring high-dose intravenous diuretics (or diuretic combinations) or episodes of low output requiring inotropes or vasoactive drugs or malignant arrhythmias causing >1 unplanned visit or hospitalization in the last 12 months; and (4) severe impairment of exercise capacity with inability to exercise or low 6 min walking test distance (<300 m) or pVO2 < 12 mL/kg/min or <50% predicted value, estimated to be of cardiac origin (McDonagh et al., 2021). Epidemiological data are still scarce, although it is estimated that 1–10% of the HF population has advanced HF (Crespo-Leiro et al., 2018).

Therapeutic Challenges

Despite strong professional recommendations through guidelines and performance measures, Guideline Directed Medical Therapy (GDMT) use among eligible patients with Heart Failure with reduced Ejection Fraction (HFrEF) remains suboptimal. In an analysis from the CHAMP-HF (Change the Management of Patients with Heart Failure) registry, 73.4%, 67%, and 33.4% of eligible patients were treated with any dose of angiotensin-converting enzyme (ACE) inhibitor/angiotensin receptor blocker (ARB)/angiotensin receptor-neprilysin inhibitor (ARNI), beta-blocker (BB), or mineralocorticoid receptor antagonist (MRA), respectively (Greene et al., 2018). There are several barriers to appropriate GDMT utilization. Elderly patients are typically more prone to adverse drug reactions, often hindering titration (Solari et al., 2022). Renal dysfunction is an ongoing challenge given eGFR and creatinine limitations with RAASi, MRA, and SGLTi (Heidenreich et al., 2022; Cheung et al., 2021). Additionally, financial concerns, including high out-of-pocket costs, can lead to patients being unable to afford all four therapies.

Other challenges to implementing GDMT, the most important being patient-related factors (comorbidities, advanced age, frailty, cognitive impairment, poor adherence, low socioeconomic status), treatment-related factors (intolerance, side-effects) and healthcare-related factors that influence availability and accessibility of HF care (Seferović et al., 2021). As a result, many patients in clinical practice are not treated with the above agents or are treated with lower-than-recommended doses (Greene et al., 2018; Thomas et al., 2019).

The use of NT-proBNP concentrations to "guide" GDMT have suggested that the approach leads to more assiduous application of GDMT along with better outcomes compared with usual care, (Lainchbury et al., 2009; Laali et al., 2018) but many patients in the GUIDE-IT trial do not receive GDMT adjustments, particularly in the long term, even in those with known elevated NT-proBNP concentrations (Fiuzat et al., 2020). In a retrospective analysis found that patients not managed on GDMT had a significantly increased risk of 2-year mortality compared to patients on GDMT. We found 2-year mortality to be approximately 20% in HFrEF patients, similar to results published in the PARADIGM-HF trial, which demonstrated a rate slightly less than 20%.

GDMT Opportunity

Heart Failure Hospitalization (HFH) presents a unique opportunity for the initiation and titration of GDMT. HFH is positively associated with initiation of GDMT as well as dose escalation of ACE inhibitor/ARB and MRA. They also demonstrate that HFH is positively associated with de-escalation and discontinuation of all classes of GDMT in those on pre-existing therapy (Greene et al., 2019). Neurohormonal antagonists, including angiotensin-converting enzyme inhibitors (ACEi), angiotensin receptor blockers, angiotensin receptor neprilysin inhibitors, beta-blockers, and mineralocorticoid receptor antagonists, and sodiumglucoseco-transporter 2 (SGLT2) inhibitors, are the mainstay of HFrEF treatment, improving the clinical course of HF. Adherence to GDMT is associated with improved outcome (35, 56). Implementation of GDMT remains a cornerstone of treatment of also the patients with advanced HF and reduced LVEF.

CONCLUSION

Heart failure is a geriatric multimorbid disease, thus treatment guidelines and recommendations need be formulated according to its unique nature. Similar to any other Multimorbid disease appropriate research need to investigate its cluster patterns, their significance and their morbidity and mortality differences. Some parts of its pathophysiology gained a lion share of research representation, but other parts are fairly under investigated, and thus under appreciated by treating physicians.

REFERENCES

Ahmad, T., Pencina, M. J., Schulte, P. J., O'Brien, E., Whellan, D. J., Piña, I. L., Kitzman, D. W., Lee, K. L., O'Connor, C. M., & Felker, G. M. (2014). Clinical implications of chronic heart failure phenotypes defined by cluster analysis. *Journal of the American College of Cardiology, 64*(17), 1765–1774. doi:10.1016/j. jacc.2014.07.979 PMID:25443696

Araiza-Garaygordobil, D., Gopar-Nieto, R., Martinez-Amezcua, P., Cabello-López, A., Alanis-Estrada, G., Luna-Herbert, A., González-Pacheco, H., Paredes-Paucar, C. P., Sierra-Lara, M. D., Briseño-De la Cruz, J. L., Rodriguez-Zanella, H., Martinez-Rios, M. A., & Arias-Mendoza, A. (2020). A randomized controlled trial of lung ultrasound-guided therapy in heart failure (CLUSTER-HF study). *American Heart Journal, 227*, 31–39. doi:10.1016/j.ahj.2020.06.003 PMID:32668323

Biegus, J., Niewinski, P., Josiak, K., Kulej, K., Ponikowska, B., Nowak, K., Zymlinski, R., & Ponikowski, P. (2021). Pathophysiology of Advanced Heart Failure: What Knowledge Is Needed for Clinical Management? *Heart Failure Clinics, 17*(4), 519–531. doi:10.1016/j.hfc.2021.06.001 PMID:34511202

Blach, A., Pangle, A., Azhar, G., & Wei, J. (2022). Disparity and multimorbidity in heart failure patients over the age of 80. *Gerontology & Geriatric Medicine, 8*, 23337214221098901. doi:10.1177/23337214221098901 PMID:35591952

Blázquez-Bermejo, Z., Farré, N., Llagostera, M., Caravaca Perez, P., Morán-Fernández, L., Fort, A., De-Juan, J., Ruiz, S., & Delgado, J. F. (2020). The development of chronic diuretic resistance can be predicted during a heart-failure hospitalization. Results from the REDIHF registry. *PLoS One, 15*(10), e0240098. doi:10.1371/journal.pone.0240098 PMID:33007024

Boyes, N. G., Marciniuk, D. D., Haddad, H., & Tomczak, C. R. (2022). Autonomic cardiovascular reflex control of hemodynamics during exercise in heart failure with reduced ejection fraction and the effects of exercise training. *Reviews in Cardiovascular Medicine, 23*(2), 72. doi:10.31083/j.rcm2302072 PMID:35229563

Bradley, T. D., & Floras, J. S. (2003). Sleep apnea and heart failure: Part I: obstructive sleep apnea. *Circulation, 107*(12), 1671–1678. doi:10.1161/01. CIR.0000061757.12581.15 PMID:12668504

Charokopos, A., Griffin, M., Rao, V. S., Inker, L., Sury, K., Asher, J., Turner, J., Mahoney, D., Cox, Z. L., Wilson, F. P., & Testani, J. M. (2019). Serum and urine albumin and response to loop diuretics in heart failure. *Clinical Journal of the American Society of Nephrology; CJASN, 14*(5), 712–718. doi:10.2215/CJN.11600918 PMID:31010938

Cheung, A. K., Chang, T. I., Cushman, W. C., Furth, S. L., Hou, F. F., Ix, J. H., Knoll, G. A., Muntner, P., Pecoits-Filho, R., Sarnak, M. J., Tobe, S. W., Tomson, C. R. V., & Mann, J. F. E. (2021). KDIGO 2021 clinical practice guideline for the management of blood pressure in chronic kidney disease. *Kidney International, 99*(3), S1–S87. doi:10.1016/j.kint.2020.11.003 PMID:33637192

Combes, A., Price, S., Slutsky, A. S., & Brodie, D. (2020). Temporary circulatory support for cardiogenic shock. *Lancet, 396*(10245), 199–212. doi:10.1016/S0140-6736(20)31047-3 PMID:32682486

Crespo-Leiro, M. G., Metra, M., Lund, L. H., Milicic, D., Costanzo, M. R., Filippatos, G., Gustafsson, F., Tsui, S., Barge-Caballero, E., De Jonge, N., Frigerio, M., Hamdan, R., Hasin, T., Hülsmann, M., Nalbantgil, S., Potena, L., Bauersachs, J., Gkouziouta, A., Ruhparwar, A., & Ruschitzka, F. (2018). Advanced heart failure: A position statement of the Heart Failure Association of the European Society of Cardiology. *European Journal of Heart Failure, 20*(11), 1505–1535. doi:10.1002/ejhf.1236 PMID:29806100

Ellison, D. H., & Felker, G. M. (2017). Diuretic treatment in heart failure. *The New England Journal of Medicine, 377*(20), 1964–1975. doi:10.1056/NEJMra1703100 PMID:29141174

Esposito, M., Bader, Y., Pedicini, R., Breton, C., Mullin, A., & Kapur, N. K. (2017). The role of acute circulatory support in ST-segment elevation myocardial infarction complicated by cardiogenic shock. *Indian Heart Journal, 69*(5), 668–674. doi:10.1016/j.ihj.2017.05.011 PMID:29054200

Fiuzat, M., Ezekowitz, J., Alemayehu, W., Westerhout, C. M., Sbolli, M., Cani, D., Whellan, D. J., Ahmad, T., Adams, K., Piña, I. L., Patel, C. B., Anstrom, K. J., Cooper, L. S., Mark, D., Leifer, E. S., Felker, G. M., Januzzi, J. L., & O'Connor, C. M. (2020). Assessment of limitations to optimization of guideline-directed medical therapy in heart failure from the GUIDE-IT trial: A secondary analysis of a randomized clinical trial. *JAMA Cardiology, 5*(7), 757–764. doi:10.1001/jamacardio.2020.0640 PMID:32319999

Fudim, M., Hernandez, A. F., & Felker, G. M. (2017). Role of volume redistribution in the congestion of heart failure. *Journal of the American Heart Association*, 6(8), e006817. doi:10.1161/JAHA.117.006817 PMID:28862947

Gimeno-Miguel, A., Gutiérrez, A. G., Poblador-Plou, B., Coscollar-Santaliestra, C., Pérez-Calvo, J. I., Divo, M. J., & Ruiz-Laiglesia, F. J. (2019). Multimorbidity patterns in patients with heart failure: An observational Spanish study based on electronic health records. *BMJ Open*, 9(12), e033174. doi:10.1136/bmjopen-2019-033174 PMID:31874886

Greene, S. J., Butler, J., Albert, N. M., DeVore, A. D., Sharma, P. P., Duffy, C. I., Hill, C. L., McCague, K., Mi, X., Patterson, J. H., Spertus, J. A., Thomas, L., Williams, F. B., Hernandez, A. F., & Fonarow, G. C. (2018). Medical therapy for heart failure with reduced ejection fraction: The CHAMP-HF registry. *Journal of the American College of Cardiology*, 72(4), 351–366. doi:10.1016/j.jacc.2018.04.070 PMID:30025570

Greene, S. J., Fonarow, G. C., DeVore, A. D., Sharma, P. P., Vaduganathan, M., Albert, N. M., Duffy, C. I., Hill, C. L., McCague, K., Patterson, J. H., Spertus, J. A., Thomas, L., Williams, F. B., Hernandez, A. F., & Butler, J. (2019). Titration of medical therapy for heart failure with reduced ejection fraction. *Journal of the American College of Cardiology*, 73(19), 2365–2383. doi:10.1016/j.jacc.2019.02.015 PMID:30844480

Hanna, A., & Frangogiannis, N. G. (2020). Inflammatory cytokines and chemokines as therapeutic targets in heart failure. *Cardiovascular Drugs and Therapy*, 34(6), 849–863. doi:10.100710557-020-07071-0 PMID:32902739

Heidenreich, P. A., Bozkurt, B., Aguilar, D., Allen, L. A., Byun, J. J., Colvin, M. M., Deswal, A., Drazner, M. H., Dunlay, S. M., Evers, L. R., Fang, J. C., Fedson, S. E., Fonarow, G. C., Hayek, S. S., Hernandez, A. F., Khazanie, P., Kittleson, M. M., Lee, C. S., Link, M. S., & Yancy, C. W. (2022a). 2022 AHA/ACC/HFSA guideline for the management of heart failure: A report of the American College of Cardiology/American Heart Association Joint Committee on Clinical Practice Guidelines. *Journal of the American College of Cardiology*, 79(17), e263–e421. doi:10.1016/j.jacc.2021.12.012 PMID:35379503

Heidenreich, P. A., Bozkurt, B., Aguilar, D., Allen, L. A., Byun, J. J., Colvin, M. M., Deswal, A., Drazner, M. H., Dunlay, S. M., Evers, L. R., Fang, J. C., Fedson, S. E., Fonarow, G. C., Hayek, S. S., Hernandez, A. F., Khazanie, P., Kittleson, M. M., Lee, C. S., Link, M. S., & Yancy, C. W. (2022b). 2022 AHA/ACC/HFSA guideline for the management of heart failure: executive summary: a report of the American College of Cardiology/American Heart Association Joint Committee on Clinical Practice Guidelines. *Journal of the American College of Cardiology*, *79*(17), 1757–1780. doi:10.1016/j.jacc.2021.12.011 PMID:35379504

Hetzer, R., Müller, J. H., Weng, Y. G., Loebe, M., & Wallukat, G. (2000). Midterm follow-up of patients who underwent removal of a left ventricular assist device after cardiac recovery from end-stage dilated cardiomyopathy. *The Journal of Thoracic and Cardiovascular Surgery*, *120*(5), 843–855. doi:10.1067/mtc.2000.108931 PMID:11044309

Ho, J. E., Redfield, M. M., Lewis, G. D., Paulus, W. J., & Lam, C. S. (2020). Deliberating the diagnostic dilemma of heart failure with preserved ejection fraction. *Circulation*, *142*(18), 1770–1780. doi:10.1161/CIRCULATIONAHA.119.041818 PMID:33136513

Horiuchi, Y., Tanimoto, S., Latif, A. M., Urayama, K. Y., Aoki, J., Yahagi, K., Okuno, T., Sato, Y., Tanaka, T., Koseki, K., Komiyama, K., Nakajima, H., Hara, K., & Tanabe, K. (2018). Identifying novel phenotypes of acute heart failure using cluster analysis of clinical variables. *International Journal of Cardiology*, *262*, 57–63. doi:10.1016/j.ijcard.2018.03.098 PMID:29622508

Itkin, G. P., & Itkin, M. G. (2021). Lymph circulation and heart failure. *Journal of Transplantology and Artificial Organs*, *23*(3), 186–191. doi:10.15825/1995-1191-2021-3-186-191

Itkin, M., Rockson, S. G., & Burkhoff, D. (2021). Pathophysiology of the lymphatic system in patients with heart failure: JACC state-of-the-art review. *Journal of the American College of Cardiology*, *78*(3), 278–290. doi:10.1016/j.jacc.2021.05.021 PMID:34266581

Jaski, B. E., Ha, J., Denys, B. G., Lamba, S., Trupp, R. J., & Abraham, W. T. (2003). Peripherally inserted veno-venous ultrafiltration for rapid treatment of volume overloaded patients. *Journal of Cardiac Failure*, *9*(3), 227–231. doi:10.1054/jcaf.2003.28 PMID:12815573

Jiritano, F., Coco, V. L., Matteucci, M., Fina, D., Willers, A., & Lorusso, R. (2020). Temporary mechanical circulatory support in acute heart failure. *Cardiac Failure Review*, *6*, 6. doi:10.15420/cfr.2019.02 PMID:32257388

Jurgens, C. Y., Moser, D. K., Armola, R., Carlson, B., Sethares, K., & Riegel, B. (2009). Symptom clusters of heart failure. *Research in Nursing & Health*, *32*(5), 551–560. doi:10.1002/nur.20343 PMID:19650069

Laali, K. K., Greves, W. J., Correa-Smits, S. J., Zwarycz, A. T., Bunge, S. D., Borosky, G. L., Manna, A., Paulus, A., & Chanan-Khan, A. (2018). Novel fluorinated curcuminoids and their pyrazole and isoxazole derivatives: Synthesis, structural studies, Computational/Docking and in-vitro bioassay. *Journal of Fluorine Chemistry*, *206*, 82–98. doi:10.1016/j.jfluchem.2017.11.013

Lainchbury, J. G., Troughton, R. W., Strangman, K. M., Frampton, C. M., Pilbrow, A., Yandle, T. G., Hamid, A. K., Nicholls, M. G., & Richards, A. M. (2009). N-terminal pro–B-type natriuretic peptide-guided treatment for chronic heart failure: Results from the BATTLESCARRED (NT-proBNP–Assisted Treatment To Lessen Serial Cardiac Readmissions and Death) trial. *Journal of the American College of Cardiology*, *55*(1), 53–60. doi:10.1016/j.jacc.2009.02.095 PMID:20117364

McDonagh, T. A., Metra, M., Adamo, M., Gardner, R. S., Baumbach, A., Böhm, M., ... Kathrine Skibelund, A. (2021). 2021 ESC Guidelines for the diagnosis and treatment of acute and chronic heart failure: Developed by the Task Force for the diagnosis and treatment of acute and chronic heart failure of the European Society of Cardiology (ESC) With the special contribution of the Heart Failure Association (HFA) of the ESC. *European Heart Journal*, *42*(36), 3599–3726. doi:10.1093/eurheartj/ehab368 PMID:34447992

McMurray, J. J., Packer, M., Desai, A. S., Gong, J., Lefkowitz, M. P., Rizkala, A. R., & Zile, M. R. (2014). Angiotensin–neprilysin inhibition versus enalapril in heart failure. *N Engl J Med, 371*, 993-1004.

Miller, L. A., Spitznagel, M. B., Alosco, M. L., Cohen, R. A., Raz, N., Sweet, L. H., Colbert, L., Josephson, R., Hughes, J., Rosneck, J., & Gunstad, J. (2012). Cognitive profiles in heart failure: A cluster analytic approach. *Journal of Clinical and Experimental Neuropsychology*, *34*(5), 509–520. doi:10.1080/13803395.2012.663344 PMID:22375800

Moser, D. K., Lee, K. S., Wu, J. R., Mudd-Martin, G., Jaarsma, T., Huang, T. Y., Fan, X.-Z., Strömberg, A., Lennie, T. A., & Riegel, B. (2014). Identification of symptom clusters among patients with heart failure: An international observational study. *International Journal of Nursing Studies*, *51*(10), 1366–1372. doi:10.1016/j.ijnurstu.2014.02.004 PMID:24636665

Pachen, M., Abukar, Y., Shanks, J., Lever, N., & Ramchandra, R. (2021). Regulation of Coronary Blood Flow by the Carotid Body Chemoreceptors in Ovine Heart Failure. *Frontiers in Physiology*, *12*, 709. doi:10.3389/fphys.2021.681135 PMID:34122147

Packer, M., & Metra, M. (2020). Guideline-directed medical therapy for heart failure does not exist: A non-judgmental framework for describing the level of adherence to evidence-based drug treatments for patients with a reduced ejection fraction. *European Journal of Heart Failure*, *22*(10), 1759–1767. doi:10.1002/ejhf.1857 PMID:32432391

Ponikowski, P., Chua, T. P., Anker, S. D., Francis, D. P., Doehner, W., Banasiak, W., Poole-Wilson, P. A., Piepoli, M. F., & Coats, A. J. (2001). Peripheral chemoreceptor hypersensitivity: An ominous sign in patients with chronic heart failure. *Circulation*, *104*(5), 544–549. doi:10.1161/hc3101.093699 PMID:11479251

Rolski, F., & Błyszczuk, P. (2020). Complexity of TNF-α signaling in heart disease. *Journal of Clinical Medicine*, *9*(10), 3267. doi:10.3390/jcm9103267 PMID:33053859

Salyer, J., Flattery, M., & Lyon, D. E. (2019). Heart failure symptom clusters and quality of life. *Heart & Lung*, *48*(5), 366–372. doi:10.1016/j.hrtlng.2019.05.016 PMID:31204015

Seferović, P. M., Polovina, M., Adlbrecht, C., Bělohlávek, J., Chioncel, O., Goncalvesova, E., Milinković, I., Grupper, A., Halmosi, R., Kamzola, G., Koskinas, K. C., Lopatin, Y., Parkhomenko, A., Põder, P., Ristić, A. D., Šakalytė, G., Trbušić, M., Tundybayeva, M., Vrtovec, B, & Coats, A. J. (2021). Navigating between Scylla and Charybdis: Challenges and strategies for implementing guideline-directed medical therapy in heart failure with reduced ejection fraction. *European Journal of Heart Failure*, *23*(12), 1999–2007. doi:10.1002/ejhf.2378 PMID:34755422

Silverberg, D. S., Wexler, D., & Iaina, A. (2002). The importance of anemia and its correction in the management of severe congestive heart failure. *European Journal of Heart Failure*, *4*(6), 681–686. doi:10.1016/S1388-9842(02)00115-0 PMID:12453537

Solari, E., Marcozzi, C., Ottaviani, C., Negrini, D., & Moriondo, A. (2022). Draining the Pleural Space: Lymphatic Vessels Facing the Most Challenging Task. *Biology (Basel)*, *11*(3), 419. doi:10.3390/biology11030419 PMID:35336793

Song, E. K., Moser, D. K., Rayens, M. K., & Lennie, T. A. (2010). Symptom clusters predict event-free survival in patients with heart failure. *The Journal of Cardiovascular Nursing*, *25*(4), 284–291. doi:10.1097/JCN.0b013e3181cfbcbb PMID:20539163

St John Sutton, M. G., Plappert, T., Abraham, W. T., Smith, A. L., DeLurgio, D. B., Leon, A. R., Loh, E., Kocovic, D. Z., Fisher, W. G., Ellestad, M., Messenger, J., Kruger, K., Hilpisch, K. E., & Hill, M. R. (2003). Effect of cardiac resynchronization therapy on left ventricular size and function in chronic heart failure. *Circulation*, *107*(15), 1985–1990. doi:10.1161/01.CIR.0000065226.24159.E9 PMID:12668512

Takeuchi, S., Kohno, T., Goda, A., Shiraishi, Y., Kawana, M., Saji, M., Nagatomo, Y., Nishihata, Y., Takei, M., Nakano, S., Soejima, K., Kohsaka, S., & Yoshikawa, T.West Tokyo Heart Failure Registry Investigators. (2022). Multimorbidity, guideline-directed medical therapies, and associated outcomes among hospitalized heart failure patients. *ESC Heart Failure*, *9*(4), 2500–2510. doi:10.1002/ehf2.13954 PMID:35561100

Taylor, C. J., Harrison, C., Britt, H., Miller, G., & Hobbs, F. R. (2017). Heart failure and multimorbidity in Australian general practice. *Journal of Comorbidity*, *7*(1), 44–49. doi:10.15256/joc.2017.7.106 PMID:29090188

Thomas, M., Khariton, Y., Fonarow, G. C., Arnold, S. V., Hill, L., Nassif, M. E., Sharma, P. P., Butler, J., Thomas, L., Duffy, C. I., DeVore, A. D., Hernandez, A., Albert, N. M., Patterson, J. H., Williams, F. B., McCague, K., & Spertus, J. A. (2019). Association of changes in heart failure treatment with patients' health status: Real-world evidence from CHAMP-HF. *JACC. Heart Failure*, *7*(7), 615–625. doi:10.1016/j.jchf.2019.03.020 PMID:31176672

Truby, L. K., & Rogers, J. G. (2020). Advanced heart failure: Epidemiology, diagnosis, and therapeutic approaches. *Heart Failure*, *8*(7), 523–536. PMID:32535126

Vargo, D. L., Kramer, W. G., Black, P. K., Smith, W. B., Serpas, T., & Brater, D. C. (1995). Bioavailability, pharmacokinetics, and pharmacodynamics of torsemide and furosemide in patients with congestive heart failure. *Clinical Pharmacology and Therapeutics*, *57*(6), 601–609. doi:10.1016/0009-9236(95)90222-8 PMID:7781259

Wilcox, C. S., Testani, J. M., & Pitt, B. (2020). Pathophysiology of diuretic resistance and its implications for the management of chronic heart failure. *Hypertension*, *76*(4), 1045–1054. doi:10.1161/HYPERTENSIONAHA.120.15205 PMID:32829662

Yu, D. S. F., Li, P. W. C., & Chong, S. O. K. (2018). Symptom cluster among patients with advanced heart failure: A review of its manifestations and impacts on health outcomes. *Current Opinion in Supportive and Palliative Care*, *12*(1), 16–24. doi:10.1097/SPC.0000000000000316 PMID:29176333

Chapter 5
Medication Non-Adherence in Geriatric Patients With Multimorbidity

Khawar Shabbir
University of Auckland, New Zealand

Adil Hamad Alharthi
King Fahad Armed Forces Hospital, Saudi Arabia

Aisha Alshehri
King Fahad Armed Forces Hospital, Saudi Arabia

Danyah Ahmed Katlan
King Fahad Armed Forces Hospital, Saudi Arabia

Alaa Shahbar
Umm Alqura University, Saudi Arabia

EXECUTIVE SUMMARY

In many cases, the prescription medications are not taken as prescribed is because of failure to adhere to the medication regimen. The reason for not adhering to drug treatment include unpleasant or inconvenient side effects of the medications; dry mouth, change in taste, fatigue or frequent urination are various reasons of stopping a mediation. Older adults are at higher risk for medication nonadherence due to prevalence of multiple comorbidities, including cognitive deficit and polypharmacy. Medication adherence can be enhanced by considering geriatric's vision, hearing, swallowing, cognition, motor impairment, and health literacy while providing counselling and education. On the positive side, a study found that increased medication adherence was associated with fewer hospitalizations and decreased cost in patients with certain chronic medical conditions (e.g., diabetes, hypertension).

DOI: 10.4018/978-1-6684-2354-7.ch005

INTRODUCTION

Medication adherence is defined as the patient's behavior agree with the physician's plan regarding the agreed treatment plan. Compliance and adherence are usually used interchangeably despite the subtle difference in the meaning. Compliance is the degree of patient's behavior corresponding with the health care provider's plan whereas adherence is the mutual work between the patient and the physician to achieve the desired outcome of the treatment plan. There are three common types of non-adherence in practice. First, the primary non-fulfillment adherence when the therapy is prescribed but has not been used by the patient. Second, the non-persistence non-adherence occurs when the patient stops the therapy in the midway of the treatment journey without consulting the physician. This type of non-adherence could be intentional or unintentional. Unintentional could be due to lack of access to therapy, poor memory, and financial burden while Intentional non-adherence is attributed to the patient's beliefs, attitudes, motivation, and expectation. Third, the non-conforming in which the medication is utilized by the patient in incorrect time, dose, or frequency. The rate of adherence is measured in literatures as a percentage of the actual consumed doses divided on the supposed doses to be utilized during a treatment period. The rate is estimated to be approximately 50% in developed countries and half of the non-adherence is intentional (Jimmy & Jose, 2011).

Medication non-adherence is linked to poor disease outcome and prognosis, increase of healthcare cost, increase hospital admission rates and death. In USA, medication non-adherence is accounted for 33 to 69% of hospital admissions linked to medication issues with a yearly cost of $100 billion (Osterberg & Blaschke, 2005). Of all hospital admissions, medication non-adherence consisted of 10% of the total hospitalizations. Non-adherence increases the yearly cost by $2000 due to increase in medical visits by 3 visits annually. The adjusted cost of medication non-adherence is the highest in cancer patients followed by osteoporosis, cardiovascular, mental health, and diabetes mellitus with adjusted costs of $144,101, $43,240, $16,124, $16,110, and $7,077, respectively (Cutler et al., 2018).

There are indirect and direct methods to detect non-adherence with advantages and disadvantages for each methos. Direct observed therapy, drug level in bodily fluids and measurement of biological markers in blood are examples for the direct methos. Direct observed therapy is the most accurate method, but patients may hide pills in the mouth cavity to throw them away later on. Measurement of drug or its metabolites in blood is objective method, despite that, metabolism may vary greatly among patients due to genetic differences. Also, Measurement of biological markers may differ due to variation of response from an individual to another. Indirect methos such as pill counts and prescription refills are often used in practice, however, they may not assess the actual received medication due to pill dumping and stocking pills without using them (Osterberg & Blaschke, 2005).

In many cases the prescription medications are not taken as prescribed because failure to adhere to the medication regimen. The reason for not adhering to drug treatment include unpleasant or inconvenient side effects of the medications like dry mouth, change in taste, fatigue or frequent urination are various reasons of stopping a mediation. Older adults are at higher risk for medication nonadherence due to prevalence of multiple comorbidities including cognitive deficit and polypharmacy. Medication adherence can be enhanced by considering geriatric's vision, hearing, swallowing, cognition, motor impairment and health literacy while providing counselling and education. On the positive side, a study found that increased medication adherence was associated with fewer hospitalizations and decreased cost in patients with certain chronic medical conditions (e.g., diabetes, hypertension).

The WHO suggests clinicians consider five dimensions when assessing medication adherence: social/economic factors (e.g., cultural), provider–patient/healthcare system factors (e.g., provider–patient relationship), condition-related factors (e.g., chronic conditions), therapy-related factors (e.g., regimen complexity), and patient-related factors (e.g., visual or hearing impairment). Clinicians can improve the likelihood of adherence by considering the use of adhering aids like special packaging, a medication record, a drug calendar, medication boxes, magnification for insulin syringes, dose-measuring devices, and spacer devices for metered-dose inhalers.

STUDIES REVIEW

After studying 163 elder patients in UAE Ibrahim NA et al found that patient and health care provider factors influence medication adherence in geriatric patients and that clinicians have a key role in promoting the adherence of geriatric patients (Ibrahim et al., 2020). Bastani et al. found that several factors affected the elderly's Medication adherence the main problem of which was delinquency (Bastani et al., 2021). Zhi Li et al. (2016) found a positive association between medication nonadherence and the number of comorbidities in elderly with hypertension. Lonzano-Hernandez et al. (2020) found that among elder patient with Multimorbidity and polypharmacy, lower functional support was related to non-adherence to treatment.

Patient Case

A 70-year-old lady Coming from a rural area is known to have diabetes, hypertension, chronic kidney disease and obesity. The patient came to you for follow up. Her blood pressure and hemoglobin A1C were uncontrolled for the last eight months despite being on three antihypertensive medications and high dose insulin. She is taking her medication from the pharmacist regularly every month. She doesn't look attentive, but she looks healthy with a low mood and her vitals are stable except for blood pressure. She denies any complaints.

Upon asking her specifically screening questions with an eye-to-eye contact while showing your interest and empathy towards her, she reveals that she is suffering from urge incontinence, foot numbness, loss of foot sensation, difficulty sleeping, chronic Constipation, poor hearing of quiet sounds and heartburn for the last six months. And in the last three months she started to have loss of interest in everything even her grandchildren visits. She started also feeling worthlessness and started thinking of death recurrently. She added that doctors are not interested in her health they are only interested in prescribing more medications and she mentioned that she feels you're the only doctor she felt interested in listening to her since a long time. Upon asking about medications, she revealed that most medications she only takes if she feels headache, but mostly she doesn't take them because she believes there are harmful to the kidney as one doctor told her, and it might cause her to need dialysis later.

DISCUSSION

This elderly lady with Multimorbidity is manifesting nonadherence due to a combination of causes:

First

Altered patient doctor relationship, it seems that most of the physicians who saw her were unaware of managing the elderly patients and how they need to show their interest and empathy to gain the patient trust and gain a proper history and adherence to follow up, and that could have caused lack of trust in the Healthcare system.

Second

Hearing difficulty which contributed to communication difficulties with her physicians and possibly pharmacists as well.

Third

Over concern and false believes caused her to be hesitant about medication adherence to prevent complications.

Fourth

Depression as underlying complication caused lack of interest and non-adherence to medication further worsening her situation.

Fifth

Educational status and health illiteracy as it found that the patient's awareness about their diseases and prescribed medications contributed to medication adherence.

Sixth

Polypharmacy which is defined as prescribing five or more medications for a patient. Polypharmacy is strongly related to medications non-adherence.

All of these factors will be discussed later in this chapter.

Recommendations Regarding the Case

In this patient, a multidisciplinary team is needed mainly the social worker, psychologist, pharmacist, ENT specialist, psychiatrist, Religion affairs and the patient's family to be involved actively as well.

Suggested plan and follow up for cognitive therapy, education about medications, diseases in elderly people. Group therapy is also suggested so the patient can see how other patients of her same age and multiple problems are looking healthy and happy on their medications. Appropriate medication adherence aids should be considered as well. She will also need to follow up with the urologist and foot specialist for possible urge incontinence and Diabetic foot complications.

FACTORS RELATED TO MEDICATION NON-ADHERENCE IN GERIATRIC PATIENTS WITH MULTIMORBIDITY

Doctor-Patient Relationship

The doctor–patient relationship is a central part of health care and the practice of medicine. A doctor–patient relationship is formed when a doctor attends to a patient's medical needs. Generally, the relationship is entered into by mutual consent between the physician and patient. This relationship is built on trust, respect, communication, and a common understanding of both the doctor and patients' sides. The trust aspect of this relationship goes is mutual: the doctor trusts the patient to reveal any information that may be relevant to the case, and in turn, the patient trusts the doctor to respect their privacy and not disclose this information to outside parties. The healthiness of a doctor–patient relationship is essential to keep the quality of the patient's healthcare high as well as to ensure that the doctor is working at their ideal (American Medical Association, 2022).

As elderly patients deal with the physical, psychological, social, economic, and lifestyle changes associated with aging, their relationship with their physician may remain an important source of support and encouragement. Communication between physician and patient can have far-reaching implications for the physical and mental health of elder patients. Effective physician-patient communication involves the exchange of both medical and psychosocial information as well as the emotional and effective care that is so important to older patients' health outcomes. The development of a trusting therapeutic relationship can be central to the health care of elder patients (Starfield et al., 2005).

Providing information to patients and successfully conveying it in a clear and comprehensible format is a central component of the medical visit. Physicians typically give their patients information in the form of explanations or instructions. They communicate a diagnosis, describe options for treatment, and discuss the advantages and disadvantages of each option. Information that is given to patients in medical visits may affect not only how satisfied patients are with their care, but also how well they subsequently adhere to medical recommendations. Adherence can ultimately determine long term health outcomes (DiMatteo et al., 2002).

Active communication using sharing in decision-making by both the patient and physician will increase patient adherence to medical therapy. Active communication increases patients' knowledge of their condition allows them to convey important information to their physicians and improves the process of care. The process of physician-patient joint decision-making about medication regimens is essential to patient adherence (Street et al., 2005). Studies show that if physicians and patients together decide what medications will be taken, how often, how long, and on what schedule, as well as how to deal with side effects and other challenges, adherence is much better than if patients are simply told what to do and left to their own to work out how they will adhere (Jahng et al., 2005).

This is particularly important with older patients, who may have problems remembering multiple medical regimens that are confusing and can conflict with one another. Physicians can help their older patients by simplifying complex treatment regimens, providing helpful strategies such as timers and special pill boxes, and providing assistance in incorporating medication-taking with other daily events. Working with patients to address the practical and logistical challenges of treatment can be essential to adherence (Ownby et al., 2006).

Hearing Difficulty

As we age, we are increasingly likely to suffer from chronic conditions. Hearing impairment is among the top three such conditions along with arthritis and hypertension. It may have become a problem for the first time in old age or may have been acquired when younger or at birth. Hearing impairment can have devastating effects on an individual's social life, independence, and emotional health. Unfortunately, older people often fail to seek help, believing it is an inevitable part of aging or fearing stigmatization. Even though there are a number of measures and devices which can significantly improve an affected individual's quality of life, there is considerable unmet need for these and as the older population rises this need will rise also. It is therefore essential that doctors recognize disabling hearing loss, treat where necessary, and refer to appropriate professionals (Murlow et al., 1990).

Hearing loss of almost any extent can be improved with a hearing aid. For conductive hearing loss this is simply a matter of amplification, despite the fact that for sensorineural hearing loss the mechanism is more complex. However, there are many factors which will interfere with a patient's satisfaction with, and benefit from, a hearing aid. Lack of motivation because of fear of stigmatization, low expectations of benefit, or failure to accept there is a problem remain significant obstacles (Kemp et al., 1989). Stephens et al. showed that despite the fact that 50% of those aged 50–65 in two villages in South Wales had a hearing disability only 7% had a hearing aid. Clinicians have an important role in identifying those who would benefit from a hearing aid and emphasizing the benefits of its use (Stephens et al., 1990).

Hearing impairment is contributed to communication difficulties. Although nonadherence to medications may be common among the elderly, fundamental reasons leading to nonadherence vary among patients. Diminished functional abilities may exert an adverse effect on adherence. Older patients may have number of co-morbid conditions like the presence of cognitive, vision and/or hearing impairment which may predispose the elderly to nonadherence. Hearing problems can impede an elderly person's ability to hear instructions about the medications.

To overcome this barrier Elders should wear their hearing aid to doctors' appointments and pharmacies to increase understanding. Written instructions can also be provided from the pharmacist using such as coding prescription vials with large letters or colored labels (Gravell, 1988).

Several Electronic Medication Adherence Aids specifically designed for elderly populations have been developed and tested in clinical trials. E.g., a weekly pill box that automatically dispenses medication at programmed intervals. It emits an audible tone reminding patients to take their medication. Optional components include a modem which can be programmed to telephone the patient or a caregiver when a dose is missed, a 'voice module' which can record a customized message with a familiar voice, and a strobe light for the hearing impaired (MacLaughlin et al., 2005).

False Beliefs and Complications Over Concern

Non-adherence is a multifactorial communication issue among the patient, physician, and healthcare system. Poor provider-patient communication can lead to poor understanding of the disease, benefit and risk of the medication, and improper medication utilization (Osterberg & Blaschke, 2005). Health care providers and patients have to discuss true and false beliefs, regarding the patient's medications and disease that may hinder the patient from reaching the desirable outcomes (Horne, et al., 2013). False beliefs can originate from previous experiences and social and cultural influences. Social medias and unreliable sources on the internet can impact the patient's perception of his disease and medications. Healthcare providers should discuss patients' beliefs to understand the patients' perspectives and to reach to a shared medical decision (Tsay, 2018).

Or instance, a patient is known to have inflammatory bowel disease has visited her doctor regarding unintentional weight loss, fatigue, and agitation over 6 months. After blood workup, she found to have suboptimal calcium, iron, and folic acid levels. She adopted a vegan lifestyle 6 months ago as a habit of eating due to her animal love and her belief of that veganism can prevent hypertension, type-2 diabetes and hypercholesteremia as she read that in a medical article. She refused using medical supplements because she thinks that they are produced from animal sources. In this scenario, we may identify some beliefs, from the patient and the care giver, which can potentially impact the outcome due to variations of perspectives. A care giver, who may not be fully aware of veganism, can think of her medical condition is due to her new adopted eating style. Also, unawareness of availability of some vegan products, that may provide the patient with the deficient minerals and vitamins, can prevent the patient and care provider from reaching a shared medical decision. Another false belief, in this case, is that all medical supplements are derived from animal sources while in fact there are plenty of plant-based supplements. Addressing beliefs with patients and care givers is crucial for the patient's adherence to the therapeutic plan and for a better outcome (Southworth & Parsi, 2018).

False beliefs can drastically impact treatment outcome in diseases that require a high adherence such as in treating HIV (human immunodeficiency virus) patients with antiretroviral treatment (ART). A study measured the false beliefs regarding treatment effectiveness, side effects, adherence, and retention in 389 HIV patients receiving ART. False beliefs were measured via questionnaires through a direct patient interview. Fifty-six percent of the patients had at least one false belief. Seventeen percent of the patients believed that HIV can be cured by pastors' prayers, 17% answered that ART can cure HIV, and 10% reckoned that they can stop ART if they are taking herbs that boost the immune function (Nozaki et al., 2013). HIV suppression and prevent of medication resistance depends on a highly medication adherence that exceeds 95%. non-resolved false beliefs can affect the patients' behaviors which may lead to failure of effective treatment and increase of health care cost. Behavioral reinforcement through discussing false beliefs and patient's understanding of the treatment, can avert non-adherence. An increase of medication adherence by more than 95% in more than 90% of the patients, who underwent cognitive-behavioral therapy, has been proven clinically (Osterberg & Blaschke, 2005).

In psychiatry, false beliefs tend to occur with the health care providers and the patients as well. A study published in 2005 reported that 56% of the participants found stopping antidepressants is difficult after a long period of use because of addiction to medications. The author of the study contributed their view to mistaken opinion despite of a previous published articles in 2000 and 1998 reporting withdraw symptoms due to permeant or temporal cease of antidepressants (Hengartner & Plöderl, 2018). False beliefs in psychiatric patients have been studied by Nejad et al, in which 56 (37.4%) of 150 participants discontinued psychiatric medication without consulting the physician. The reported false beliefs were addiction to all type of psychotropic medications, no difference in efficacy between psychiatric medications, indifference to taking or omitting medications, ineffectiveness of psychiatric medications, opium is more efficacious than psychotropic medications and medications treat only comatic symptoms. A higher rate of medication refusal in psychiatric patients during treatment lead to relapse of psychiatric symptoms. Patient education on the psychiatric illness and psychotropic medications could boost the adherence rate and decrease unnecessary visits and cost for relapsed symptoms (Nejad & Pouya, 2004).

Another common issue in geriatric is Polypharmacy which is defined as prescribing five or more medications for a patient. Beliefs about medication used in geriatric lead to polypharmacy which is in return lead to non-adherence, unnecessary side effects and adverse drug reactions. In a study that evaluated the geriatric patients' beliefs, the researchers found that 96.3% of the patients are convinced by the need of all of medications prescribed. Geriatric patients may become comfortable with the notion of long-term medication use. Most of the patients reported positive relationships with the primary care physicians. Therefore, the doctor-patient relationship can positively change the patients' behaviors towards accepting deprescribing of unnecessary medications (Clyne et al., 2017).

Depression

Depression is characterized with persistent lack of interest, energy, and concentration. Disturbed sleep and appetite are common as well in depressed individuals (Institute of Health Metrics and Evaluation, 2022). Approximately 15% of adults aged 60 and over suffer from a mental disorder (World Health Organization, 2017). In geriatrics, it has been found that depression is the most common mental health problem (Canadian Coalition for Seniors' Mental Health, 2006). As per the WHO Depression occurs in 7% of the general older population and it accounts for 5.7% of Years Lived with Disability (YLDs) in adults above 60 years (Institute of Health Metrics and Evaluation, 2022). In addition, depression was found to be common in nursing home residents, with prevalence ranging from 15% up to 65 percent (Vankova et al., 2021).

The association between depressive symptoms and poor adherence to medications has been widely recognized. In a meta-analysis, investigators found that depressed individuals with chronic medical conditions were 3 times more likely to be non-adherent to their medications when compared to non-depressed patients (Wing et al., 2002). A study done by Youn-Jung Son et al. found that depression and self-efficacy were statistically significant predictors of medication adherence in older patients with hypertension. Authors concluded that implementing systematic approaches are required to resolve these barriers to improve control (Son & Won, 2017). The detection and management of depression can improve medication adherence and are found to be important in the management of hypertension (Kretchy et al., 2014).

Cooperation of the interprofessional team in the screening of depressive symptoms has the potential to improve the quality of care (Vankova et al., 2021). In order to overcome this barrier Yuda et al, suggested a stepwise approach for managing the burden of being elderly, with hypertension and mental health problems in order to improve adherence. The approach includes: 1. identifying elderly with high risk for mental problems through screening as early detection and early intervention might have a role in controlling the problem. 2. Identifying the barriers to adherence which includes access, affordability, poor knowledge, false beliefs. 3. Develop a strategy to overcome the barriers and treat the medical conditions including the mental illnesses. 4. increased awareness and knowledge and create a supportive environment. This will lead to better adherence which in turn will provide a higher quality of life (Turana et al., 2021).

Educational Status

Various risk factors associated with non-adherence in the elderly exists in literature. These include but not limited to medication factors, health care system factors and patient factors. Patient factors include age, educational level, physical and mental status as well as health literacy (Osterberg & Blaschke, 2005). In the United States it has been found that an excess cost of over 170 billion dollars annually is caused by non-adherence (Sabaté & Sabaté, 2003). In geriatrics, the problem is even wider. It is estimated that around 10% of geriatric hospitalizations are due to medication non-adherence (MacLaughlin et al., 2005), and the rate of non-adherence is as high as 75% (Félix & Henriques, 2021).

Non-adherence among geriatrics accounts for adverse outcomes. Medication wastage, increased cost of healthcare, and worsening in patients' medical conditions are consequences of medication non-adherence which in turn can lead to increased disability or even death (Osterberg & Blaschke, 2005). R. Shruthi et al. studied the level of medication compliance as well as the factors contributing to compliance in geriatrics with chronic illnesses using structured questionnaires as per modified Morisky Medication Adherence Scale (MMAS) in 251 patients. The study found that the level of compliance positively correlated with the educational status of the study subjects and their awareness about the diseases and prescribed medications (Shruthi et al., 2016).

Moreover, JIN, Hyekyung et al, performed a cross sectional multicenter survey study. One hundred and sixty participants aged 65 years and older were included. The participants' functional health literacy (FHL) which is associated with adherence was evaluated. The authors found that the education level, the satisfaction with patient counseling, and explanation of medication are associated with medication adherence of elderly patients. Other factors included were health-related problems and dosing frequency (Jin et al., 2016).

In contrast a cross-sectional study included 422 patients targeting outpatient geriatrics with chronic diseases in Riyadh, Saudi Arabia were assessed for medication adherence. The authors measured different factors impacting medication adherence which includes patient behavior, cost, comorbidity, and pill burden. Data were collected using a structured questionnaire and the GMAS validated instrument scale (General Medication Adherence Scale). The study found good level of adherence in geriatrics when compared with other international figures. Authors suggested that patient education about their disease and the strong beliefs about the medications prescribed are crucial factors to promote adherence (Alhabib et al., 2022).

Overcoming the lack of knowledge in geriatrics comes first when looking into topics of needs in this age group (Leung et al., 2006). The importance of health education has been emphasized by World Health Organization (WHO) to support health care needs and health promotion for geriatrics (Rana et al., 2010).

Lack of general educational status can be overcome by patient education about their medical condition as well as their prescribed medications. Patient education play important role that can significantly improve adherence to medications used for treating different conditions with different disease severities (Gold & McClung, 2006). Comprehensive assessment of patients' medications and their disease and/or medication related knowledge is a critical initial step to identify medication related issues (Bazargan et al., 2017).

Patient education could enhance their empowerment and medication adherence. It is considered a basic right of the patients. Healthcare professionals are responsible to provide information to the patients as they play a crucial role to educate their patients and hence improve the compliance (Tan, 2020). Inter-professional collaboration is required to follow and modify complicated medication regimens (Bazargan et al., 2017).

Pharmacists play an important role in promoting medication adherence through identifying and preventing medication related problems considering elderly patients' individual characteristics which includes educational background and other specific patient-related health problems or comorbidities. Moreover, pharmacists play a clinical role in designing evidence-based medication regimens that are patient-specific (Patel & Krishnaswami, 2015).

Due to the frequent contact with patients, pharmacists are in ideal position to promote medication adherence, providing sufficient information about the importance of the prescribed medication and ensure patient satisfaction with the counseling. The Federal Study of Adherence to Medications in the Elderly, studied the pharmacists' effectiveness in increasing adherence to medication. In this study 200 patients ³ 65 years were included if they were taking ³ 4 medications. Adherence, blood pressure, and cholesterol were monitored and found to be improved in participants at a comprehensive pharmacy care program (Lee et al., 2006). Comprehensive collaborative programs should be implemented to support patient education support and to provide patients counselling on medication adherence (Lee et al., 2006).

Polypharmacy

Polypharmacy is commonly referred to the use of five or more drugs, including prescription, over-the-counter, complementary and alternative medications. Accurate medication history may be more challenging to gather when a patient's medication increases, which makes it more difficult to evaluate and prescribe medications. The probability of adverse drug reactions increases when more medications are being used (57,58).

Polypharmacy is linked to inappropriate prescribing. The more medications a patient takes, the more likely that those medications are not prescribed correctly and the more decline the patient's overall function (Pharmaceutical Society of Australia, 2019; Rossi, 2018).

Elderly patients usually have complicated medication needs. Elderly patients are using a lot of medication because they often have multiple comorbidities and are often dependent on others like health care staff or family to administer their medication. Elderly patients have greater vulnerability to the side effects and adverse reactions of medication, due to the underlying factors which include reduced body water, increased body fat, reduced protein binding, and renal and hepatic impairment. Drug interactions are also more common because of the multiple medications often prescribed to Elderly patients for the management of their comorbidities (McLean & Le Couteur, 2004; Huang & Mallet, 2013). Polypharmacy and medication adherence in the elderly are significant public-health considerations worldwide and are an important focus of integrated care. Polypharmacy may be a barrier to adherence because of the associated complex medication regimens, increased risk of adverse drug events and high medication costs (Beer et al., 2011).

Optimal medication management in older people requires a multidisciplinary approach to improve medication adherence and ensure the best quality of life. There are many recommendations to reduce polypharmacy, one of the most important recommendations is the recommendations of The International Group for Reducing Inappropriate Medication Use and Polypharmacy (IGRIMUP) which included:

1. Review the medication of all older people with an eye to deprescribing, particularly those who are vulnerable to the adverse effects of medication.
2. Before initiating a potentially 'appropriate' medication, consider the validity of the evidence based on patient characteristics and preferences.
3. Beyond the established lists, take into account the probable withdrawal of each medication.
4. Medical education needs a stronger focus on inappropriate medication use and polypharmacy.
5. Medical training should review methods to stop treatments and provide equal attention to drug side effects and benefits.
6. When patients have multimorbidity, the single disease model should be rejected. The single disease approach with adherence to clinical guidelines for each illness makes polypharmacy and inappropriate medication use unavoidable.
7. In elderly complicated cases, decisions should consistently take expected survival and quality of life into account, giving patient and family preferences top consideration (Mangin, et al., 2018).

The use of electronic health records (EHR) is another person-centered approach to reduce the risk associated with polypharmacy. An accessible electronic medical database would assist physicians in prescribing new drugs, reviewing medication efficacy, and to deprescribe when co-morbid conditions improve. This method can potentially prevent avoidable ADR that may result from polypharmacy via drug-drug interactions. Another important aspect of the electronic medical record system is that it contains the results of the administrative and clinical encounters of a patient, therefore EHR interoperability with other provider systems will help prevent extended hospitalization and delayed referrals for older persons due to the compilation of medical history (Hoerbst & Ammenwerth, 2010).

REFERENCES

Alhabib, M. Y., Alhazmi, T. S., Alsaad, S. M., AlQahtani, A. S., & Alnafisah, A. A. (2022). Medication adherence among geriatric patients with chronic diseases in Riyadh, Saudi Arabia. *Patient Preference and Adherence, 16*, 2021–2030. doi:10.2147/PPA.S363082 PMID:35966222

American Medical Association. (2022). *Patient-physician relationships.* AMA. https://www.ama-assn.org/delivering-care/ethics/patient-physician-relationships

Bastani, P., Bikineh, P., Mehralian, G., Sadeghkhani, O., Rezaee, R., Kavosi, Z., & Ravangard, R. (2021). Medication adherence among the elderly: Applying grounded theory approach in a developing country. *Journal of Pharmaceutical Policy and Practice, 14*(1), 1–8. doi:10.118640545-021-00340-9 PMID:34193278

Bazargan, M., Smith, J., Yazdanshenas, H., Movassaghi, M., Martins, D., & Orum, G. (2017). Non-adherence to medication regimens among older African American adults. *BMC Geriatrics, 17*(1), 1–12. doi:10.118612877-017-0558-5 PMID:28743244

Beer, C., Hyde, Z., Almeida, O. P., Norman, P., Hankey, G. J., Yeap, B. B., & Flicker, L. (2011). Quality use of medicines and health outcomes among a cohort of community dwelling older men: An observational study. *British Journal of Clinical Pharmacology, 71*(4), 592–599. doi:10.1111/j.1365-2125.2010.03875.x PMID:21395652

Canadian Coalition for Seniors' Mental Health. (2006). National guidelines for seniors' mental health: The assessment and treatment of depression. Toronto, ON: Canadian Coalition for Seniors'. *Mental Health.*

Clyne, B., Cooper, J. A., Boland, F., Hughes, C. M., Fahey, T., & Smith, S. M. (2017). Beliefs about prescribed medication among older patients with polypharmacy: A mixed methods study in primary care. *The British Journal of General Practice, 67*(660), e507–e518. doi:10.3399/bjgp17X691073 PMID:28533200

Cutler, R. L., Fernandez-Llimos, F., Frommer, M., Benrimoj, C., & Garcia-Cardenas, V. (2018). Economic impact of medication non-adherence by disease groups: A systematic review. *BMJ Open*, *8*(1), e016982. doi:10.1136/bmjopen-2017-016982 PMID:29358417

DiMatteo, M. R., Giordani, P. J., Lepper, H. S., & Croghan, T. W. (2002). Patient adherence and medical treatment outcomes a meta-analysis. *Medical Care*, *40*(9), 794–811. doi:10.1097/00005650-200209000-00009 PMID:12218770

Félix, I. B., & Henriques, A. (2021, October). Medication adherence and related determinants in older people with multimorbidity: A cross-sectional study. *Nursing Forum*, *56*(4), 834–843. doi:10.1111/nuf.12619 PMID:34076260

Gold, D. T., & McClung, B. (2006). Approaches to patient education: Emphasizing the long-term value of compliance and persistence. *The American Journal of Medicine*, *119*(4), S32–S37. doi:10.1016/j.amjmed.2005.12.021 PMID:16563940

Gravell, R. (1988). *Communication problems in elderly people: practical approaches to management*. Croom Helm.

Hengartner, M. P., & Plöderl, M. (2018). False beliefs in academic psychiatry: The case of antidepressant drugs. *Ethical Human Psychology and Psychiatry*, *20*(1), 6–16. doi:10.1891/1559-4343.20.1.6

Hoerbst, A., & Ammenwerth, E. (2010). Electronic health records. *Methods of Information in Medicine*, *49*(04), 320–336. doi:10.3414/ME10-01-0038 PMID:20603687

Horne, R., Chapman, S. C., Parham, R., Freemantle, N., Forbes, A., & Cooper, V. (2013). Understanding patients' adherence-related beliefs about medicines prescribed for long-term conditions: A meta-analytic review of the Necessity-Concerns Framework. *PLoS One*, *8*(12), e80633. doi:10.1371/journal.pone.0080633 PMID:24312488

Huang, A. R., & Mallet, L. (2013). Prescribing opioids in older people. *Maturitas*, *74*(2), 123–129. doi:10.1016/j.maturitas.2012.11.002 PMID:23201325

Ibrahim, N. A., Edis, Z., & Al-Owais, K. S. (2020). Adherence of geriatric patients and their beliefs toward their medicines in the United Arab Emirates. *Journal of Pharmacy & Bioallied Sciences*, *12*(1), 22. doi:10.4103/jpbs.JPBS_93_19 PMID:32801597

Institute of Health Metrics and Evaluation. (2019). Global Health Data Exchange (GHDx). http://ghdx.healthdata.org/gbd-results-tool?params=gbd-api-2019-permalink/d780dffbe8a381b25e1416884959e88b

Jahng, K. H., Martin, L. R., Golin, C. E., & DiMatteo, M. R. (2005). Preferences for medical collaboration: Patient–physician congruence and patient outcomes. *Patient Education and Counseling*, *57*(3), 308–314. doi:10.1016/j.pec.2004.08.006 PMID:15893213

Jimmy, B., & Jose, J. (2011). Patient medication adherence: Measures in daily practice. *Oman Medical Journal*, *26*(3), 155–159. doi:10.5001/omj.2011.38 PMID:22043406

Jin, H., Kim, Y., & Rhie, S. J. (2016). Factors affecting medication adherence in elderly people. *Patient Preference and Adherence*, *10*, 2117–2125. doi:10.2147/PPA.S118121 PMID:27799748

Kemp, B., Brummel-Smith, K., & Plowman, V. J. (1989). Geriatric rehab program focuses on research, training, and service. *Journal of Rehabilitation*, *55*(4), 9–12.

Kretchy, I. A., Owusu-Daaku, F. T., & Danquah, S. A. (2014). Mental health in hypertension: Assessing symptoms of anxiety, depression, and stress on anti-hypertensive medication adherence. *International Journal of Mental Health Systems*, *8*(1), 1–6. doi:10.1186/1752-4458-8-25 PMID:24987456

Lee, J. K., Grace, K. A., & Taylor, A. J. (2006). Effect of a pharmacy care program on medication adherence and persistence, blood pressure, and low-density lipoprotein cholesterol: A randomized controlled trial. *Journal of the American Medical Association*, *296*(21), 2563–2571. doi:10.1001/jama.296.21.joc60162 PMID:17101639

Leung, A., Chi, I., & Lui, Y. H. (2006). A Cross-Cultural Study in Older Adults' Learning Experience. *Asian Journal of Gerontology & Geriatrics*, *1*, 78–83.

Li, Z., Zhao, Y. P., & Hu, X. Y. (2016). The association between multimorbidity and medication non-adherence in elderly with hypertension in western China. *Hu Li Za Zhi*, *63*(5), 65. PMID:27699741

Lozano-Hernández, C. M., López-Rodríguez, J. A., Leiva-Fernández, F., Calderón-Larrañaga, A., Barrio-Cortes, J., Gimeno-Feliu, L. A., Poblador-Plou, B., & Cura-González, I. (2020). Social support, social context, and nonadherence to treatment in young senior patients with multimorbidity and polypharmacy followed-up in primary care. MULTIPAP Study. *PLoS One*, *15*(6), e0235148. doi:10.1371/journal.pone.0235148 PMID:32579616

MacLaughlin, E. J., Raehl, C. L., Treadway, A. K., Sterling, T. L., Zoller, D. P., & Bond, C. A. (2005). Assessing medication adherence in the elderly: Which tools to use in clinical practice? *Drugs & Aging*, *22*(3), 231–255. doi:10.2165/00002512-200522030-00005 PMID:15813656

Mangin, D., Bahat, G., Golomb, B. A., Mallery, L. H., Moorhouse, P., Onder, G., Petrovic, M., & Garfinkel, D. (2018). International Group for Reducing Inappropriate Medication Use & Polypharmacy (IGRIMUP): Position statement and 10 recommendations for action. *Drugs & Aging, 35*(7), 575–587. doi:10.100740266-018-0554-2 PMID:30006810

McLean, A. J., & Le Couteur, D. G. (2004). Aging biology and geriatric clinical pharmacology. *Pharmacological Reviews, 56*(2), 163–184. doi:10.1124/pr.56.2.4 PMID:15169926

Murlow, C. D., Aguilar, C., Endicott, J. E., Tuley, M. R., Velez, R., & Charlip, W. S. (1990). Quality of life changes and hearing impairment. *Annals of Internal Medicine, 113*(3), 188–194. doi:10.7326/0003-4819-113-3-188 PMID:2197909

Nejad, A. G., & Pouya, F. (2004). False beliefs and medication non-compliance in psychiatric patients. *Neuroscience Journal, 9*(2), 124–128. PMID:23377366

Nozaki, I., Kuriyama, M., Manyepa, P., Zyambo, M. K., Kakimoto, K., & Bärnighausen, T. (2013). False beliefs about ART effectiveness, side effects and the consequences of non-retention and non-adherence among ART patients in Livingstone, Zambia. *AIDS and Behavior, 17,* 122–126. doi:10.100710461-012-0221-2 PMID:22714115

Osterberg, L., & Blaschke, T. (2005). Adherence to medication. *The New England Journal of Medicine, 353*(5), 487–497. doi:10.1056/NEJMra050100 PMID:16079372

Ownby, R. L., Hertzog, C., Crocco, E., & Duara, R. (2006). Factors related to medication adherence in memory disorder clinic patients. *Aging & Mental Health, 10*(4), 378–385. doi:10.1080/13607860500410011 PMID:16798630

Patel, S., & Krishnaswami, A. (2015). *The role of pharmacists in the care of older adults with multiple chronic conditions in a multidisciplinary, team-based setting.* Academic Press.

Rana, A. K. M. M., Kabir, Z. N., Lundborg, C. S., & Wahlin, A. (2010). Health Education Improves Both Arthritis-related Illness and Self-rated Health: An Intervention Study Among Older People in Rural Bangladesh. *Public Health, 124*(12), 705–712. doi:10.1016/j.puhe.2010.07.005 PMID:21056439

Rossi, S. (2018). *AMH Aged Care companion.* Adelaide: Australian Medicines Handbook Pty Ltd. Available at www.amh.net.au

Sabaté, E., & Sabaté, E. (Eds.). (2003). *Adherence to long-term therapies: evidence for action.* World Health Organization.

Shruthi, R., Jyothi, R., Pundarikaksha, H. P., Nagesh, G. N., & Tushar, T. J. (2016). A study of medication compliance in geriatric patients with chronic illnesses at a tertiary care hospital. *Journal of Clinical and Diagnostic Research: JCDR, 10*(12), FC40. doi:10.7860/JCDR/2016/21908.9088 PMID:28208878

Son, Y. J., & Won, M. H. (2017). Depression and medication adherence among older Korean patients with hypertension: Mediating role of self-efficacy. *International Journal of Nursing Practice, 23*(3), e12525. doi:10.1111/ijn.12525 PMID:28194846

Southworth, E., & Parsi, K. (2018). How Should a Physician Counsel a Vegan Patient With IBD Who Might Benefit From Supplements? *AMA Journal of Ethics, 20*(11), 1025–1032. doi:10.1001/amajethics.2018.1025 PMID:30499430

Starfield, B., Lemke, K. W., Herbert, R., Pavlovich, W. D., & Anderson, G. (2005). Comorbidity and the use of primary care and specialist care in the elderly. *Annals of Family Medicine, 3*(3), 215–222. doi:10.1370/afm.307 PMID:15928224

Stephens, S. D., Callaghan, D. E., Hogan, S., Meredith, R., Rayment, A., & Davis, A. C. (1990). Hearing disability in people aged 50-65: Effectiveness and acceptability of rehabilitative intervention. *British Medical Journal, 300*(6723), 508–511. doi:10.1136/bmj.300.6723.508 PMID:2107929

Street, R. L. Jr, Gordon, H. S., Ward, M. M., Krupat, E., & Kravitz, R. L. (2005). Patient participation in medical consultations: Why some patients are more involved than others. *Medical Care, 43*(10), 960–969. doi:10.1097/01.mlr.0000178172.40344.70 PMID:16166865

Tan, C. S. (2020). The need of patient education to improve medication adherence among hypertensive patients. *Malaysian Journal of Pharmacy, 6*(1), 1–5. doi:10.52494/MOEL1486

Tsay, A. J. (2018). The internet, ethics, and false beliefs in health care. *AMA Journal of Ethics, 20*(11), 1003–1006. doi:10.1001/amajethics.2018.1003

Turana, Y., Tengkawan, J., Chia, Y. C., Shin, J., Chen, C. H., Park, S., Tsoi, K., Buranakitjaroen, P., Soenarta, A. A., Siddique, S., Cheng, H.-M., Tay, J. C., Teo, B. W., Wang, T.-D., & Kario, K. (2021). Mental health problems and hypertension in the elderly: Review from the HOPE Asia Network. *Journal of Clinical Hypertension, 23*(3), 504–512. doi:10.1111/jch.14121 PMID:33283971

Vankova, H., Holmerova, I., & Volicer, L. (2021). Geriatric depression and inappropriate medication: Benefits of interprofessional team cooperation in nursing homes. *International Journal of Environmental Research and Public Health, 18*(23), 12438. doi:10.3390/ijerph182312438 PMID:34886164

Wing, R. R., Phelan, S., & Tate, D. (2002). The role of adherence in mediating the relationship between depression and health outcomes. *Journal of Psychosomatic Research, 53*(4), 877–881. doi:10.1016/S0022-3999(02)00315-X PMID:12377297

World Health Organization. (2017, December 12). *Mental health of older adults.* WHO.

Chapter 6

Multimorbidity Case Studies in Dementia Patients:
Epilepsy, Diabetes, and Cardiovascular Disease

Aikaterini Christogianni
Loughborough University, UK

Suhaiza Hanim Suroya
Loughborough University, UK

EXECUTIVE SUMMARY

Co-/multi-morbidities are prevalent in the elderly. Some noteworthy examples include the elderly with dementia, for example, elderly with Alzheimer's disease, Parkinson's disease dementia and vascular dementia diagnoses. Based on high prevalence rates, the elderly with dementia is likely to experience more than one disease. Usual co-/multi-morbidities in the elderly with dementia are epilepsy, diabetes, and cardiovascular diseases. For this reason, healthcare providers are tremendously challenged with demands for treatment and therapy plans to improve the quality of life and overall well-being of the elderly and their families. This Chapter discusses these co-/multi-morbidities and aims to inspire the translation of this knowledge into specialised services and therapy plans for the elderly.

DOI: 10.4018/978-1-6684-2354-7.ch006

INTRODUCTION

Cognitive impairment is common in ~ 10-20% of the elderly population and a world public health concern (Etgen et al., 2010). Even though this health problem is transitioning from normal ageing cognitive processes to mild cognitive deficits, it could be benign and remain mild or lead to severe dementia (Lee et al., 2008). Therefore, outpatient clinics, hospitals, and primary care units evaluate the symptom complaints with extensive screening methods to differentiate between demented and non-demented patients. Healthcare systems worldwide have increased their detection methodologies to provide the necessary care for the elderly with dementia (Borson & Chodosh, 2014). Thus, many care plans and assistance are available for the patients and their families. Although there is a radical change and improvement in how health care policies favour early dementia detection and care plans, healthcare systems may be overwhelmed when the elderly with dementia have additional health problems that require attention, therapy, and support.

The healthcare systems might experience limitations related to the knowledge, skill sets, clinical system resources, and barriers to understanding that an elder with dementia might have another medical condition (Borson & Chodosh, 2014). It is interesting to evaluate how professionals and health systems face such complex challenges and provide the right treatment plans for the patients (Borson & Chodosh, 2014). For this reason, it has been suggested that redesigning and retraining clinical staff members may organise comprehensive care which can be tailored to the individual patient (Borson & Chodosh, 2014). The management strategies ought to include decision-making curriculums in treatment plans to associate co-/multi-morbidities and medications with patient health outcomes progress and sensitivity to the adverse effects of medications (Hommet et al., 2008).

Therefore, the purpose of the Chapter is to identify the diagnosis, monitoring, and treatment challenges of elderly with dementia when they are challenged with more than one disease/diagnosis; and to discuss the long-term management issues in healthcare systems.

BACKGROUND

Healthcare systems constitute the financial and organisational planning of care distribution. They aim to improve health efficiently and effectively according to patients' needs and available resources. The healthcare systems, such as organisations, institutions, public and private hospitals, primary and secondary health units, including medical doctors, nurses, and clinical staff, require a solid infrastructure to function correctly, for example, supplies of medical equipment, medication, and enough funding resources to assist with patients' medical conditions (Demirkan, 2013). Healthcare should provide equitable access to care and support for the elderly population and prioritise treatment according to the case (Demirkan, 2013).

Dementia is one of the most significant global health challenges in the ageing population (Livingston et al., 2017). Even though research has shown that some life factors may influence and predict the presence of dementia, the healthcare systems' priority is to delay the progression of the disease (Livingston et al., 2017). Most people who visit healthcare providers exhibit mild cognitive impairment with manageable symptom manifestations. However, whether the intervention is pharmacological, psychological, environmental, or social, it cannot cure the disease. The older the patients get, the higher the chance of co-/multi-morbidities appearing (Livingston et al., 2017).

Epilepsy is a chronic neurological disease that is manifested with recurrent and unpredictable seizure episodes due to abnormal neuronal activity in the brain (Moshé et al., 2015). The disease causes a loss of autonomy daily with consequences on a cognitive, psychological, and social level (Moshé et al., 2015). The burden increases when epileptic patients face more diseases/illnesses. For example, epileptic patients with dementia might struggle with both diseases' clinical signs and symptoms. Patients with dementia are more likely to experience seizures or epilepsy than patients without dementia (Sherzai et al., 2014). Also, older people with dementia are frequently hospitalised with seizures (Sherzai et al., 2014). As these patients grow older essential risk factors may increase the likelihood of the seizures because of stenosis or thrombosis of the blood vessels in the brain that cause cerebrovascular disease (Liu et al., 2016).

Having epilepsy may cause hospital readmissions, prolonged hospital stays, higher readmission rates, multiple transfers between hospitals, and in-hospital mortality rates, especially when there are co-/multi-morbidities. The elderly with epilepsy may be challenged with conditions such as septicemia, delirium, urinary tract infections, and aspiration pneumonitis, especially when they have a dementia diagnosis (Lehrer et al., 2021). Although emergency and surgical treatments are frequent, healthcare professionals, epilepsy specialists, and general neurologists might be challenged with time barriers and limitations in their resources to respond to the patients' needs (Moshé et al., 2015).

In diabetes, patients are in danger of failing in body organ functions, such as eye problems, kidney disease, nerve damage, heart disease, etc. (Mellitus, 2005). Diabetes mellitus (DM) is a metabolic disease characterised by chronic hyperglycemia because of impaired insulin secretion in the pancreatic beta cells (Mellitus, 2005). An endocrine hormone, amylin, is implicated in neuronal decay in people with diabetes, which could be why these patients might develop Parkinson's disease later (Miller, 2022). Elderly with diabetes are at high-risk mortality rates because of complications with organ failure, hypercholesterolemia, hypertension and deficits in the function of plasma glucose and Hgb A1C values (Meneilly & Tessier, 2001). These patients might be challenged when they experience co-/multi-morbidities. For example, patients who experience diabetes and Parkinson's disease are frequently challenged with cardiovascular, genitourinary, gastrointestinal and respiratory dysfunction (Borghammer et al., 2017).

Healthcare professionals and clinicians are often challenged with elderly with diabetes because they may be underweight or overweight, have poor food intake, and suffer from several cognitive and psychological symptoms such as confusion, concentration issues and mood changes (Meneilly & Tessier, 2001). The elderly with diabetes are more impacted than younger people with this disease and they are more likely to receive multiple medications and medical attention. The diabetes-related complications in the elderly could be hard to manage in healthcare; for example, complications may involve the clinical signs and symptoms of diabetic neuropathic cachexia, diabetic amyotrophy and malignant otitis externa, which are mainly characterised by painful peripheral neuropathy and infections (Meneilly & Tessier, 2001). Although the clinicians provide medical care to the elder with diabetes, the patients can never be cured, but their symptoms can be less intensive (Meneilly & Tessier, 2001).

The elderly with cardiovascular diseases might be challenged with high treatment burdens and body functional difficulties, impacting life expectancy and increased use of health services. As people grow old, the collagen in their arterial walls increases and the elastin in the central arteries becomes less (Jackson & Wenger, 2011). As a result, the decreased vascular compliance and elasticity may exhibit increased systolic and decreased diastolic blood pressure (Jackson & Wenger, 2011). The elderly might be challenged with worsening of their cardiovascular activity, and thus, they may benefit from care plans arranged by the healthcare. In the case of multimorbidity, for example, when patients suffer from dementia, the healthcare systems might benefit from diagnosing long-term health conditions associated with heart diseases on time; and defining additional physical or mental health impairments that reduce the quality of life in the elderly (Jackson & Wenger, 2011).

In a nutshell, the elderly with co-/multi-morbidities might be challenged with the difficulty of their complex symptoms, the physical and mental health conditions that might define the level of care and support in healthcare. Healthcare systems may face difficulties managing all the symptoms and providing treatments and additional services. Healthcare might be challenged with being continuously alerted to the patients' needs and making decisions about which needs are a priority for treatment and which needs are not a priority to be treated later (Jackson & Wenger, 2011). As a result, managing an elder's health conditions might require time and effort to develop guidance and individualised care plans. Encouraging family members, caregivers, and patients to identify what is important to them may reduce symptom burden and the risk of prolonged hospitalisations. Therefore, reviewing the progression of the patients' diseases might be one good strategy to improve their quality of life (Jackson & Wenger, 2011).

CASE STUDIES IN ELDERLY WITH DEMENTIA

Case Study 1: Alzheimer's Disease and Epilepsy

Alzheimer's disease (AD) is the most frequent cause of dementia worldwide, with more than 11% of the elderly population affected (Alzheimer's Association, 2022a). Neuroimaging brain studies have indicated reduced brain weight, cortical atrophy, ventricular enlargement (DeCarli et al., 1990), neurofibrillary tangles, and senile plaques in AD patients (DeCarli, 2001; Selkoe, 1994). The clinical manifestation of this brain disruption is severe and exhibits debilitating cognitive dysfunction, often accompanied by psychiatric disturbances and various abnormal behaviours, such as delirium, depression, anxiety, hallucinations, and delusions (National Health Service, 2021).

AD is mainly characterised by disruption of the brain's neuronal function that causes gradual progressive deterioration of the cognitive functions and affects behaviour and mental health. One of the most critical risk factors in AD is age; therefore, care homes and health clinics might benefit from early detection assessments. The diagnosis is based on patient and family claims about clinical signs and symptoms; for example, the patient might show memory loss for recent conversations, apathy during social interactions and confusion while they are in familiar surroundings, e.g., their home. Clinical criteria, which are the clinicians' and the neurologists' guides for the AD diagnosis, are included in the Diagnostic and Statistical Manual of Mental Disorders (DSM-5TR) guide (American Psychiatric Association, 2022). Also, the results from neuropsychological testing complete the puzzle of the patients' cognitive impairment signs and provide information about their brain neurological issues. However, computed tomography (CT), magnetic resonance imaging techniques (MRI), positron emission tomography, single-photon emission, and functional MRI assist in clinical diagnosis. These are necessary neuroimaging assessments for the AD diagnosis because they detect structural and pathological changes in the brain. The accurate AD diagnosis depends on the disease stage and the reliability of the diagnostic criteria.

The next step is monitoring the patients and ensuring their safety as they progress to severe cognitive deterioration. Monitoring methods are essential to establish the well-being of the patients, for example, wireless health care services that include in-home health monitoring such as global positioning systems (GPS), geographic information systems, radio frequency identification devices and biosensors, e.g., blood pressure monitors (Lin et al., 2006). Even though each stage of dementia challenges healthcare providers with emergency visits in hospitals, inaccurate diagnosis, aetiology and severity of the symptoms, the monitoring methods produce tracing information packages for families, caregivers, health search teams and ambulances that are essential for the safety of these patients (Lin et al., 2006).

In epilepsy, the clinical context of the seizures can be described with electroencephalogram (EEG), diffusion tensor imaging (DTI), CT and MRI testing procedures (Cendes et al., 2016). There is evidence of epileptogenic brain lesions that differentiate in mesial temporal lobe and neocortical lesions (Cendes et al., 2016). Furthermore, there is evidence of hippocampal and anterior temporal lobe atrophy indications in the brain (Cendes et al., 2016). It is prevalent to develop epilepsy in AD and share neuropathological features between the two diseases, e.g., amyloid plaques and tau neurofibrils (Horváth et al., 2018). Animal models that presented high Amyloid β-proteins in the brain were associated with subclinical epileptiform even in the absence of neuronal loss, which might show that Amyloid β-proteins may be neurotoxic in both dementia and epilepsy (Johnson et al., 2020). It is important to note that the seizures may create vasovagal or cardiogenic syncope and paroxysmal movement disorders (Shih et al., 2018).

Epilepsy monitoring is essential to track the seizures. EEG and MRI are frequently used to collect information about the seizures and plan future surgeries if needed (Shih et al., 2018). Specialised epilepsy nurses are trained in caring for epilepsy patients during the seizures. They may recognise any dangerous or unsafe situations and complications during the epileptic episodes (Shih et al., 2018). Severe epilepsy may be linked to severely impaired cognition (Caramelli & Castro, 2005). The prognosis of cognitive performance, especially in language functions, the autonomy reduction, and the injury risk during the seizures, are of specific interest in the clinical management strategies. In addition, nonepileptic psychogenic events such as depression and anxiety are treated with psychotherapy or other psychological therapies (Shih et al., 2018). Although, it is prevalent for patients with epilepsy to take antidepressant medications, such as selective serotonin reuptake inhibitors (SSRIs) (Albano et al., 2006).

Patients with epilepsy suffer from a plethora of symptoms which are manifested with seizures, confusion, stiff muscles, uncontrollable movements that might affect the bowel movement, and loss of awareness of their surroundings (Devinsky, 2004). These symptoms may also cause psychological burdens, such as depression, anxiety, suicidal thoughts, and fear of what might happen during the seizures (Devinsky, 2004). Cognitive dysfunction is prevalent in individuals with epilepsy, such as memory, attention, and information processing difficulties that may impact dramatically everyday functioning (Devinsky, 2004; Holmes, 2015). Furthermore, AD and epilepsy share common cognitive symptoms such as memory, attention, language, and learning difficulties, which complicate the treatment management in the elderly (Van Rijckevorsel, 2006). The high rates of cognitive difficulties may underly affect communication issues between the elderly and families, carers, and healthcare providers. Having AD is one significant risk factor of epilepsy for the elderly. However, the diagnosis of either one of the medical conditions might be difficult in healthcare because of non-specific clinical signs that the elderly present, especially when these are short-term and they seem common symptoms in elder people, for example, regular falls, memory disturbances and motor deficits (Devinsky, 2004; S. K. Lee, 2019).

Having AD and epilepsy may severely foreshadow and confuse clinical care. It may also pose severe implications in disease care and management because of the overlapping nature of the symptoms. There are many more challenges when the health care providers stretch the already overburdened resources to treat AD and epilepsy together (Savva & Stephan, 2010). Patients with epilepsy are challenged by a lack of medical staff availability, lack of accessibility to services and health care, primarily in low-income countries (Mahendran et al., 2017). Therefore, the clinical staff members may train in how crucial it is to ascertain patient-specific requirements in utilising general and emergency services to ensure the well-being and safety of these patients (Keenan et al., 2014; Sampson et al., 2009). Clinical staff members may be more alert to the elderly falling and having accidents, especially when they do not witness such events. Also, understanding the myoclonic jerks and confusion of the patients who might indicate the presence of a seizure could be essential in preventing accidents in the elderly. Furthermore, understanding the adverse effects of medications and multi-treatments that may create pharmacokinetic characteristics could be essential in symptom management. Since severe cognitive deficits might be present in these individuals, understanding the patients' needs is necessary to lead a less stressful life.

Case Study 2: Parkinson's Disease and Diabetes Mellitus

Parkinson's disease is a progressive chronic neurodegenerative disorder that affects 2% of the elderly above 65 years, with ~65% experiencing Parkinson's disease dementia (PDD) (Alzheimer's Association, 2022b). The disease affects the brain region that controls body movements by exhibiting early signs of tremors, shakiness, muscle stiffness, rigidity, mental health issues, and cognitive impairments, for example, thinking, reasoning, confusion, memory, and concentration problems. PDD patients have DM in 80% of the cases when they encounter risk factors such as low-density lipoprotein cholesterol that causes plaque inside arteries (Wang et al.,

2020). PDD and DM are at high risk of appearing together and exhibiting vascular, inflammatory, and metabolic issues (Wang et al., 2020), with overlapping symptoms the memory and thinking impairments. These may worsen when the patients are unable to perform daily tasks.

It is imperative that PDD is recognised and accurately diagnosed to have appropriate and correct patient treatments. The clinical diagnosis of PDD is based on cognitive impairment characteristics according to the DSM-5-TR (American Psychiatric Association, 2022) and is different from other dementias, for example, AD (Poewe et al., 2008). However, the PDD diagnosis requires that the cognitive impairment appears after the motor symptoms manifest. During diagnostic assessments, the cognitive deficits that seem to dominate are problems in attention, memory, language and visuospatial difficulties (Poewe et al., 2008). This being said, the diagnostic evaluation is rather generic, referring to cognitive and motor slowing, executive dysfunction, and impairment in memory retrieval. Nevertheless, demographic evaluations of people diagnosed with PDD have concluded that key risk factors in developing PDD are the age, the severity of the Parkinson's symptoms and the disease duration (Poewe et al., 2008).

Healthcare professionals, clinicians, commissioners and providers follow healthcare guidelines that recommend the pharmacological and non-pharmacological management of motor and cognitive symptoms in patients with PDD in all age groups. Cholinesterase inhibitors and rivastigmine might assist with the dementia symptoms (Poewe et al., 2008). Additional therapy plans might include cognitive remediation therapy and behavioural management in the early stages of PDD as long as the elderly can cope with engaging during the therapy sessions.

As soon as elderly are diagnosed with dementia, their health issues and life expectancy seem to deteriorate. For example, pre-existing diabetes in PDD may be associated with increased disability levels and death rates (de Pablo-Fernández et al., 2021). When diabetes is diagnosed later in life after receiving the Parkinson's disease diagnosis it may contribute to faster illness and reduced survival rates (de Pablo-Fernández et al., 2021). In addition, when PDD patients are diagnosed with DM, they are likely to experience frequent falls, wheelchair dependence, and care home admission, especially when they are elderly, which might threaten their overall health outcomes. The elderly with DM may develop cardiovascular issues, glucose toxicity, changes in insulin metabolism and inflammation, which might be life-threatening because of ageing. Therefore, novel medicinal strategies are necessary to reduce PDD development in people with DM (Ninomiya, 2014).

The pathophysiology of cognitive impairment in DM includes deficiencies in insulin signalling, autonomic function, neuroinflammatory pathways, and mitochondrial metabolism (Meneilly & Tessier, 2001). Even though several promising therapies for the treatment of DM have been identified in preclinical studies, they still remain to be proven in clinical interventions. The biggest concern is that elderly are usually unaware of having DM (Meneilly & Tessier, 2001). Diabetic symptoms such as excessive thirst might be confused with other overlapping illnesses or normal ageing (Meneilly & Tessier, 2001).

The challenge in healthcare systems in PDD and DM is the administration of multiple medications (polypharmacy), which is associated with adverse outcomes such as mortality, falls, and hospitalisations (Masnoon et al., 2017). Results of inappropriate prescribing may lead to an increased risk of overmedicating and end up in nursing/care homes. Additional issues cannot be controlled when the elderly are challenged with many medical conditions, for example, substance abuse and alcoholism (Hendrie et al., 2013). Thus, prolonged hospitalisations are expected in such cases. Moreover, the progression and cost of treatments, examination results, medicines, discharge plans and follow-up appointments might be significantly affected. In addition, understanding that the elderly may have many medical conditions could be a struggle in PDD with DM. Continuous care in later stages in life might be necessary to control blood sugar daily and live a safe life. Medical professionals and clinicians might pay attention to these complex health problems in the elderly, organise care, build patient safety in the hospital, emergency rooms, and care homes.

The elderly who are mentally ill and have DM and PDD may confound healthcare and self-care management. Care pathways are needed in medical and mental health settings. The creation of care platforms and critical steps to integrate the care pathways for the elderly might provide guidance and recognise each condition accurately. Managing the problematic issues of hypoglycaemia in PDD patients who have DM might be the most important thing, along with acknowledging the diabetic complications in patients who cannot communicate their needs to their caregivers due to dementia. Creating awareness could be important for families/ caregivers and healthcare systems treating and caring for PDD patients. In terms of mental health issues, for example, depression, anxiety, psychosis and apathy, clinicians and health care providers might follow courses and seminars on how the symptoms worsen when the patients cannot perform daily tasks. These symptoms may reveal the severity of PDD and DM.

Case Study 3: Vascular Dementia and Cardiovascular Disease

Vascular dementia (VD) is the second most common dementia in the elderly population, with prevalence rates of 15% in dementia cases and ~2.7% in the elderly population (Hébert & Brayne, 1995; Román, 2003). It results from ischemic haemorrhagic brain episodes because of either cardiovascular disease (CD) or cerebrovascular disease (Hébert & Brayne, 1995; Román, 2003). In CD, hypertension in the brain creates the primary lesions and strokes, which increase the risk of memory problems, executive function deficits, disorganised thoughts, behaviours, and emotions (Román, 2003). The condition assumes that stroke occurs first, and cognitive impairment comes post-stroke. However, there are some VD types, such as stroke-related, post-stroke, single-infarct and multi-infarct, and subcortical dementia, depending on how narrow, thick, and stiff the blood vessels are when blood clots block them. Research has shown that cardiovascular conditions, e.g., myocardial infarction, peripheral artery disease, coronary atherosclerosis, and even coronary bypass surgery or carotid endarterectomy, could cause vascular dementia (Paciaroni & Bogousslavsky, 2013). The common symptoms of VD and CD are problems in executive functions, e.g., word-finding difficulties, misplacing things, and perceptual speed depending on the patient (Leritz et al., 2011).

The diagnosis of VD is determined by blood vessel abnormalities caused by strokes, tumours, or brain traumatic injuries. The brain imaging procedures which are recommended by healthcare systems worldwide are brain scans such as MRI and CT scans. The MRI technology uses a magnetic field and radio waves that produce detailed brain images (Van Straaten et al., 2004). The MRI is one of the most preferred methods to identify strokes and blood vessel abnormalities in the brain that are strong indicators of dementia (Van Straaten et al., 2004). The CT scan uses X-rays and translates them into detailed cross-sectional images of the brain. (Van Straaten et al., 2004) The CT scan identifies brain regions that show shrinkage; it detects areas that have been affected by stroke and changes in the blood vessels that might result from any traumatic brain injury. Additionally, to the brain scans, neuropsychological tests such as language, memory, and problem-solving skills testing complete the diagnosis puzzle and contribute to the neurological reports and diagnosis.

Monitoring the cerebrovascular disease that causes vascular dementia focuses on investigating and controlling the risk parameters that might contribute to worsening symptoms. The risk factors that constitute adverse health outcomes in vascular dementia might be reductions in cholesterol and increases in blood sugar. Depending on the case, the treatment plans focus on preventing disease decline due to pathognomonic issues. In addition, the healthcare systems coordinate care plans, for example, which services to use, manage all co-/multi-morbidities, involve families and caregivers in the decision making, and plan according to patients' needs (National Institute for Health and Care Excelllence, 2018).

Old and elderly patients with CD exhibit reduced cardiac output and abnormalities of systemic vascular function because of their age (Cohen et al., 2009). The more advanced people are in age, the higher the probability that the body's homeostatic functions maintain the hemodynamic regulation in the body; as a result, the blood perfusion in the brain is significantly affected (Cohen et al., 2009). The proximal aorta, part of the body's largest artery, stiffens as people age due to hypertension, causing heart failure and brain damage (de Roos et al., 2017; Jackson & Wenger, 2011). A cardiac MRI scan is the critical assessment in CD, for example, coronary heart disease, congenital heart disease, inherited heart conditions, heart valve failure, cardiac and systemic vascular abnormalities, and tumours inside and around the heart. After diagnosis, monitoring occurs with routine checks on the cardiovascular condition, often with scheduled medical appointments. Also, mapping the disease progression and medication to avoid heart attacks, heart surgery, operations, or procedures.

Small vessel disease and strokes indicate reduced blood supply to the brain, resulting in either one of the medical conditions (Jackson & Wenger, 2011). Therefore, it is common for the elderly to have VD and CD, especially the elderly with hypertension and the ones who follow lifestyles that increase the risk factors to receive any of the two diagnoses. Unfortunately, the medical professionals and clinical staff may misinterpret cognitive symptoms as normal ageing and underdiagnose the patients' actual conditions (Leritz et al., 2011). Even though the healthcare systems might administer care, this may be inadequate, unable to provide correct treatments to meet the patients' needs, thus creating complications from unnecessary treatment therapies. Consequently, improvement of the knowledge and clinical practice might be necessary. Screening and diagnosing procedures might improve with meticulous examinations of brain activity and neuropsychological testing. In addition, spreading the awareness about co-/multi-morbidities in vascular dementia might assist in detecting even subtle cognitive changes and have a critical impact on patient care. Therefore, it is important to understand the complications of VD and CD when they occur together and provide quality improvement training for medical professionals about these diseases.

The elderly with VD and CD might require regular reassessments to establish a clear clinical picture during the progression of both diseases. Their cognitive symptoms might affect how they communicate their wishes and needs to healthcare staff, family members, and caregivers. During the experience of severe symptoms, there is no decisional capacity especially regarding risks; therefore, care is essential. Elderly with VD and CD are not able to remember taking their medication, eating, and drinking nutritious food, being careful while walking to avoid falls and accidents indoors and outdoors, in case of an emergency such as a fire in their residence, using an emergency exit, due to poor or lack of judgment and understanding a situation. Removing serious harms, e.g., items, or objects that are placedclose to the patients might improve their quality of life and keep them safe. They should not be left alone in a residence/care home but always wear alert bracelets with contact details. These patients are highly vulnerable, and may not be able to show that they have experienced a heart attack or other heart failure symptoms; as a result, they are in danger of high mortality rates. The healthcare staff members ought to be meticulously trained in these medical conditions and offer their support, make decisions in the best interest of the patients, and use technological approaches to always locate patients in their surroundings and ensure regular medication intake according to prescription.

SOLUTIONS AND RECOMMENDATIONS

More than 44 million people have dementia worldwide, with the highest rates being reported in people up to 95 years of age, and the costs to treat those patients yearly increase (Meads et al., 2020; O'Shea & O'Reilly, 2000; Xu et al., 2017). For example, in the last few decades in the UK, the cost to treat people with dementia in healthcare has surpassed £26 billion per year and is expected to rise to £40 billion per year by 2040 (Meads et al., 2020). It is also estimated that in developed countries, the cost of each dementia patient in healthcare corresponds to more than £8000 per year, which is relatively high, especially for families which are required to pay, and they do not have insurances to cover these expenses (O'Shea & O'Reilly, 2000). Nonetheless, part of the increases in care costs is due to the neuropsychiatric and behavioural issues dementia patients have while at hospitals, care homes, emergency rooms and in their own homes (Meads et al., 2020). These issues are crucial to monitor for prevention purposes for the reason that dementia patients may experience agitation, frustration, anger, delusions, begin to shout and attack their families and caregivers, and even harm themselves or whoever is around them (Meads et al., 2020). Therefore the dementia care costs may rise due to staff training, such as psychiatric and behavioural courses, which are estimated to be ~£450 per carer per training session depending on the country (Meads et al., 2020).

However, in complex healthcare systems and countries suffering from financial difficulties, the cost burden to treat dementia patients is different. For example, there might be professional and non-professional carers for dementia patients, from which the ones who do not have or do not require nursing training provide zero costs in healthcare systems (e.g. in underdeveloped countries) (Eggenberger et al., 2013). In addition, the care costs might be less for patients with dementia that live at home and their families care for them (Michalowsky et al., 2019; O'Shea & O'Reilly, 2000). Furthermore, the cost burden depends on the type of therapy and treatment each patient follows. For example, primary, secondary and medical treatments, such as acetylcholinesterase inhibitors, memantine, and antipsychotic drugs, are cost-effective in comparison to non-pharmacological interventions, such as psychosocial interventions, which might be costly and do no improve the dementia symptoms (Knapp et al., 2013; O'Shea & O'Reilly, 2000).

Although 5 to 8% of the elderly population are challenged with dementia symptoms that require attention from healthcare, there are still public and private resources and support services to assist with the dementia symptoms (O'Shea & O'Reilly, 2000). However, in some countries, such as Ireland, these services remain underdeveloped and limited, and the care homes constitute only 1% of the care facilities and costs (O'Shea & O'Reilly, 2000). Therefore, in such cases, the care and financial burdens are natural to stay with the families (O'Shea & O'Reilly, 2000).

One of the solutions already proposed in healthcare is the implementation of the Dementia Care Management programs, which manage chronic diseases in dementia, such as co-/multi-morbidities (Michalowsky et al., 2019). In these training and learning programs, the care staff members learn to follow medical and care guidelines about treatment and therapy options for dementia (Michalowsky et al., 2019). The clinical training includes care guidelines before the patients show signs that they cannot function independently, and it is necessary for them to move into care homes (Michalowsky et al., 2019). Families may benefit from the knowledge of the nurses and clinicians who have completed management training programs and learn how to support their patients at home. As a result, the families may be involved in the patient care and keep their patients committed to the treatment processes. This is particularly important in countries where care homes are limited, and the caregivers who assist the patients at home are not adequately trained (Xu et al., 2017).

Healthcare is restricted by specific challenges relating to the industrial factors that can help high-impact countries handle these issues. The proportion of elderly patients diagnosed with co-/multi-morbidities is high, and this number has the potential to remarkably go higher in some decades. However, many community care services in low-income countries suffer from little equipment and undereducated clinical staff members, which might pose fewer benefits in the care and support the elderly over the years. Undoubtedly, all clinical specialists require unique skill sets which can enable them to assist the elderly needs. The healthcare systems require the training of the workforce, especially the medical doctors and nurses who are responsible for screening, diagnosis, monitoring, and treatment interventions. In addition, the healthcare systems may pay special attention to the cultural and linguistic competence of the clinical staff members because these parameters may affect how they understand the patients' concerns, thoughts, actions, beliefs, and values about their health (Anderson et al., 2003). The healthcare providers may be ambitious about their preventive care for the elderly and discuss the risk factors, the management and prevention techniques with families and caregivers. Also, individualising and tailoring the health, medical, social, and support care according to the case could be beneficial to the patient's own goals and priorities. Moreover, the healthcare systems might include guidance and strategies for the family members and caregivers to know what to expect and to prepare when making decisions for their loved ones while they are at the hospital, care home, or their own home and they are following treatments or therapeutic interventions.

Healthcare may organise detailed discharge plans and reports about the course and cost of treatment, examination results, medicines, agreements with home care and follow-up appointments to avoid high rates of primary care consultations, prescriptions, and hospitalisations (Schjødt et al., 2022). Another critical factor to consider is that it would be optimal to provide this information to the patients and their families, to increase the patient self-care awareness, and build their safety and quality of life satisfaction indoors and in care homes. Furthermore, developing research to occupy and integrate information technology needs might increase security and safety in the elderly. The vital clinical and medical patient details, such as medical records, pharmacy, hospital, clinic visits and medical history, should be easily accessible to doctors, medical workers, and carers, with applications or devices that continuously monitor the patients (Ganesan & Vijaya Chamundeeswari, 2020). Artificial intelligence and machine learning may involve stakeholder values and investments to develop software applications for dementia patients to improve quality of life, cost, expenditures, social activities and mental health in the elderly with co-/multi-morbidities (Teipel et al., 2016).

The incorporated healthcare, allocating resources and planning care tailored to the elderly needs should be well planned and cater to any recurrent issues. Therefore, prescription and medication for co-/multi-morbidities such as cardiovascular and non-steroidal anti-inflammatory medication should be prescribed to patients cautiously after a detailed medical investigation (Delgado et al., 2020). Besides treatment plans, the improvement and integration of social workers in the healthcare systems might be a great asset (Ai & Carrigan, 2007) to meet the "high rates of emergency care, longer hospitalisations, increased frequency of falls, substance abuse and alcoholism where these groups require an integrated model of healthcare" (Hendrie et al., 2013).

FUTURE RESEARCH DIRECTIONS

Future research might focus on technological interventions that might improve the quality of life in the elderly with co-/multi- morbidities, especially those with psychiatric symptoms and social withdrawal (Livingston et al., 2017). Since psychological well-being might be impacted in people with dementia who have more than one disease/disorder, investigations into the positive factors that might ameliorate the negative impact of the symptoms could be necessary. Managing the neuropsychiatric symptoms might include investigations of mood changes, for example, depression, anxiety, psychosis, and behavioural changes such as agitation, aggression, and apathy. Moreover, creating decision-making plans about how patients might receive care and participate in decisions about their health, wishes, and needs might be essential to establish a sense of self-esteem and worthiness.

Further research might focus on pharmacological management of the severe symptoms and how to reduce brain damage and inflammation (Livingston et al., 2017). In addition, increasing the diagnostic rates, for example, early detection of pathogenic changes, might be effective for modifying treatments in dementia patients. Timely detection of co-/multi-morbidities might benefit the interventions and support the patients, families, and caregivers. Therefore, identifying the risk groups to exhibit dementia symptoms might be crucial and increase the quality of health received during medical, neuropsychological and neuropsychiatric testing.

More research would be beneficial in identifying the prevalence and incidence rates of co-/multi-morbidities that might affect the socioeconomic issues in families and healthcare systems. Moreover, multimorbidity reduces the quality of life and increases mortality rates and healthcare treatments in the elderly. Identifying the best validated neuropsychological tools in the elderly would assist in diagnosing cognitive impairments and differentiate those impairments from other diseases. Also, establish the treatment burden in healthcare and how medical training of the clinical staff member would benefit the elderly and their health issues.

CONCLUSION

This Chapter sought to describe some of the co-/multi-morbidities in the elderly with severe cognitive impairments and the healthcare systems issues. In AD, PDD and VD, the elderly are challenged with severe daily issues that affect their quality of life. The inability to communicate their needs and wishes poses a burden on families, caregivers, and healthcare systems that have to decide about the care and support of these patients. As difficult as it may seem, the healthcare staff members can organise the personalised care according to the case. However, to succeed in this endeavour, they ought to be clinically trained to an expert level. The elderly in hospitals or care homes might not be able to communicate when they experience medical symptoms. This is of particular importance as it may increase accidents and risks that might be life-threatening to the patients. In case of seizures, motor disability or heart failure, these patients will probably not be able to help themselves in time of need. Therefore, healthcare providers specialising in each condition may create safety and ensure that these patients receive their medication regularly and live good lives.

REFERENCES

Ai, A. L., & Carrigan, L. T. (2007). Social-strata-related cardiovascular health disparity and comorbidity in an aging society: Implications for professional care. *Health & Social Work*, *32*(2), 97–105. doi:10.1093/hsw/32.2.97 PMID:17571643

Albano, C., Cupello, A., Mainardi, P., Scarrone, S., & Favale, E. (2006). Successful treatment of epilepsy with serotonin reuptake inhibitors: Proposed mechanism. *Neurochemical Research*, *31*(4), 509–514. doi:10.100711064-006-9045-7 PMID:16758359

Alzheimer's Association. (2022a). *Facts and Figures*. Alzheimer's Association. https://www.alz.org/alzheimers-dementia/facts-figures

Alzheimer's Association. (2022b). *Parkinson's Disease Dementia*. Alzheimer's Association. https://www.alz.org/alzheimers-dementia/what-is-dementia/types-of-dementia/parkinson-s-disease-dementia

American Psychiatric Association. (2022). Diagnostic and Statistical Manual of Mental Disorders (DSM-5-TRTM) (Fifth Edit). APA

Anderson, L. M., Scrimshaw, S. C., Fullilove, M. T., Fielding, J. E., Normand, J., & Services, T. F. (2003). Culturally competent healthcare systems: A systematic review. *American Journal of Preventive Medicine*, *24*(3), 68–79. doi:10.1016/S0749-3797(02)00657-8 PMID:12668199

Borghammer, P., Knudsen, K., Fedorova, T. D., & Brooks, D. J. (2017). Imaging Parkinson's disease below the neck. *NPJ Parkinson's Disease*, *3*(1), 1–10. doi:10.103841531-017-0017-1 PMID:28649615

Borson, S., & Chodosh, J. (2014). Developing dementia-capable health care systems: A 12-step program. *Clinics in Geriatric Medicine*, *30*(3), 395–420. doi:10.1016/j.cger.2014.05.001 PMID:25037288

Caramelli, P., & Castro, L. H. M. (2005). Dementia associated with epilepsy. *International Psychogeriatrics*, *17*(s1), S195–S206. doi:10.1017/S1041610205002024 PMID:16240490

Cendes, F., Theodore, W. H., Brinkmann, B. H., Sulc, V., & Cascino, G. D. (2016). Neuroimaging of epilepsy. *Handbook of Clinical Neurology*, *136*, 985–1014. doi:10.1016/B978-0-444-53486-6.00051-X PMID:27430454

Cohen, R. A., Poppas, A., Forman, D. E., Hoth, K. F., Haley, A. P., Gunstad, J., Jefferson, A. L., Tate, D. F., Paul, R. H., Sweet, L. H., Ono, M., Jerskey, B. A., & Gerhard-Herman, M. (2009). Vascular and cognitive functions associated with cardiovascular disease in the elderly. *Journal of Clinical and Experimental Neuropsychology*, *31*(1), 96–110. doi:10.1080/13803390802014594 PMID:18608677

de Pablo-Fernández, E., Courtney, R., Rockliffe, A., Gentleman, S., Holton, J. L., & Warner, T. T. (2021). Faster disease progression in Parkinson's disease with type 2 diabetes is not associated with increased α-synuclein, tau, amyloid-β or vascular pathology. *Neuropathology and Applied Neurobiology*, *47*(7), 1080–1091. doi:10.1111/nan.12728 PMID:33969516

de Roos, A., van der Grond, J., Mitchell, G., & Westenberg, J. (2017). Magnetic resonance imaging of cardiovascular function and the brain: Is dementia a cardiovascular-driven disease? *Circulation*, *135*(22), 2178–2195. doi:10.1161/CIRCULATIONAHA.116.021978 PMID:28559496

DeCarli, C. (2001). The role of neuroimaging in dementia. *Clinics in Geriatric Medicine*, *17*(2), 255–279. doi:10.1016/S0749-0690(05)70068-9 PMID:11375135

DeCarli, C., Kaye, J. A., Horwitz, B., & Rapoport, S. I. (1990). Critical analysis of the use of computer-assisted transverse axial tomography to study human brain in aging and dementia of the Alzheimer type. *Neurology*, *40*(6), 872–883. doi:10.1212/WNL.40.6.872 PMID:2189080

Delgado, J., Bowman, K., & Clare, L. (2020). Potentially inappropriate prescribing in dementia: A state-of-the-art review since 2007. *BMJ Open*, *10*(1), e029172. doi:10.1136/bmjopen-2019-029172 PMID:31900263

Demirkan, H. (2013). A smart healthcare systems framework. *IT Professional*, *15*(5), 38–45. doi:10.1109/MITP.2013.35

Devinsky, O. (2004). Diagnosis and treatment of temporal lobe epilepsy. *Reviews in Neurological Diseases*, *1*(1), 2–9. PMID:16397445

Eggenberger, E., Heimerl, K., & Bennett, M. I. (2013). Communication skills training in dementia care: A systematic review of effectiveness, training content, and didactic methods in different care settings. *International Psychogeriatrics*, *25*(3), 345–358. doi:10.1017/S1041610212001664 PMID:23116547

Etgen, T., Sander, D., Huntgeburth, U., Poppert, H., Förstl, H., & Bickel, H. (2010). Physical activity and incident cognitive impairment in elderly persons: The INVADE study. *Archives of Internal Medicine*, *170*(2), 186–193. doi:10.1001/archinternmed.2009.498 PMID:20101014

Ganesan, R., & Vijaya Chamundeeswari, V. (2020). Composite algorithm for pervasive healthcare system–a solution to find optimized route for closest available health care facilities. *Multimedia Tools and Applications*, *79*(7), 5125–5148. doi:10.100711042-018-6136-9

Hébert, R., & Brayne, C. (1995). Epidemiology of vascular dementia. *Neuroepidemiology*, *14*(5), 240–257. doi:10.1159/000109800 PMID:7477666

Hendrie, H. C., Lindgren, D., Hay, D. P., Lane, K. A., Gao, S., Purnell, C., Munger, S., Smith, F., Dickens, J., Boustani, M. A., & Callahan, C. M. (2013). Comorbidity profile and healthcare utilization in elderly patients with serious mental illnesses. *The American Journal of Geriatric Psychiatry : Official Journal of the American Association for Geriatric Psychiatry*, *21*(12), 1267–1276. doi:10.1016/j.jagp.2013.01.056 PMID:24206938

Holmes, G. L. (2015). Cognitive impairment in epilepsy: The role of network abnormalities. *Epileptic Disorders*, *17*(2), 101–116. doi:10.1684/epd.2015.0739 PMID:25905906

Hommet, C., Mondon, K., Camus, V., De Toffol, B., & Constans, T. (2008). Epilepsy and dementia in the elderly. *Dementia and Geriatric Cognitive Disorders*, *25*(4), 293–300. doi:10.1159/000119103 PMID:18311076

Horváth, A., Szűcs, A., Hidasi, Z., Csukly, G., Barcs, G., & Kamondi, A. (2018). Prevalence, semiology, and risk factors of epilepsy in Alzheimer's disease: An ambulatory EEG study. *Journal of Alzheimer's Disease*, *63*(3), 1045–1054. doi:10.3233/JAD-170925 PMID:29710705

Jackson, C. F., & Wenger, N. K. (2011). Cardiovascular disease in the elderly. *Revista Española de Cardiología (English Ed.)*, *64*(8), 697–712. doi:10.1016/j.rec.2011.05.003 PMID:21723657

Johnson, E. C. B., Ho, K., Yu, G.-Q., Das, M., Sanchez, P. E., Djukic, B., Lopez, I., Yu, X., Gill, M., Zhang, W., Paz, J. T., Palop, J. J., & Mucke, L. (2020). Behavioral and neural network abnormalities in human APP transgenic mice resemble those of App knock-in mice and are modulated by familial Alzheimer's disease mutations but not by inhibition of BACE1. *Molecular Neurodegeneration*, *15*(1), 1–26. doi:10.118613024-020-00393-5 PMID:32921309

Keenan, T. D. L., Goldacre, R., & Goldacre, M. J. (2014). Associations between age-related macular degeneration, Alzheimer disease, and dementia: Record linkage study of hospital admissions. *JAMA Ophthalmology*, *132*(1), 63–68. doi:10.1001/jamaophthalmol.2013.5696 PMID:24232933

Knapp, M., Iemmi, V., & Romeo, R. (2013). Dementia care costs and outcomes: A systematic review. *International Journal of Geriatric Psychiatry, 28*(6), 551–561. doi:10.1002/gps.3864 PMID:22887331

Lee, J.-Y., Lee, D. W., Cho, S.-J., Na, D. L., Jeon, H. J., Kim, S.-K., Lee, Y. R., Youn, J.-H., Kwon, M., & Lee, J.-H. (2008). Brief screening for mild cognitive impairment in elderly outpatient clinic: Validation of the Korean version of the Montreal Cognitive Assessment. *Journal of Geriatric Psychiatry and Neurology, 21*(2), 104–110. doi:10.1177/0891988708316855 PMID:18474719

Lee, S. K. (2019). Epilepsy in the elderly: Treatment and consideration of comorbid diseases. *Journal of Epilepsy Research, 9*(1), 27–35. doi:10.14581/jer.19003 PMID:31482054

Lehrer, H., Lin, J.-Y., Kwon, C.-S., Agarwal, P., Mazumdar, M., & Jette, N. (2021). The co-occurrence of dementia in those with epilepsy is associated with 30-day readmission–A population-based study. *Epilepsy & Behavior, 122*, 108126. doi:10.1016/j.yebeh.2021.108126 PMID:34153638

Leritz, E. C., McGlinchey, R. E., Kellison, I., Rudolph, J. L., & Milberg, W. P. (2011). Cardiovascular disease risk factors and cognition in the elderly. *Current Cardiovascular Risk Reports, 5*(5), 407–412. doi:10.100712170-011-0189-x PMID:22199992

Lin, C.-C., Chiu, M.-J., Hsiao, C.-C., Lee, R.-G., & Tsai, Y.-S. (2006). Wireless health care service system for elderly with dementia. *IEEE Transactions on Information Technology in Biomedicine, 10*(4), 696–704. doi:10.1109/TITB.2006.874196 PMID:17044403

Liu, S., Yu, W., & Lü, Y. (2016). The causes of new-onset epilepsy and seizures in the elderly. *Neuropsychiatric Disease and Treatment, 12*, 1425. doi:10.2147/NDT.S107905 PMID:27382285

Livingston, G., Sommerlad, A., Orgeta, V., Costafreda, S. G., Huntley, J., Ames, D., Ballard, C., Banerjee, S., Burns, A., Cohen-Mansfield, J., Cooper, C., Fox, N., Gitlin, L. N., Howard, R., Kales, H. C., Larson, E. B., Ritchie, K., Rockwood, K., Sampson, E. L., ... Mukadam, N. (2017). Dementia prevention, intervention, and care. *Lancet, 390*(10113), 2673–2734. doi:10.1016/S0140-6736(17)31363-6 PMID:28735855

Mahendran, M., Speechley, K. N., & Widjaja, E. (2017). Systematic review of unmet healthcare needs in patients with epilepsy. *Epilepsy & Behavior, 75*, 102–109. doi:10.1016/j.yebeh.2017.02.034 PMID:28843210

Masnoon, N., Shakib, S., Kalisch-Ellett, L., & Caughey, G. E. (2017). What is polypharmacy? A systematic review of definitions. *BMC Geriatrics*, *17*(1), 230. doi:10.118612877-017-0621-2 PMID:29017448

Meads, D. M., Martin, A., Griffiths, A., Kelley, R., Creese, B., Robinson, L., McDermid, J., Walwyn, R., Ballard, C., & Surr, C. A. (2020). Cost-effectiveness of dementia care mapping in care-home settings: Evaluation of a randomised controlled trial. *Applied Health Economics and Health Policy*, *18*(2), 237–247. doi:10.100740258-019-00531-1 PMID:31701483

Mellitus, D. (2005). Diagnosis and classification of diabetes mellitus. *Diabetes Care*, *28*(S37), S5–S10. PMID:15618111

Meneilly, G. S., & Tessier, D. (2001). Diabetes in elderly adults. *The Journals of Gerontology. Series A, Biological Sciences and Medical Sciences*, *56*(1), M5–M13. doi:10.1093/gerona/56.1.M5 PMID:11193234

Michalowsky, B., Xie, F., Eichler, T., Hertel, J., Kaczynski, A., Kilimann, I., Teipel, S., Wucherer, D., Zwingmann, I., Thyrian, J. R., & Hoffmann, W. (2019). Cost-effectiveness of a collaborative dementia care management—Results of a cluster-randomized controlled trial. *Alzheimer's & Dementia*, *15*(10), 1296–1308. doi:10.1016/j.jalz.2019.05.008 PMID:31409541

Miller, Y. (2022). Advancements and future directions in research of the roles of insulin in amyloid diseases. *Biophysical Chemistry*, *281*, 106720. doi:10.1016/j.bpc.2021.106720 PMID:34823073

Moshé, S. L., Perucca, E., Ryvlin, P., & Tomson, T. (2015). Epilepsy: New advances. *Lancet*, *385*(9971), 884–898. doi:10.1016/S0140-6736(14)60456-6 PMID:25260236

National Health Service. (2021). *Symptoms-Alzheimer's disease*. NHS. https://www.nhs.uk/conditions/alzheimers-disease/symptoms/

National Institute for Health and Care Excelllence. (2018). Dementia: assessment, management and support for people living with dementia and their carers. In *NICE guideline [NG97]*. https://www.nice.org.uk/guidance/ng97/chapter/recommendations

Ninomiya, T. (2014). Diabetes mellitus and dementia. *Current Diabetes Reports*, *14*(5), 1–9. doi:10.100711892-014-0487-z PMID:24623199

O'Shea, E., & O'Reilly, S. (2000). The economic and social cost of dementia in Ireland. *International Journal of Geriatric Psychiatry*, *15*(3), 208–218. doi:10.1002/(SICI)1099-1166(200003)15:3<208::AID-GPS95>3.0.CO;2-X PMID:10713578

Paciaroni, M., & Bogousslavsky, J. (2013). Connecting cardiovascular disease and dementia: Further evidence. [). Am Heart Assoc.]. *Journal of the American Heart Association*, *2*(6), e000656. doi:10.1161/JAHA.113.000656 PMID:24351703

Poewe, W., Gauthier, S., Aarsland, D., Leverenz, J. B., Barone, P., Weintraub, D., Tolosa, E., & Dubois, B. (2008). Diagnosis and management of Parkinson's disease dementia. *International Journal of Clinical Practice*, *62*(10), 1581–1587. doi:10.1111/j.1742-1241.2008.01869.x PMID:18822028

Román, G. C. (2003). Vascular dementia: distinguishing characteristics, treatment, and prevention. *Journal of the American Geriatrics Society, 51*(5s2), S296–S304.

Sampson, E. L., Blanchard, M. R., Jones, L., Tookman, A., & King, M. (2009). Dementia in the acute hospital: Prospective cohort study of prevalence and mortality. *The British Journal of Psychiatry*, *195*(1), 61–66. doi:10.1192/bjp.bp.108.055335 PMID:19567898

Savva, G. M., & Stephan, B. C. M. (2010). Epidemiological studies of the effect of stroke on incident dementia: A systematic review. *Stroke*, *41*(1), e41–e46. doi:10.1161/STROKEAHA.109.559880 PMID:19910553

Schjødt, K., Erlang, A. S., Starup-Linde, J., & Jensen, A. L. (2022). Older hospitalised patients' experience of involvement in discharge planning. *Scandinavian Journal of Caring Sciences*, *36*(1), 192–202. doi:10.1111cs.12977 PMID:33694211

Selkoe, D. J. (1994). Cell biology of the amyloid beta-protein precursor and the mechanism of Alzheimer's disease. *Annual Review of Cell Biology*, *10*(1), 373–403. doi:10.1146/annurev.cb.10.110194.002105 PMID:7888181

Sherzai, D., Losey, T., Vega, S., & Sherzai, A. (2014). Seizures and dementia in the elderly: Nationwide Inpatient Sample 1999–2008. *Epilepsy & Behavior*, *36*, 53–56. doi:10.1016/j.yebeh.2014.04.015 PMID:24857809

Shih, J. J., Fountain, N. B., Herman, S. T., Bagic, A., Lado, F., Arnold, S., Zupanc, M. L., Riker, E., & Labiner, D. M. (2018). Indications and methodology for video-electroencephalographic studies in the epilepsy monitoring unit. *Epilepsia*, *59*(1), 27–36. doi:10.1111/epi.13938 PMID:29124760

Teipel, S., Babiloni, C., Hoey, J., Kaye, J., Kirste, T., & Burmeister, O. K. (2016). Information and communication technology solutions for outdoor navigation in dementia. *Alzheimer's & Dementia*, *12*(6), 695–707. doi:10.1016/j.jalz.2015.11.003 PMID:26776761

Van Rijckevorsel, K. (2006). Cognitive problems related to epilepsy syndromes, especially malignant epilepsies. *Seizure*, *15*(4), 227–234. doi:10.1016/j. seizure.2006.02.019 PMID:16563807

Van Straaten, E. C. W., Scheltens, P., & Barkhof, F. (2004). MRI and CT in the diagnosis of vascular dementia. *Journal of the Neurological Sciences*, *226*(1–2), 9–12. doi:10.1016/j.jns.2004.09.003 PMID:15537511

Wang, T., Yuan, F., Chen, Z., Zhu, S., Chang, Z., Yang, W., Deng, B., Que, R., Cao, P., Chao, Y., Chan, L., Pan, Y., Wang, Y., Xu, L., Lyu, Q., Chan, P., Yenari, M. A., Tan, E.-K., & Wang, Q. (2020). Vascular, inflammatory and metabolic risk factors in relation to dementia in Parkinson's disease patients with type 2 diabetes mellitus. *Aging (Albany NY)*, *12*(15), 15682–15704. doi:10.18632/aging.103776 PMID:32805719

Xu, J., Wang, J., Wimo, A., Fratiglioni, L., & Qiu, C. (2017). The economic burden of dementia in China, 1990–2030: Implications for health policy. *Bulletin of the World Health Organization*, *95*(1), 18–26. doi:10.2471/BLT.15.167726 PMID:28053361

ADDITIONAL READING

Aldridge, Z., & Harrison Dening, K. (2021). Managing comorbid conditions and dementia. *Journal of Community Nursing*, *35*(2).

Ben Hassen, C., Fayosse, A., Landré, B., Raggi, M., Bloomberg, M., Sabia, S., & Singh-Manoux, A. (2022). Association between age at onset of multimorbidity and incidence of dementia: 30 year follow-up in Whitehall II prospective cohort study. *BMJ (Clinical Research Ed.)*, 376. doi:10.1136/bmj-2021-068005 PMID:35110302

Cunningham, N. A., Cowie, J., & Methven, K. (2022). Right at home: Living with dementia and multi-morbidities. *Ageing and Society*, *42*(3), 632–656. doi:10.1017/ S0144686X2000104X PMID:35177874

Delgado, J., Jones, L., Bradley, M. C., Allan, L. M., Ballard, C., Clare, L., Fortinsky, R. H., Hughes, C. M., & Melzer, D. (2021). Potentially inappropriate prescribing in dementia, multi-morbidity and incidence of adverse health outcomes. *Age and Ageing*, *50*(2), 457–464. doi:10.1093/ageing/afaa147 PMID:32946561

Franco, Y., Jang, Y., Saenz, J. L., & Ho, J. Y. (2022). The Relationship Between Multimorbidity and Types of Chronic Diseases and Self-Rated Memory. *Research on Aging*, 01640275221087612. PMID:35387519

Kim, W. J., Lee, S. J., Lee, E., Lee, E. Y., & Han, K. (2022). Risk of Incident Dementia According to Glycemic Status and Comorbidities of Hyperglycemia: A Nationwide Population-Based Cohort Study. *Diabetes Care*, *45*(1), 134–141. doi:10.2337/dc21-0957 PMID:34711638

Subramaniam, H. (2019). Co-morbidities in dementia: Time to focus more on assessing and managing co-morbidities. []. Oxford University Press.]. *Age and Ageing*, *48*(3), 314–315. doi:10.1093/ageing/afz007 PMID:31063580

Zheng, B., Su, B., Udeh-Momoh, C., Price, G., Tzoulaki, I., Vamos, E. P., Majeed, A., Riboli, E., Ahmadi-Abhari, S., & Middleton, L. T. (2022). Associations of Cardiovascular and Non-Cardiovascular Comorbidities with Dementia Risk in Patients with Diabetes: Results from a Large UK Cohort Study. *The Journal of Prevention of Alzheimer's Disease*, 1–6. doi:10.14283/jpad.2022.8 PMID:35098977

KEY TERMS AND DEFINITIONS

Alzheimer's Disease: A common brain disease that causes dementia, symptoms associated with executive functioning impairment, personality changes, hallucinations, and confusion due to the disruption of brain cells, for example, the formation of beta-amyloid plaques and neurofibrillary tangles.

Cardiovascular Disease: A medical condition that causes severe implications in the heart, blood vessels, and arteries, for example, atherosclerosis, and possible blood clots, which strain the heart and increase the risk of heart attacks and heart failure.

Dementia: A deteriorating and progressive brain disorder which is mainly characterised by loss of cognitive functioning and impacts greatly daily life, behavioural and emotional functioning with most common symptom the memory loss.

Diabetes: A lifelong chronic medical condition that causes increases in blood sugar levels due to minimal or no insulin production in the pancreas, and as a result, the body is unable to break down glucose into energy.

Epilepsy: A one lifelong neurological disorder characterised by a wide range of unpredictable seizures that are manifested with uncontrollable jerking, shaking, collapsing, and fainting in most of the cases due to abnormal brain activity.

Healthcare Systems: Consists of health services that include clinical staff members, facilities, and supplies, for example, medical equipment and medications, to provide and commission care in patients.

Multimorbidity: The presence of two or more health diseases/disorders that are either physiological or psychiatric in an individual.

Parkinson's Disease: This is a progressive neurological disorder that exhibits movement malfunctions, for example, involuntary shaking, tremor, slow body movements, stiff, inflexible muscles, balance difficulties, depression, anxiety, insomnia, speech difficulties, concentration, and memory problems, due to abnormal brain activity, for example decreases in dopamine neurotransmitter, presence of Lewy bodies and increases in Alpha-synuclein protein.

Vascular Dementia: A type of dementia caused by decreased blood flow in the brain, due to diseased blood vessels in cortical and subcortical brain areas, causing progressive cognitive impairments such as problems with planning, organising, decision making, problem-solving, speech difficulties, concentration, memory, language and visuospatial deficits, apathy, depression, and anxiety.

Chapter 7
Sarcopenia in Older People

Karen Cordovil
 https://orcid.org/0000-0003-1573-7796
Oswaldo Cruz Foundation, Brazil

Masato Hada
Independent Researcher, Japan

Zagami Francesco
Tabaka Mission Hospital, Kenya

Adil Al-Harthi
King Fahad Armed Forces Hospital, Saudi Arabia

Taha Hussein Musa
Southeast University, China

EXECUTIVE SUMMARY

Sarcopenia is a generalized loss of muscle mass affecting muscle function and strength with age. The cause of sarcopenia is multifactorial and physiopathological mechanisms, including the decline of neuron numbers, changes in muscle metabolism, oxidative damage, reduced response to nutrients, and inflammation throughout proinflammatory cytokines that increase myofibrillar protein degradation and decrease protein synthesis. This chapter presents two case reports about sarcopenia and its associated multimorbidity impact on elderly patients. Sarcopenia in the elderly, when it advances to generalized muscle wasting, is mainly associated with multimorbidity which becomes a diagnostic, therapeutic, and palliative challenge to the physician; in these cases, a multidisciplinary approach is best for appropriate diagnosis and management results in a high-quality patient care setting.

DOI: 10.4018/978-1-6684-2354-7.ch007

INTRODUCTION

Sarcopenia is defined as a generalized loss of muscle mass affecting muscle function and strength with age (Cruz-Jentoft & Sayer, 2019; Mori, et al., 2019). The Drafting Group of the European Working Group on Sarcopenia (EWGSOP2) has classified sarcopenia as acute and chronic, and has given recommendations to develop realize an algorithm to identify people with sarcopenia risk, and recommended mensuration of specific cutoff points to identify and characterize the sarcopenia (Cruz-Jentoft et al., 2019).

The cause of sarcopenia is multifactorial and physiopathological mechanisms include the decline of neuron numbers, changes in muscle metabolism, oxidative damage, reduced response to nutrients, and inflammation throughout proinflammatory cytokines that increase myofibrillar protein degradation and decreasing protein synthesis (Boirie, 2009; Walrand et al., 2011). It is well documented in the current literature that sarcopenia is present in many other chronic illnesses and infectious diseases (de Almeida et al., 2020; Dozio et al., 2021; Peterson & Mozer, 2017). Sarcopenia affects more the elderly and is related to a higher frequency of hospital admissions, as well as morbidity and mortality (Ekiz, Kara & Özçakar, 2020; Ekiz et al., 2020; Mehta et al., 2020).

Currently, there are several techniques in the evaluation of sarcopenia according to the guidelines and consensus for the diagnosis and treatment of sarcopenia (Cruz-Jentoft et al., 2019). Performing a non-invasive assessment of muscle mass is recognized as the standard, but should be performed by highly trained personnel, especially for patients with poorly defined cut-off values of muscle mass reduction (Cruz-Jentoft et al., 2019).

A method widely used in research and clinical practice to determine muscle mass because it is non-invasive and provides a reproducible estimate of appendicular skeletal muscle mass (ASM) is dual-energy X-ray absorptiometry (DXA) (Cruz-Jentoft & Sayer, 2019; Cruz-Jentoft et al., 2019). Despite this, as a disadvantage, DXA can be influenced by the degree of hydration of the patient, it is not portable, the brands available on the market still need to present more reliable results in its measurement, and may not support obese and tall people (Cruz-Jentoft et al., 2019; Martone et al., 2019; Tosato et al., 2017).

Another method considered transportable and cheaper is bioelectrical impedance analysis (BIA), which uses a DXA-mediated pattern-fitted lean mass conversion equation in a representative population (Cruz-Jentoft et al., 2019; Martone et al., 2019; Tosato et al., 2017). As a disadvantage, it can be influenced by the individual's degree of hydration, and its derivation patterns are based on older European populations (Cruz-Jentoft et al., 2019; Martone et al., 2019; Tosato et al., 2017).

According to with criteria diagnosis of EWGSOP2, sarcopenia can be identified by low muscle strength, with confirmation by the low muscle quantity or quality and low physical performance (Cruz-Jentoft et al., 2019; De Francesco, Vella & Belfiore, 2020).

An attractive way to present clinical situations for virtual discussion (learning by induced feedback) which starting from our field experience, transfer the clinical intuition in a pathophysiological pathway to clinical goal reach.

DIAGNOSIS OF SARCOPENIA

Diagnostic criteria are essential for recognizing sarcopenia and frailty in clinical practice. The prevalence of sarcopenia is highly dependent on the applied diagnostic criteria (Bijlsma et al., 2013). The tools for diagnosis of a decreased muscle mass or function require a high specificity with a high internal and external validity (Mijnarends et al., 2013).

Therefore, using different diagnostic criteria may lead to different conclusions and may have different implications for treatment. Twenty-six studies used muscle mass for the definition of sarcopenia, while two studies included mass, strength, and performance, as recommended by the European Sarcopenia Consensus (Pagotto & Silveira, 2014). Two setting-specific diagnostic criteria were created for the Asian Working Group for Sarcopenia (AWGS2019) (Chen et al., 2020).

The first is a hospital or research setting, where severe sarcopenia is diagnosed using low muscle mass plus low muscle strength or low physical performance. The second is a primary health care or preventive services setting, where sarcopenia is diagnosed using calf circumference, SARC-F, or SARC-CalF, defined by low muscle strength, or reduced physical performance (Pagotto & Silveira, 2014; Chen et al., 2020).

CT scanning is considered a gold standard, especially in patients undergoing a CT scan for other purposes, data for quantification of muscle mass can be easily extracted for diagnosing sarcopenia. The limitation of the tool is the use of cut-off points in different studies, high medical costs, and the radiation burden (Baracos & Arribas, 2018). However, depending on local availability and expertise, MRI, DXA, and BIA can be cautiously used as alternatives (Ackermans et al., 2022). However, depending on local availability and expertise, MRI is considered a safe alternative it does not use ionizing radiation and it provides additional information on muscle quality. While the complexity, costs, and contra-indications of MRI render it less suitable for the assessment of muscle mass in clinical practice (Kim, Wilson & Lee, 2010).

DXA might be a reasonable alternative for assessing muscle mass because radiation exposure is low, but the cost of DXA is high (Yin et al., 2021). BIA is the best diagnostic tool for muscle mass quantification, it is cheap, harmless, and easily accessible (Ackermans et al., 2022). The fasting insulin and AST/ALT ratio exhibit good diagnostic performance for sarcopenia (Yin et al., 2021).

Diet Managements of Sarcopenia

There is growing evidence that links nutrition to muscle mass, strength, and function in older, therefore it has an important role in the prevention and management of sarcopenia. The food and energy intake was a decline with increasing age, as energy needs decreased (Wakimoto & Block, 2001). Food intake falls by 25% between 40 and 70 years of age (Nieuwenhuizen, et al., 2010). Older people are less hungry and thirsty, consume small meals, and eat few snacks between meals than younger (Nieuwenhuizen, et al., 2010). It occurs alongside appetite changes and has been described as the 'anorexia of aging' (Malafarina et al., 2013).

Specific age-related changes include loss of acuity in taste, smell, and sight, changes in the secretion and peripheral action of appetite hormones, gastrointestinal motility, chewing and swallowing difficulties, and other effects of chronic disease that can affect food intake (Hedman, Nydahl & Faxén-Irving, 2016).

Protein is a crucial nutrient in older age, provides amino acids that are needed for muscle protein synthesis, and absorbed amino acids that are needed for muscle protein synthesis after feeding (Kim, Wilson & Lee, 2010). Supplementation with leucine, isoleucine, and valine was used to improve athletic performance and attenuate muscle loss (Borack & Volpi, 2016).

Loss of muscle mass and vitamin D deficiency often occur together and are interrelated; both are linked to common clinical outcomes, including weakness, falls, and frailty in older age (Halfon, Phan & Teta, 2015). The potential mechanisms that link vitamin D status to muscle function are complex and include both genomic and non-genomic roles (Robinson, Cooper & Sayer, 2017). The vitamin D receptor (VDR) was expressed in skeletal muscle (Hamilton, 2010), and polymorphisms of the VDR are related to differences in muscle strength (Robinson, Cooper & Sayer, 2017).

Markers of oxidative damage have been shown to predict impairments in physical function in older (Semba, et al., 2007). Damage in DNA, lipids, and proteins may occur when reactive oxygen species (ROS) are present in cells in excess. The actions of ROS are normally counterbalanced by antioxidant defense mechanisms that include the enzymes superoxide dismutase and glutathione peroxidase and exogenous antioxidants derived from the diet, such as selenium, carotenoids, tocopherols, flavonoids, and other plant polyphenols (Li et al., 2014). The increases in the production of C-reactive protein (CRP), tumor necrosis factor-a (TNF-a), and interleukin 6 (IL-6) have an important role in many chronic conditions (Li et al., 2014) and also implicated in age-related diseases (Jeffery, Shum & Hubbard, 2013) Dairy products are important due to their whey protein content, which is relatively high in branched-chain amino acids (Bos, Gaudichon & Tomé, 2000) and antioxidant properties (Jeffery et al., 2013).

Some anti-oxidant-rich foods are also rich in inorganic nitrates, such as green leafy vegetables. Dietary nitrate ingestion appears to enhance exercise capacity and performance in young individuals, and beetroot juice has become popular among some endurance athletes (Siervo et al., 2016). In the body, nitrate is converted to nitrite and nitric oxide is pleiotropic and has effects on various muscle performance-related functions related to muscle contraction efficiency (Robinson et al., 2018).

Poor diet quality was related to sarcopenia presence in Koreans aged 75 and older (Na et al., 2020). The sarcopenia in the high-altitude population was significantly lower than those in the plain population, and the incidences of sarcopenia in the high-altitude population over 60 years old were 17.2% in men and 36.0% in women, which were significantly higher than those in the plain population (Ye et al., 2020). To improve the diet quality of the elderly, it is necessary to develop dietary improvement guidelines (Ye, et al., 2020). Protein supplementation that includes 20 g of whey protein, essential amino acids, leucine, beta-hydroxy-beta-methyl butyrate, and 800 IU vitamin D improves muscle quality in sarcopenic elderly people (Yanai, 2015). A dietary pattern characterized by high intakes of fish, soybean products, potatoes, most vegetables, mushrooms, seaweeds, and fruits and low rice intake was inversely associated with sarcopenia in community-dwelling older Japanese (Yokoyama et al., 2021).

A combination therapy that includes both nutritional and exercises therapy improves gait speed and knee extension strength more than either exercise alone or nutrition therapy alone. A combined physical activity intervention, and exercise regime along with protein intake > 1gr/kg/d is the safest strategy to follow to manage sarcopenia and T2DM concurrently (Argyropoulou et al., 2022). ROS have both physiological and pathological roles, interventions based on simple suppression of their activities may be unlikely to improve age-related declines in muscle mass and function (Jackson, 2009).

Therapeutic

It is agreed that the therapeutic approach for patients with sarcopenia and multimorbidities can be supported by a change in lifestyle (Bernabeu-Wittel et al., 2020). As discussed earlier, a healthy diet plays a key role in preventing sarcopenia with multimorbidity (Bernabeu-Wittel et al., 2020). As a therapeutic approach, protein supplementation, a high-protein diet, vitamin D, and omega 3, would also be very promising strategies in the fight against sarcopenia in individuals with poly pathologies (Curcio et al., 2020).

Concerning physical exercise, has been related to a decrease in muscle mass loss, inflammation, and oxidative stress, especially in patients with heart failure and sarcopenia (Dennison, Sayer, & Cooper, 2017). In addition, several therapeutic possibilities can be used to prevent, treat or recover sarcopenic patients with poly pathologies (Curcio et al., 2020).

In cardiac patients, drug therapy would use, for example, spironolactone, an aldosterone antagonist, to stop the progression of sarcopenia (Fattirolli & Pratesi, 2015). In heart failure, the use of beta-blockers would be important to help reduce the risk of loss of body mass (Fattirolli & Pratesi, 2015).

Another example was from a prospective, multicenter observational study with 444 patients with multimorbidity, the prevalence of frail elderly, sarcopenic, or both was 62%, 21.8%, and 18%, with significantly increased levels of oxidative stress markers and the presence of shortening of the absolute length of telomeres, with lower survival risks (Bernabeu-Wittel et al., 2020). These findings demonstrate the possible therapeutic applicability of markers of oxidative stress and telomere length shortening levels in clinical practice involving sarcopenic patients with multimorbidities (Bernabeu-Wittel et al., 2020). More recent therapeutic approaches include stem cell transplantation, mitochondrial biogenesis, restoration of mitochondrial functions, and other therapies that synergistically combine physical exercise (Lo et al., 2020).

The therapeutic secret of the treatment of sarcopenia in patients with various pathologies is to carry out the clinical and pharmacological treatment in harmony with each other and to act with clinical treatment with not only multi-professional but interdisciplinary support in the fight against sarcopenia (Mankhong et al., 2020).

DIFFICULTIES IN SARCOPENIA WITH MULTIMORBIDITY

Sarcopenia has a greater risk of appearing with advancing age and has a tripod of well-defined risk factors: a sedentary lifestyle, adiposity, and multimorbidity (Landi et al., 2013). According to current literature, multimorbidity has been defined as the presence of two or more long-term pathological conditions and has been directly related to the constant process of progressive aging of individuals, and many risk factors such as environmental agents, lifestyle and genetic factors could be involved (Dodds et al., 2020).

Sarcopenia with multimorbidity is a severe problem that requires a holistic view to provide health care and represents a significant factor in the assessment of the risk of falls and fractures (Aspray & Hill, 2019). Among the common types of comorbidity, especially in the elderly who have sarcopenia, are osteoporosis, heart failure, and metabolic diseases, among others (Brown et al., 2011).

In a study with 499,000 participants in a biobank in England, individuals with multimorbidities represented 44.5% of the sample and were also twice as likely to have sarcopenia when compared with individuals without multimorbidity (OR 1.96 - 95% CI: 1.91; 2.02) (Dodds et al., 2020). These results also showed that the multimorbidities that were more likely to develop sarcopenia were musculoskeletal/trauma (OR 2.17 - 95% CI: 2.11; 2.23), endocrine/diabetes (OR 1.49 - 95% CI: 1.45;1.55) and neurological/psychiatric (OR 1.39 - 95% CI: 1.34;1.43) (Dodds et al., 2020).

The main difficulty in the treatment of patients with sarcopenia with multimorbidity is early screening in the establishment of pathological conditions that appear in the long term (Dodds et al., 2020). Another limiting factor is that although many studies point to new therapies to combat sarcopenia, many have not yet shown consistent benefits, especially in the long term (Lo et al., 2020).

Challenges

From a public health point of view, sarcopenia is still a global health problem and a new clinical practice challenge for developed as well as developing countries, based on its current and expected prevalence, its clinical, cost, and economic consequences. Clinically, osteoporosis and sarcopenia are common in older age and have been reported to be associated with significant mortality, increased risk of physical limitation, and a variety of chronic diseases.

Osteoporosis is a skeletal disease characterized by low bone mass, was reported also associated with an increased risk of fragility fractures was remain the main clinical consequence that leads to a significant burden on health. In addition, lack of exercise and adequate, balanced nutrition is the major impact on health-related quality of life compared with those without self-reported musculoskeletal diseases.

The WHO showed the number of people around the world estimated at 1.2 billion by 2025 and 2 billion by 2050 with sarcopenia. The estimated prevalence of sarcopenia, WHO suggests that sarcopenia affects more than 50 million people today, and will affect more than 200 million people over the next 40 years. Owing to an increase in the rates of disability, disability, and premature, poor mobility, frailty, and hospitalization rate.

Despite the high social and economic cost of osteoporosis, researchers find out still there is an enormous gap a substantial treatment gap and a projected increase in the economic burden driven by the aging population, followed by a lack of awareness of sarcopenia and its risk, lack of research productivity to prevent or delay adverse health outcomes and decrease the burden for patients and healthcare systems.

This might be exponentially able to intervene earlier in the life course to prevent their occurrence of prevalence among the populations. Other scientific report shows that despite the strong association of sarcopenia with morbidity and mortality rate no unifying mechanism has yet been proposed as to why muscle-wasting conditions are associated with functional declines. Beside others, challenges include pharmacological interventions to prevent fractures, and change in healthcare policy is warranted. However, another small study recommended paying attention to assessing the quality of life in sarcopenic subjects, specifically for mobility or physical function.

CASE 1

Elderly Bedridden with Advanced Dementia Frailty and Sarcopenia

An 85-year-old lady was brought from home because her daughter noticed recurrent vomiting. She's not tolerating feeding and is bedridden with a clinical picture of advanced dementia with poor activity in daily living taken care of at home by her daughter. She looks underweight with generalized muscle wasting. Clinical evidence noted the presence of abdominal distention that is soft and lax but tender all over.

In our first case, the patient had dementia, different studies showed a relationship between sarcopenia and dementia. Both sarcopenia and dementia share some common risk factors most importantly age, which both are common in the elder population and more common in the very old population. Both are associated with multimorbidity as well.

Different studies have also shown that there is a relationship between sarcopenia and cognitive impairment but studies have wide variations in their results due to different definitions of sarcopenia as some studies did not include muscle mass loss which is included in the new consensus definition of sarcopenia (Bai et al., 2021).

A study that investigated the relationship between sarcopenia and different stages of Alzheimer's dementia found that sarcopenia is common in all elders generally but more in those who have Alzheimer's dementia. The study also found that moderate Alzheimer's dementia has more muscle loss and loss of muscle function, than elders with normal cognitive capabilities. They also found that early and mild Alzheimer's disease have a loss of muscle function but not muscle mass which is called dynapenia (Age-related loss of muscle function) that could be a manifestation of frailty, and that could be used as a noncognitive early manifestation of Alzheimer's disease (Ogawa et al., 2018).

Many studies have shown that people with Alzheimer's disease have sarcopenic muscle characteristics. Sarcopenia is not only associated with age, but with BMI and mini-mental test scores as well. It has been also noticed that Alzheimer's disease patients exhibit increased eating behaviors concordant with weight loss, and this weight loss precedes Alzheimer-related cognitive impairment (Ogawa et al., 2018). This motivated scientists to examine the relationship between Alzheimer's disease and weight loss which resulted in a few hypotheses about the association. One important hypothesis is that altered central regulation of body weight causes weight loss in Alzheimer's disease. In a study injecting Beta Amyloid in the hypothalamus of experimental rats resulted in more weight loss compared to the rats of the same age, it also showed that the weight loss is more related to lean body weight than visceral fat.

Further studies on experimental rats showed that after injecting beta-Amyloid, weight reduction occurs as fast as four weeks in both diabetic and non-diabetic rats. The above experiments indicate an alteration in the central regulation of body weight in Alzheimer's disease (Minaglia et al., 2019).

It is noticed in the literature that experimental studies done on the relation between dementia and frailty is far more than those done on the relation between dementia and sarcopenia, more longitudinal studies are needed to understand the association and the underlying pathophysiology among sarcopenic dementia patients, and whether it's relation is a bidirectional one or not, I.e. does sarcopenia lead to dementia making sarcopenia a dementia precursor state just like frailty or not.

Our case also has abdominal distention in the presence of generalized muscle wasting, this could be due to multiple causes more likely colonic distention due to stool impaction, or the accumulation of ascetic fluid, but abdominal distention could be due to obesity as well. Obesity in the presence of sarcopenia is called sarcopenic obesity, which is a well-known entity with increased prevalence in old age, this phenomenon needs to be further investigated biochemically and genetically to know the reasons why these elder patients end up in sarcopenic obesity, rather than sarcopenia or Obesity alone, some researchers suggest to further understand the cross talk between adipose tissue and muscle tissue to understand its unique phenomena (Kalinkovich & Livshits, 2017).

A bidirectional cross talk between adipocytes and mayocites is hypothesized, mwhich is influenced by myokines secreted from myocites that alter the normal, adispose tissue metabolism, on the other hand adipokines secreted by white adipose tissue that is known to alter muscle tissue by increasing intramuscular fat accumulation and further promoting muscle wasting. Observational studies showed that sarcopenic obesity has serious consequences on the elderly in the form of frailty, falls, mortality, increased cardiovascular and atherosclerotic risk as well indicating that sarcopenic obesity has a more hazardous consequence on the elder than obesity alone (Zamboni et al., 2022). Further understanding of sarcopenic obesity and its unique underlying mechanisms will help us formulate therapeutic and preventive strategies to reduce its consequences.

Our patient has advanced dementia, there is a unique relationship between sarcopenia and advanced dementia. An advanced stage of weight loss in which muscle and fat loss are observed, called cachexia, which is thought of as a final stage of sarcopenia in advanced dementia, of the possible etiologies of advanced dementia related to cachexia is anorexia of aging, dysphasia, cognitive impairment, increase energy expenditure, inflammatory and metabolic dysregulation, and altered central weight control.

The logical thinking is that advanced dementia needs high protein intake to counteract Its catabolic state, so different methods of tube feeding to overcome anorexia and dysphagia, known collectively as artificial nutrition and hydration (ANH).

Retrospective studies on advanced dementia tube feeding all agree that it didn't show an improvement in quality of life, an increase in physical performance, or an improvement in mortality. Most of the studies also showed that ANH did not reduce bedsores, aspiration pneumonia, nor improve malnutrition (Minaglia et al., 2019). Concerning percutaneous endoscopic gastrostomy (PEG) feeding, a study is done in an advanced center where PEG tube complication screening is done routinely, they found that the quality of life benefit of PEG tube feeding compared to those without tube Feeding is less than 5%, in comparison to its complications which are higher than 15% (Minaglia et al., 2019).

The above retrospective studies show that advanced dementia-related cachexia is an irreversible condition that does not improve by dietary supplementation, this proves that the cachexia is not only due to anorexia, dysphagia, or cognitive impairment, but other important etiologies are attributed to it. Retrospective studies on advanced dementia patients living in hospice and elder care settings showed that palliative care guidelines and end-of-life protocols are not fully activated for all of the patients and some patients are investigated and managed in a similar way to the non-advanced dementia patients (Minaglia et al., 2019).

In advanced dementia complications and decisions should be within the palliative and end-of-life guidelines, which should be done after discussion among the palliative care team, and the patient or caregiver, psychological stress of the grieving relatives should be put into consideration. The aims and goals should be comfort care rather than longevity and improving performance in order to reduce the patients suffering from pain, shortness of breath, or other disturbing symptoms.

CASE 2

Elderly with Multiple Strokes Difficulty Swallowing on Tube Feeding and Sarcopenia

An 85 year old gentleman with multiple strokes, wheelchair-bound, presented with progressive weight loss and sarcopenia for the last three years. Patients started feeding via a nasogastric tube in the last four months.

In our second case, we noticed that the sarcopenic patient was diagnosed with a stroke previously, when sarcopenia is not due to aging by itself, it's called secondary sarcopenia, which is divided into disease-related and nutrition related. Stroke is a type of disease-related sarcopenia which is known as stroke-related sarcopenia (Hollingworth et al., 2021). Stroke-related sarcopenia is a common disease because it identifies two common diseases in the elder population namely stroke and sarcopenia, and stroke is not only a common disease in the elder, but it's one of the common causes of muscle disability in the elderly population.

Prevalence of stroke-related sarcopenia differs widely, depending on the definition used for sarcopenia, and depending on the population characteristics, one retrospective study investigating the incidence of stroke-related sarcopenia in developing countries, namely Egypt and China using the Asian working group of sarcopenia 2019 (AWGS-2019) found the prevalence of sarcopenia is about 20 to 30% compared to the developed countries, this is a large prevalence which could be due to reduced access to health service, reduced health education or increased pre-morbid conditions, etc. In comparison to primary or age-related sarcopenia, stroke-related sarcopenia is characterized by faster muscle loss specifically (Mohammed & Li, 2022).

Previously it was told that brain pathology was the main reason for sarcopenia among stroke survivors but later imaging studies showed that sarcopenia doesn't only develop in the paretic limb but it's also found in the non-paretic limp as well in the form of muscle loss and intramuscular fat infiltration, so there must be other factors involved in its pathogenesis (Li, Yue & Liu, 2020). Among the important factors related to its pathogenesis is immobility, most stroke survivors are unable to mobilize appropriately, due to the paraplegia and disability causing reduced physical performance.

A study done on elder patients found that 10 days bedrest causes a reduction in protein synthesis and increased protein catabolism that results in a reduction of 16% in muscle strength (Li, Yue & Liu, 2020). Studies have shown that early strengthening exercise, reduce sarcopenia and improves outcome in stroke survivors. Another important factor is nerve denervation, studies have shown that in muscle cross-sectional area showed by imaging that the motor unit number is reduced as fast as four hours after the stroke in the paretic limp and two weeks in the nonparetic limp as well. One important factor causing stroke-related sarcopenia is nutrition, due to the common occurrence of dysphasia in stroke survivors, which is around 50% that leads to nutritional challenges in these patients, which could be a strong contribution to sarcopenia.

Other causes of reduced nutrition in stroke survivors are post-stroke cognitive impairment, and alteration in the central appetite centers. Another factor is sympathetic activation and inflammation. It is found that most stroke survivors have over sympathetic activation some hypothesis behind this are psychological stress, pain and loss of preganglionic central inhibition. This sympathetic over activation can lead to inflammation, and possibly immunosuppression, experimental studies showed that stroke-related sarcopenia patients have higher levels of cytokines specifically, tumor necrosis factor-alpha (TNFa) and its messenger RNA compared to the non-stroke elders. It is also found when given beta blockers to experimental mice with stroke-related sarcopenia to reduce sympathetic over-activation (Li, Yue & Liu, 2020). It was found that the level of cytokines is reduced but this intervention did not affect the level of muscle loss.

Multiple intervention studies on humans were done for stroke-related sarcopenia management and prevention, and they found that early strengthening exercise and nutritional replacement reduce the occurrence of sarcopenia among stroke survivors. It is also worth mentioning that pre-stroke sarcopenia is common in older patient so educating healthcare providers about primary sarcopenia and promoting sarcopenia screening measures in highly suspected individuals like elders living in home care facilities or those with reduced physical capabilities for early discovery of primary sarcopenia, and thus reducing its hazardous consequence on elder patients.

CONCLUSION

Sarcopenia in the elderly mostly presents with frailty, and when it advances to generalized muscle wasting, is mostly associated with multimorbidity, which becomes a diagnostic, therapeutic, and palliative challenge to the physician, in these cases a multidisciplinary approach is best to reach the appropriate diagnosis in a high-quality patient care setting.

REFERENCES

Ackermans, L. L., Rabou, J., Basrai, M., Schweinlin, A., Bischoff, S. C., Cussenot, O., Cancel-Tassin, G., Renken, R. J., Gómez, E., Sánchez-González, P., Rainoldi, A., Boccia, G., Reisinger, K. W., Ten Bosch, J. A., & Blokhuis, T. J. (2022). Screening, diagnosis and monitoring of sarcopenia: When to use which tool? *Clinical Nutrition ESPEN*, *48*, 36–44. doi:10.1016/j.clnesp.2022.01.027 PMID:35331514

Argyropoulou, D., Geladas, N. D., Nomikos, T., & Paschalis, V. (2022). Exercise and Nutrition Strategies for Combating Sarcopenia and Type 2 Diabetes Mellitus in Older Adults. *Journal of Functional Morphology and Kinesiology*, *7*(2), 48. doi:10.3390/jfmk7020048 PMID:35736019

Aspray, T. J., & Hill, T. R. (2019). Osteoporosis and the ageing skeleton. *Biochemistry and cell biology of ageing: Part II clinical science*, 453-476.

Bai, A., Xu, W., Sun, J., Liu, J., Deng, X., Wu, L., Zou, X., Zuo, J., Zou, L., Liu, Y., Xie, H., Zhang, X., Fan, L., & Hu, Y. (2021). Associations of sarcopenia and its defining components with cognitive function in community-dwelling oldest old. *BMC Geriatrics*, *21*(1), 292. doi:10.118612877-021-02190-1 PMID:33957882

Baracos, V. E., & Arribas, L. (2018). Sarcopenic obesity: Hidden muscle wasting and its impact for survival and complications of cancer therapy. *Annals of Oncology: Official Journal of the European Society for Medical Oncology*, *29*, ii1–ii9. doi:10.1093/annonc/mdx810

Bernabeu-Wittel, M., Gómez-Díaz, R., González-Molina, Á., Vidal-Serrano, S., Díez-Manglano, J., Salgado, F., Soto-Martín, M., & Ollero-Baturone, M. (2020). Oxidative stress, telomere shortening, and apoptosis associated to sarcopenia and frailty in patients with multimorbidity. *Journal of Clinical Medicine*, *9*(8), 2669. doi:10.3390/jcm9082669 PMID:32824789

Bijlsma, A. Y., Meskers, C. G. M., Ling, C. H. Y., Narici, M., Kurrle, S. E., Cameron, I. D., Westendorp, R. G. J., & Maier, A. B. (2013). Defining sarcopenia: The impact of different diagnostic criteria on the prevalence of sarcopenia in a large middle-aged cohort. *Age (Dordrecht, Netherlands)*, *35*(3), 871–881. doi:10.100711357-012-9384-z PMID:22314402

Boirie, Y. (2009). Physiopathological mechanism of sarcopenia. *JNHA-. The Journal of Nutrition, Health & Aging*, *13*(8), 717–723. doi:10.100712603-009-0203-x PMID:19657556

Borack, M. S., & Volpi, E. (2016). Efficacy and safety of leucine supplementation in the elderly. *The Journal of Nutrition, 146*(12), 2625S–2629S. doi:10.3945/jn.116.230771 PMID:27934654

Bos, C., Gaudichon, C., & Tomé, D. (2000). Nutritional and physiological criteria in the assessment of milk protein quality for humans. *Journal of the American College of Nutrition, 19*(sup2), 191S-205S.

Brown, P., McNeill, R., Leung, W., Radwan, E., & Willingale, J. (2011). Current and future economic burden of osteoporosis in New Zealand. *Applied Health Economics and Health Policy, 9*(2), 111–123. doi:10.2165/11531500-000000000-00000 PMID:21271750

Chen, L. K., Woo, J., Assantachai, P., Auyeung, T. W., Chou, M. Y., Iijima, K., Jang, H. C., Kang, L., Kim, M., Kim, S., Kojima, T., Kuzuya, M., Lee, J. S. W., Lee, S. Y., Lee, W.-J., Lee, Y., Liang, C.-K., Lim, J.-Y., Lim, W. S., ... Arai, H. (2020). Asian Working Group for Sarcopenia: 2019 consensus update on sarcopenia diagnosis and treatment. *Journal of the American Medical Directors Association, 21*(3), 300–307. doi:10.1016/j.jamda.2019.12.012 PMID:32033882

Cruz-Jentoft, A. J., Bahat, G., Bauer, J., Boirie, Y., Bruyère, O., Cederholm, T., ... Zamboni, M. (2019). Sarcopenia: Revised European consensus on definition and diagnosis. *Age and Ageing, 48*(1), 16–31. doi:10.1093/ageing/afy169 PMID:30312372

Cruz-Jentoft, A. J., & Sayer, A. A. (2019). Sarcopenia. *Lancet, 393*(10191), 2636–2646. doi:10.1016/S0140-6736(19)31138-9 PMID:31171417

Curcio, F., Testa, G., Liguori, I., Papillo, M., Flocco, V., Panicara, V., Galizia, G., Della-Morte, D., Gargiulo, G., Cacciatore, F., Bonaduce, D., Landi, F., & Abete, P. (2020). Sarcopenia and heart failure. *Nutrients, 12*(1), 211. doi:10.3390/nu12010211 PMID:31947528

de Almeida, L. L., Ilha, T. A., de Carvalho, J. A., Stein, C., Caeran, G., Comim, F. V., Moresco, R. N., Haygert, C. J. P., Compston, J. E., & Premaor, M. O. (2020). Sarcopenia and its association with vertebral fractures in people living with HIV. *Calcified Tissue International, 107*(3), 249–256. doi:10.100700223-020-00718-y PMID:32683475

De Francesco, E. M., Vella, V., & Belfiore, A. (2020). COVID-19 and diabetes: The importance of controlling RAGE. *Frontiers in Endocrinology, 11*, 526. doi:10.3389/fendo.2020.00526 PMID:32760352

Dennison, E. M., Sayer, A. A., & Cooper, C. (2017). Epidemiology of sarcopenia and insight into possible therapeutic targets. *Nature Reviews. Rheumatology*, *13*(6), 340–347. doi:10.1038/nrrheum.2017.60 PMID:28469267

Dodds, R. M., Granic, A., Robinson, S. M., & Sayer, A. A. (2020). Sarcopenia, long-term conditions, and multimorbidity: Findings from UK Biobank participants. *Journal of Cachexia, Sarcopenia and Muscle*, *11*(1), 62–68. doi:10.1002/jcsm.12503 PMID:31886632

Dozio, E., Vettoretti, S., Lungarella, G., Messa, P., & Corsi Romanelli, M. M. (2021). Sarcopenia in chronic kidney disease: Focus on advanced glycation end products as mediators and markers of oxidative stress. *Biomedicines*, *9*(4), 405. doi:10.3390/biomedicines9040405 PMID:33918767

Ekiz, T., Kara, M., & Özçakar, L. (2020). Fighting against frailty and sarcopenia– As well as COVID-19? *Medical Hypotheses*, *144*, 109911. doi:10.1016/j.mehy.2020.109911 PMID:32505075

Ekiz, T., Kara, M., Özcan, F., Ricci, V., & Özçakar, L. (2020). Sarcopenia and COVID-19: a manifold insight on hypertension and the renin angiotensin system. *American journal of physical medicine & rehabilitation*.

Fattirolli, F., & Pratesi, A. (2015). Cardiovascular prevention and rehabilitation in the elderly: Evidence for cardiac rehabilitation after myocardial infarction or chronic heart failure. *Monaldi Archives for Chest Disease*, *84*(1-2). Advance online publication. doi:10.4081/monaldi.2015.731 PMID:27374045

Halfon, M., Phan, O., & Teta, D. (2015). Vitamin D: A review on its effects on muscle strength, the risk of fall, and frailty. *BioMed Research International*, *2015*, 2015. doi:10.1155/2015/953241 PMID:26000306

Hamilton, B. (2010). Vitamin D and human skeletal muscle. *Scandinavian Journal of Medicine & Science in Sports*, *20*(2), 182–190. PMID:19807897

Hedman, S., Nydahl, M., & Faxén-Irving, G. (2016). Individually prescribed diet is fundamental to optimize nutritional treatment in geriatric patients. *Clinical Nutrition (Edinburgh, Lothian)*, *35*(3), 692–698. doi:10.1016/j.clnu.2015.04.018 PMID:25998583

Hollingworth, T. W., Oke, S. M., Patel, H., & Smith, T. R. (2021). Getting to grips with sarcopenia: Recent advances and practical management for the gastroenterologist. *Frontline Gastroenterology*, *12*(1), 53–61. doi:10.1136/flgastro-2019-101348 PMID:33489069

Jackson, M. J. (2009). Strategies for reducing oxidative damage in ageing skeletal muscle. *Advanced Drug Delivery Reviews*, *61*(14), 1363–1368. doi:10.1016/j.addr.2009.07.018 PMID:19737589

Jeffery, C. A., Shum, D. W., & Hubbard, R. E. (2013). Emerging drug therapies for frailty. *Maturitas*, *74*(1), 21–25. doi:10.1016/j.maturitas.2012.10.010 PMID:23141547

Kalinkovich, A., & Livshits, G. (2017). Sarcopenic obesity or obese sarcopenia: A cross talk between age-associated adipose tissue and skeletal muscle inflammation as a main mechanism of the pathogenesis. *Ageing Research Reviews*, *35*, 200–221. doi:10.1016/j.arr.2016.09.008 PMID:27702700

Kim, J. S., Wilson, J. M., & Lee, S. R. (2010). Dietary implications on mechanisms of sarcopenia: Roles of protein, amino acids and antioxidants. *The Journal of Nutritional Biochemistry*, *21*(1), 1–13. doi:10.1016/j.jnutbio.2009.06.014 PMID:19800212

Landi, F., Liperoti, R., Russo, A., Giovannini, S., Tosato, M., Barillaro, C., Capoluongo, E., Bernabei, R., & Onder, G. (2013). Association of anorexia with sarcopenia in a community-dwelling elderly population: Results from the il SIRENTE study. *European Journal of Nutrition*, *52*(3), 1261–1268. doi:10.100700394-012-0437-y PMID:22923016

Li, K., Huang, T., Zheng, J., Wu, K., & Li, D. (2014). Effect of marine-derived n-3 polyunsaturated fatty acids on C-reactive protein, interleukin 6 and tumor necrosis factor α: A meta-analysis. *PLoS One*, *9*(2), e88103. doi:10.1371/journal.pone.0088103 PMID:24505395

Li, W., Yue, T., & Liu, Y. (2020). New understanding of the pathogenesis and treatment of stroke-related sarcopenia. *Biomedicine and Pharmacotherapy*, *131*, 110721. doi:10.1016/j.biopha.2020.110721 PMID:32920517

Lo, J. H. T., Yiu, T., Ong, M. T. Y., & Lee, W. Y. W. (2020). Sarcopenia: Current treatments and new regenerative therapeutic approaches. *Journal of Orthopaedic Translation*, *23*, 38–52. doi:10.1016/j.jot.2020.04.002 PMID:32489859

Malafarina, V., Uriz-Otano, F., Gil-Guerrero, L., & Iniesta, R. (2013). The anorexia of ageing: Physiopathology, prevalence, associated comorbidity and mortality. A systematic review. *Maturitas*, *74*(4), 293–302. doi:10.1016/j.maturitas.2013.01.016 PMID:23415063

Mankhong, S., Kim, S., Moon, S., Kwak, H. B., Park, D. H., & Kang, J. H. (2020). Experimental models of sarcopenia: Bridging molecular mechanism and therapeutic strategy. *Cells*, *9*(6), 1385. doi:10.3390/cells9061385 PMID:32498474

Martone, A. M., Marzetti, E., Calvani, R., Picca, A., Tosato, M., Bernabei, R., & Landi, F. (2019). Assessment of sarcopenia: From clinical practice to research. *Journal of Gerontology and Geriatrics*, *67*(1), 39–45.

Mehta, P., McAuley, D. F., Brown, M., Sanchez, E., Tattersall, R. S., & Manson, J. J. (2020). COVID-19: Consider cytokine storm syndromes and immunosuppression. *Lancet*, *395*(10229), 1033–1034. doi:10.1016/S0140-6736(20)30628-0 PMID:32192578

Mijnarends, D. M., Meijers, J. M., Halfens, R. J., ter Borg, S., Luiking, Y. C., Verlaan, S., Schoberer, D., Cruz Jentoft, A. J., van Loon, L. J. C., & Schols, J. M. (2013). Validity and reliability of tools to measure muscle mass, strength, and physical performance in community-dwelling older people: A systematic review. *Journal of the American Medical Directors Association*, *14*(3), 170–178. doi:10.1016/j.jamda.2012.10.009 PMID:23276432

Minaglia, C., Giannotti, C., Boccardi, V., Mecocci, P., Serafini, G., Odetti, P., & Monacelli, F. (2019). Cachexia and advanced dementia. *Journal of Cachexia, Sarcopenia and Muscle*, *10*(2), 263–277. doi:10.1002/jcsm.12380 PMID:30794350

Mohammed, M., & Li, J. (2022, November). Stroke-Related Sarcopenia among Two Different Developing Countries with Diverse Ethnic Backgrounds (Cross-National Study in Egypt and China). [). Multidisciplinary Digital Publishing Institute.]. *Health Care*, *10*(11), 2336. PMID:36421660

Mori, H., Kuroda, A., Ishizu, M., Ohishi, M., Takashi, Y., Otsuka, Y., Taniguchi, S., Tamaki, M., Kurahashi, K., Yoshida, S., Endo, I., Aihara, K., Funaki, M., Akehi, Y., & Matsuhisa, M. (2019). Association of accumulated advanced glycation end-products with a high prevalence of sarcopenia and dynapenia in patients with type 2 diabetes. *Journal of Diabetes Investigation*, *10*(5), 1332–1340. doi:10.1111/jdi.13014 PMID:30677242

Na, W., Kim, J., Chung, B. H., Jang, D. J., & Sohn, C. (2020). Relationship between diet quality and sarcopenia in elderly Koreans: 2008–2011 Korea National Health and Nutrition Examination Survey. *Nutrition Research and Practice*, *14*(4), 352–364. doi:10.4162/nrp.2020.14.4.352 PMID:32765815

Nieuwenhuizen, W. F., Weenen, H., Rigby, P., & Hetherington, M. M. (2010). Older adults and patients in need of nutritional support: Review of current treatment options and factors influencing nutritional intake. *Clinical Nutrition (Edinburgh, Lothian)*, *29*(2), 160–169. doi:10.1016/j.clnu.2009.09.003 PMID:19828215

Ogawa, Y., Kaneko, Y., Sato, T., Shimizu, S., Kanetaka, H., & Hanyu, H. (2018). Sarcopenia and muscle functions at various stages of Alzheimer disease. *Frontiers in Neurology*, *9*, 710. doi:10.3389/fneur.2018.00710 PMID:30210435

Pagotto, V., & Silveira, E. A. (2014). Methods, diagnostic criteria, cutoff points, and prevalence of sarcopenia among older people. *TheScientificWorldJournal*, *2014*, 2014. doi:10.1155/2014/231312 PMID:25580454

Peterson, S. J., & Mozer, M. (2017). Differentiating sarcopenia and cachexia among patients with cancer. *Nutrition in Clinical Practice*, *32*(1), 30–39. doi:10.1177/0884533616680354 PMID:28124947

Robinson, S., Cooper, C., & Sayer, A. A. (2017). Nutrition and sarcopenia: a review of the evidence and implications for preventive strategies. *Clinical Nutrition and Aging*, 3-15.

Robinson, S. M., Reginster, J. Y., Rizzoli, R., Shaw, S. C., Kanis, J. A., Bautmans, I., Bischoff-Ferrari, H., Bruyère, O., Cesari, M., Dawson-Hughes, B., Fielding, R. A., Kaufman, J. M., Landi, F., Malafarina, V., Rolland, Y., van Loon, L. J., Vellas, B., Visser, M., Cooper, C., ... Rueda, R. (2018). Does nutrition play a role in the prevention and management of sarcopenia? *Clinical Nutrition (Edinburgh, Lothian)*, *37*(4), 1121–1132. doi:10.1016/j.clnu.2017.08.016 PMID:28927897

Semba, R. D., Ferrucci, L., Sun, K., Walston, J., Varadhan, R., Guralnik, J. M., & Fried, L. P. (2007). Oxidative stress and severe walking disability among older women. *The American Journal of Medicine*, *120*(12), 1084–1089. doi:10.1016/j.amjmed.2007.07.028 PMID:18060930

Siervo, M., Oggioni, C., Jakovljevic, D. G., Trenell, M., Mathers, J. C., Houghton, D., Celis-Morales, C., Ashor, A. W., Ruddock, A., Ranchordas, M., Klonizakis, M., & Williams, E. A. (2016). Dietary nitrate does not affect physical activity or outcomes in healthy older adults in a randomized, cross-over trial. *Nutrition Research (New York, N.Y.)*, *36*(12), 1361–1369. doi:10.1016/j.nutres.2016.11.004 PMID:27890482

Tosato, M., Marzetti, E., Cesari, M., Savera, G., Miller, R. R., Bernabei, R., Landi, F., & Calvani, R. (2017). Measurement of muscle mass in sarcopenia: From imaging to biochemical markers. *Aging Clinical and Experimental Research*, *29*(1), 19–27. doi:10.100740520-016-0717-0 PMID:28176249

Wakimoto, P., & Block, G. (2001). Dietary intake, dietary patterns, and changes with age: An epidemiological perspective. *The Journals of Gerontology. Series A, Biological Sciences and Medical Sciences*, *56*(suppl_2), 65–80. doi:10.1093/gerona/56.suppl_2.65 PMID:11730239

Walrand, S., Guillet, C., Salles, J., Cano, N., & Boirie, Y. (2011). Physiopathological mechanism of sarcopenia. *Clinics in Geriatric Medicine, 27*(3), 365–385. doi:10.1016/j.cger.2011.03.005 PMID:21824553

Yanai, H. (2015). Nutrition for sarcopenia. *Journal of Clinical Medicine Research, 7*(12), 926–931. doi:10.14740/jocmr2361w PMID:26566405

Ye, L., Wen, Y., Chen, Y., Yao, J., Li, X., Liu, Y., Song, J., & Sun, Z. (2020). Diagnostic reference values for sarcopenia in Tibetans in China. *Scientific Reports, 10*(1), 3067. doi:10.103841598-020-60027-0 PMID:32080301

Yin, M., Zhang, H., Liu, Q., Ding, F., Deng, Y., Hou, L., Wang, H., Yue, J., & He, Y. (2021). Diagnostic performance of clinical laboratory indicators with sarcopenia: Results from the west China health and aging trend study. *Frontiers in Endocrinology, 12*, 785045. doi:10.3389/fendo.2021.785045 PMID:34956096

Yokoyama, Y., Kitamura, A., Seino, S., Kim, H., Obuchi, S., Kawai, H., Hirano, H., Watanabe, Y., Motokawa, K., Narita, M., & Shinkai, S. (2021). Association of nutrient-derived dietary patterns with sarcopenia and its components in community-dwelling older Japanese: A cross-sectional study. *Nutrition Journal, 20*(1), 1–10. doi:10.118612937-021-00665-w PMID:33461556

Zamboni, M., Mazzali, G., Brunelli, A., Saatchi, T., Urbani, S., Giani, A., Rossi, A. P., Zoico, E., & Fantin, F. (2022). The Role of Crosstalk between Adipose Cells and Myocytes in the Pathogenesis of Sarcopenic Obesity in the Elderly. *Cells, 11*(21), 3361. doi:10.3390/cells11213361 PMID:36359757

Chapter 8
Ear, Nose, and Throat Complications and Challenges in the Elderly With Multimorbidity

Samuel Oluyomi Ayodele

iD https://orcid.org/0000-0002-1703-6427
Obafemi Awolowo Teaching Hospital Complex, Nigeria

EXECUTIVE SUMMARY

Elderly patients will not only present to specialists with specific ear, nose, and throat (ENT) complaints but will also seek treatment for comorbidities that have significant impacts on their quality of life; as well as the prognosis of the specific disease being managed the specialist with an increased demand on health care resources. While the principles of management of ENT disorders in the elderly are not so different from what is obtainable for other age groups, it is very important to take note of the specific differences and apply individualized treatment plan for better outcome. ENT diseases in the elderly may also present with unexpected or uncommon symptoms and this will mean that management must be carried out with caution. Medication dosage, performance scale, extent of surgical operations, and other treatment modalities are considerable in management of elderly ones. Subtle complaints from the elderly should not be over looked or managed by unqualified personnel. They should be referred early to specialists for proper management.

DOI: 10.4018/978-1-6684-2354-7.ch008

INTRODUCTION

An Ear, Nose and Throat (ENT) Specialist otherwise known as an Otolaryngologist—Head and Neck Surgeon plays a very important role in the evaluation, diagnosis and treatment of ENT/ Head and Neck related diseases for various age groups, (AAO—HNSF, 2006). An informed population of elderly patients will not only present to specialists with specific illnesses (for example, hearing problems, middle ear infection, sinusitis, and upper respiratory tract infections, head and neck tumours among others) but will also seek treatment for medical conditions/comorbidities that have a significant impact on their quality of life of the individual patient as well as the prognosis of the specific disease being managed by an ENT specialist, (AAO—HNSF, 2006).

Multimorbidity among the elderly has been found to be a public health matter of concern worldwide. It can be defined as the co-occurrence of a minimum of two chronic diseases in an individual. It is generally associated with increased mortality, poor quality of life, and an increased demand on health-care resources, (Sara, Chowdhury, & Haque, 2018). Coincidentally, there has been a considerable increase in the elderly population requiring hospital visit and many of the co-morbidities only surfaced at their old ages, (AAO—HNSF, 2006) (Sara et al., 2018). Common comorbidities seen among ENT elderly patients include but not limited to systemic hypertension, arthritis, type II diabetes mellitus, and cardiopulmonary diseases, thyroid disorders, hyperlipidemia, vitamin D deficiency and renal disorders, (Adegbiji, Aremu, & Aluko, 2019; Mohammad & Muhammad, 2017; Sreenivas, Natashya, & Sumy, 2021). ENT complications as well as challenges associated with managing an elderly patient presenting with ENT features with background co-morbidities have become a center of a never-ending discussion in various specialties.

PECULIARITIES OF OLD AGE AND MULTIMORBIDITY

Geriatric otorhinolaryngologic diseases or disorders are common clinical problems encountered in ENT practices generally. Due to the events of aging, cognitive impairment and associated comorbid diseases, there may be alteration of the disease presentation. That is, all these may make it difficult for elderly patients to provide an accurate history with resultant difficulty in arriving at accurate diagnosis for the best and appropriate treatment, (Adegbiji et al., 2019).

Generally, illnesses in the elderly usually present with unexpected or uncommon symptoms and medical therapy may be hard to administer because of possible drug-drug interaction resulting from a combination of essential medications. Old age with the presence of multimorbidity must also be put into consideration when performing surgical procedures in the elderly. Although, age should not always be an obstacle to carrying out indicated surgical procedure on them, (AAO—HNSF, 2006). While not inherently impaired, the reserve capacity of the older individual to compensate for stress, metabolic derangement, and drug metabolism is increasingly limited because with aging, organs in the body, such as the heart, kidneys, liver, lungs, and brain losses mass and functional disability occurs faster with associated longer time to remediate, necessitating early preventive interventions, (Oskvig, 1999). Other than comorbidities, other factors that a likely to influence elderly patients response to ENT diseases and treatment includes but not limited to the wear and tear occurred throughout the their active age from exposure to loud noise (especially occupational noise), overuse of the voice, and cumulative effect of infections (be it viral, bacterial or fungal origin) or infestations as well as the effect of substance use like hard drugs, alcohol, and tobacco etc. Some older people are affected more than others, (Kaylie, 2022). Frailty is the most problematic manifestation of old age, is a consequence of cumulative decline in many physiological systems during a lifetime. This cumulative decline depletes homoeostatic reserves until minor stressor events trigger disproportionate changes in health status, (Clegg, Young, Iliffe, Rikkert, & Rockwood, 2013). In most aging societies managing frailty has become a priority for health systems, (Orfila et al., 2022).

Common reasons for presentation of elderly patients into an ENT emergency room includes trauma from falls, impaction of foreign bodies like denture, steaks etc., ENT infection/inflammation, vocal disorders, head and neck benign/ malignant tumors and aesthetic problems linked to degenerative changes in the body, and immunosuppressed problems and so on. Common diseases identified in various studies were sinonasal tumor, earwax impaction, otitis externa, pharyngotonsillitis and pharyngeal tumor. This leads to the common clinical presentation of pain of various degrees, hearing loss, tinnitus, balance disorders nasal blockage and discharge, nasal bleeding, dysphagia, breathing difficulties among others, (Adegbiji et al., 2019) (Clegg et al., 2013) (Lunedo, Sass, Gomes, Kanashiro, & Bortolon, 2008). It is worthy of note that there is really no specific or special treatment outline for ENT management of elderly other than what is used across board. However, treatment outcomes may differ if management of elderly patients are not individualized and comorbidities not considered in the management plan.

THE EAR

A wide range of age-specific changes as well as common ear diseases occur in elderly patients. In studies that looked at ontological diseases among the elderly patients revealed a high prevalence of ear diseases with a figure as high as 49.3% of the participants suffering from various ear diseases out of which 37% hearing impaired cases was detected. In addition, 9.4% and 2.9% of the elderly patients presented with otitis media and otitis externa respectively, (Alenezi et al., 2017) (Sogebi, 2013). The prevalence and severity of an atrophy of the tensor veli palatini muscle and calcifications of the Eustachian tube (ET) cartilage were revealed and noted to increase with age in a research work where the temporal bones of younger adult were compared with that of the elderly patients, (Tsuji et al., 2000). Another study also found that the functional compliance of the ET worsens with aging. The prevalence of Eustachian tube dysfunction (ETD) is therefore likely to be more and difficult to treat among the elderly, (Ologe, Segun-Busari, Abdulraheem, & Afolabi, 2005).

In terms of both complications and prognosis of otologic surgeries among the elderly, there has been diverse findings in numerous studies. However, studies have shown that age is not a contraindication to ear surgeries. Specifically, no significant difference has been found in the success of graft take after tympanoplasty when elder patients were compared with other younger patients, (Ologe et al., 2005).

Cerumen Auris

Cerumen impaction is one of the common causes of earache, sensation of blockage, tinnitus. and conductive hearing loss in elderly patients worldwide. Risk factors that increases production and impaction of cerumen particularly among the elderly include the presence of ear canal long strands of hairs, constant use of hearing aids, narrowing of the external auditory canal (EAC) following bony growths secondary to exophysis or osteoma formation, persistently increased pH of the EAC especially among those living with diabetes, (Ologe et al., 2005) (Meador, 1995).

In a hospital based study, (Ologe et al., 2005) 30% of elderly patient were found to have impacted cerumen auris over a period of one year with a dramatic improvement in hearing ability in 75% of the ears after cerumen removal. This has helped to avert serious psychosocial withdrawal effects due to the resultant conductive hearing loss. It is also very important to note that removal of cerumen should be carefully carried out by an ENT trained health worker. Due to the possible friability of the EAC skin, inexperienced hands can evoke an inadvertent damage to the canal or ear drum exposing the patient to otitis externa and/or media, (Ologe et al., 2005).

Hearing Ability

It is an established fact that hair cells and neurons in the inner ear do not regenerate or increase in number. The inner ear is known to be sensitive to gradual alterations resulting from age and a gradual loss in the number of hair cells with increasing age has also been reported, (Iwasaki & Yamasoba, 2015) (Albernaz, 2014). While some individuals maintain good hearing ability throughout their lifetime, presbycusis is also common among the elderly due to the general auditory changes that result from increasing age. Presbycusis can also be described as a direct consequence of the worsening rigidity of the inner ear membranes/ outer hair cells, the decreased speed of transmission of vestibulocochlear nerve impulses and the degeneration of the auditory pathway in the central nervous system. Other auditory disorders can be tied to vascular, autoimmune, or metabolic diseases as comorbidities, (Albernaz, 2014). Finding on pure tone audiometry is usually in keeping with descending audiometric curves at high frequencies which is commonly seen in presbycusis, (Mohammad & Muhammad, 2017). Studies have consistently shown a 30% to 70% incidence of age-related hearing loss but widely variable assessment of the degree of impairment induced by the hearing loss. In a nutshell, the degree of hearing loss increases with increasing age and is more prevalent in geriatric patients, (Mohammad & Muhammad, 2017) (Albernaz, 2014). In a research work on the hearing outcomes and complications of cochlear implantation (CI) in elderly patients, Kanai et al (2021) submitted that age alone should not be a contraindication to CI surgery which is known to be a very safe procedure for elderly patients when comorbidities are managed appropriately. They found that a CI can provide good speech recognition in elderly patients and that they are likely to continue to use the CI for a long period of time, considering their average life expectancy. Kanai et al (2021) also noted that the proportion of patients with comorbidities was higher in the elderly when compared to the younger ones. There were very low incidence of CI complications leading to deterioration of general health status or requiring removal of the CI in elderly patients.

Vestibular Activity

Balance disorders, though probably as common as auditory problems in elderly persons, are complex and have not been as fully studied. A large percentage of balance disorders can be attributed to cardiovascular disease, neurologic disease, or medication effects, but a significant number can nonetheless be ascribed to disorders of the peripheral vestibular system. Research done on temporal bone have shown that there is an age-related decline in both vestibular sensory and ganglion cells. Type I hair cells show a significant decline in the cristae, whereas type II hair cells are lost in both the cristae and the macular organs. There is also a decline of vestibular ganglion cells with age, (Tsuji et al., 2000).

About 20% of elderly patient has experienced vestibular disorder which presented early with intermittent, recurrent and simile harmless symptoms. The usual differential diagnosis of vestibular disorders includes benign paroxysmal positional vertigo (BPPV), Meniere's disease, vestibular neuritis, labyrinthitis acoustic neuroma.

BPPV is the most common cause of vertigo worldwide, with an increased prevalence in elderly patents due to degenerative changes in the inner ear. In addition to age, other risk factors includes osteoporosis and osteopenia, (Sogebi, Ariba, Otulana, & Osalusi, 2014) (Le & Marrone, 2017). The vestibular disorders in elderly can lead to fear of falling, which in turn lead to sedentary lifestyle with resultant decreasing strength and balance and further exacerbates fall risk in a vicious cycle, (Iwasaki & Yamasoba, 2015) (Le & Marrone, 2017).

Although the standard and most effective test to evaluate BPPV is the Dix-Hallpike maneuver, however, there are several contraindications and protective measures which should be occasionally taken note of when managing an elderly patient. The risk of vascular compromise and stroke should be always considered in elderly patients with vascular disease. It would be appropriate to use slow mild movements and avoid sudden fast movements and hyperextension of the head in handling them, (Balatsouras, Koukoutsis, Fassolis, Moukos, & Apris, 2018). Care should also be taken in patients with comorbidities like cervical spinal stenosis, cervical radiculopathy kyphoscoliosis, limited cervical motion, lower back pain and dysfunction, morbid obesity, and advanced rheumatoid arthritis, which may exist more frequently in older people with balancing disorder, (Balatsouras et al., 2018).

Sreenivas et al (2021) revealed that the presence of comorbidities will worsen the status of BPPV, causing more frequent otolith detachment and multiple episodes of vertigo even after several successful repositioning maneuver. Hence, patients presenting with vestibular disorder should have careful and detailed history, neurotologic examination, laboratory testing, imaging and treated for the comorbidities along with the management of vertigo (Albernaz, 2014). The careful selection of a drug regimen depends on an equally careful diagnosis (Albernaz, 2014). Though, labyrinthine sedatives are part of the treatment medications but vertigo still tends to recur. This also reinforce the need for specialized comprehensive geriatric care and practice, (Sogebi et al., 2014). Dietary changes should also be useful in correcting metabolic problems secondary to poor eating habits. In addition, vestibular rehabilitation is very useful in the treatment of vestibular disorders preventing falls and maintaining a good quality of life, particularly in elderly patients, (Albernaz, 2014).

Ear Infections

Infection is a significant cause of morbidity among our elderly patients. Of these, chronic suppurative otitis media (CSOM) is distinctively most common while acute otitis media, and malignant otitis externa only occur commonly in the presence of immunocompromised state, (Ologe et al., 2005). It is advisable that early detection of ear infection, proper and adequate evaluation and focused treatment will greatly enhance the ontological wellbeing of older people and alleviate the burdens of chronicity of ear infection and improve quality of life of the elderly, (Ologe et al., 2005). One of the important means of preventing ear infection is to continually manage the predisposing comorbidities like Type II diabetes mellitus and immunosuppression. Medical treatment may be a little prolonged with antibiotics use based on microscopy, culture, and sensitivity results.

THE NOSE AND PARANASAL SINUSES

There are modifications and alterations in the structure and functions of the nose and paranasal sinuses following aging which predisposes older people to diseases and recurrent needs to present at ENT Clinics. Generally, the nasal cavity and the adjoining sinuses serves there main function: respiration, olfaction and immunity. The septal cartilage of the nose continues to weaken and may deviate from the midline in the elderly, resulting into septal collapse, drooping of the nasal tip and reduction in the cavities of the nose. There is a resultant restriction in nasal airflow, particularly around the anterior nasal valve, (Edelstein, 1996). As this process progresses with age, it can result into recurrent complaints of nasal blockage and other nasal symptoms like facial pressure, recurrent nasal crusting, hyposmia (reduction in the sense of smell) or parosmia (distortion in the sense of smell) etc. Elderly people are also exposed to allergens and can develop symptoms suggestive of allergic rhinitis like any other person in their environment. Comorbidities and chronic use of medications have their various effects on the disease pattern and management process of elderly clients, (Kaylie, 2022). Although studies done on the effect of type II diabetes mellitus on chronic rhinosinusitis (CRS) showed that Type II diabetes is not a determinant or predictor of sinonasal outcome in CRS patients, (Zhang et al., 2014) (Ayodele, Olarinoye, Alabi, & Ologe, 2020).

Again, it is worthy of note that the process and pattern of evaluation, diagnosis, and treatment of nasal problems in elderly does not totally deviate from that of the other age groups. Be that as it may, there are some specific considerations in the elderly. Basically, management of diseases of the nose needs to be individualized and medications should be dose specific for patients in their age bracket to measure up with their metabolic capability and possibilities of treatment failure or adverse/side effects and drug interactions. Therefore, the use of over-the-counter medications is completely prohibited among the elderly and early referral to an ENT specialist centre is advised.

Rhinosinusitis

Elderly patients with rhinosinusitis typically present with complaints recurrent nasal blockage, nasal congestion, and postnasal drips. Other associated symptoms include facial headaches, a constant need to clear the throat, pharyngitis, decreased sense of smell and taste, cough, fatigue, dental pain fever, halitosis, and otologic symptoms like ear fullness and tinnitus. Sometimes, the clinical features might be subtle and the condition difficult to diagnosed. The most important clinical clue to the diagnosis of acute rhinosinusitis is the continuation of symptoms after usual exposure to cold has subsided. In cases of CRS, there is often a distinct lack of symptoms, although most patients will have nasal obstruction and purulent post-nasal drip, (Knutson & Slavin, 1995) These clinical features tends to occur for a long time with a need to go in and out of the hospital constantly. Due to the chronicity, they present more with dryness of the nasal cavities filled with crust and debris other than the usual thick mucopurulent discharge and redness of the nasal mucosa found in CRS. Dehydration from poor fluid intake or side effects of medications while treat chronic comorbidities has been implicated, (Edelstein, 1996) The diagnosis is confirmed with a computed tomography scan (CTS) of the paranasal sinuses and diagnostic nasal endoscopy, (Fokkens et al., 2020) Based on diverse factors, some present with nasal polyps (CRSwNP) and some without (CRSsNP). Knutson and Slavin (1995) noted that CRS in elderly patients present itself with more of subtle clinical features. They noted that in cases where CRS is associated with lower airway problems, if sinusitis is properly managed, the treatment of asthma will surely improve.

The goal of treatment is to eradicate infection with clearance of the infected material from the nose and sinuses. While the use of an appropriate antibiotic is necessary, the use of ancillary therapy is also of great importance, and it includes steam inhalation nasal irrigation with isotonic saline, decongestants, and topical corticosteroid. They are given in order to reduce nasal obstruction, increase the size of sinus ostia, promote improved mucociliary function, decrease mucosal inflammation and thin secretions, (Knutson & Slavin, 1995) Early endoscopic assisted with minimally invasive access surgical intervention is advisable in the elderly especially in those who failed to respond to aggressive medical treatment. Functional endoscopic sinus surgery will help to provide relief and improved quality of life by opening up the blocked sinuses and reactivate mucociliary functions, (Knutson & Slavin, 1995) A result of endoscopic sinus surgery for CRS revealed that elderly patients made up of 15% of the patient population with a higher incidence of complications but with a final outcomes that were comparable to those of the other age groups, (Jiang & Hsu, 2001). Structural abnormalities which is likely predisposing them to sinus infection and relapse of treatment could be addressed surgically as well.

Sense of Smell and Taste

Olfactory sensitivity has been found to reduce gradually with aging. This can be related to degeneration of the sensory cell loss in the olfactory mucosa, along with a general deterioration in both peripheral and central olfactory pathways, (Boyce & Shone, 2006). Even in the absence of multimorbidity, the olfactory receptor neurons undergo apoptosis at a baseline rate peculiar to each person with ability for regular replacement of apoptotic cells, (Boyce & Shone, 2006). Consecutively, the decline in the sense of smell also affects the sense of taste so that foods sometimes do not taste the same way, (Kaylie, 2022). Unfortunately, when elderly people suffer smell and taste disorders, they are likely not taken serious and their symptoms overlooked. Distortion of smell function is a risk factor for increased exposure to accidental gas poisonings and explosions that can endanger their safety. Decreased smell and taste can also result into appetite suppression resulting in nutritional problems and damaged immunity which can further result to declining health state and deteriorated quality of life, (Boyce & Shone, 2006) There is also a tendency for elderly ones to have a higher content of salt and sugar in their daily diet which can worsen their comorbid conditions, (Boyce & Shone, 2006) (Winkler, Garg, Mekayarajjananonth, Bakaeen, & Khan, 1999).

Management of distortion of smell and taste will involve detailed counseling and reassurance to allay fear about the possible causes, consequences, and treatment plan. Relatives, family members or near neighbors will be advised to give a closer monitoring to prevent ingestion of spoiled food or in cases of burning of home appliances. Visual stimulating gas detector will be good for those using gas cookers. Elderly patients can develop loss of appetite following the declining taste and smell perception, (Winkler et al., 1999). They should therefore be encouraged to add seasonings (natural flavor enhancers as supplement) to their food instead of relying on excessive consumption of salt and sugar to give their food flavor. Adequate nutrition, tongue cleaning and smoking cessation are recommended for those with dental problems (Winkler et al., 1999). Research works on flavor enhancement in management of elderly people with smell and taste disorder revealed an improvement in their immune status and increase in the rate of salivary IgA (Boyce & Shone, 2006) (Winkler et al., 1999).

THE THROAT

Common problems seen in the laryngopharyngeal region in the elderly includes acute and chronic laryngitis, pharyngitis, laryngopharyngeal reflux disease, nonspecific dysphonia, swallowing disorders, and laryngeal lesions. Voice disorders, for example, affect all ages, but some findings have been linked with higher risks in the extreme of ages. A large national database study, (Roy, Kim, Courey, & Cohen, 2016), on voice disorder showed that the prevalence rate of dysphonia in the treatment-seeking elderly population was 1.3% among those aged 60 to 69 years and 2.5% among patients above 70 years. In another study that studied non–treatment seeking elderly participants reported that 47% had a voice disorder during their lifetime and 29% were actively experiencing hoarseness, (Roy, Stemple, Merrill, & Thomas, 2007.) Similarly, another study found about 20% of elder patients presenting with voice disorders associated with problems with quality of life changes, (Stachler et al., 2018).

Voice Disorders

A basic description of age-related voice changes is related to the alteration in the pitch, frequency and loudness of voice. With increase in age, the fundamental frequency of the male voice increases while that of female gender decreases. Estimated subglottic pressure increases with increasing age. The voice onset time also was found to become prolonged with age, (Higgins & Saxman, 1991). The tissues in the larynx may become more stiffen, affecting the pitch and quality of the voice with resultant hoarseness. Studies (Higgins & Saxman, 1991; Tafiadis et al., 2019; Woo, Casper, Colton, & Brewer, 1992) on the histologic changes in aging vocal cords have shown fatty degeneration of the muscles of the larynx, and fiber density and elastin fibers in the vocal folds decrease. There is increasing ossification of the larynx with aging which also alters the elastic and biomechanical properties of the vocal cords. Woo et al (1992) reviewed the case notes of elderly patients who presented to their clinic with complaints of hoarseness. They found cases of vocal cord abnormalities following aging and others with resultant effects from their comorbid conditions like those related to central nervous system dysfunction (such as stroke, Parkinson's disease), neoplastic vocal cord lesions, granulomatous diseases, or vocal cord paralysis.

Swallowing Problems

Total swallowing time and time to initiation of oropharyngeal swallowing has been noticed to be prolonged with advanced age. A series of elderly volunteers without swallowing problems were examined by laryngoscopy and fluoroscopy and were found to require a much larger pharyngeal bolus to initiate swallowing, (Shaker et al., 1994). Normal aging does not appear to result in problems with the coordination of swallowing and protective deglutitive vocal cord closure; however, pressure sensitivity in the supraglottic region of elder people appears to decrease with aging and the loss of sensory function may contribute both to difficulty in swallowing and aspiration in the elderly, (Aviv, 1997). Age related changes in the lining of the pharynx has also been related with gradual loss of pharyngeal phase of swallowing mechanism resulting into aspiration. If aspiration become severe or persistent, it could cause bronchopneumonia, (Kaylie, 2022).

THE HEAD AND NECK

The effect of aging on head and neck region and surgical treatment of head and neck tumours has been reported in research papers. The most common surgical complications that have been assessed include mortality rate, postoperative haemorrhage, postoperative urinary tract infection, pneumonia, pulmonary embolus, myocardial infarction, and postoperative wound infection. Disease progression and treatment outcome have shown controversial findings among the elderly when compared with other age ranges. In a series of patients with recurrence of tongue cancer post radiotherapy, age at tumor presentation was found to be significant in determining outcome. Older men were statistically more likely to have shorter survival than age-matched women or the younger ones, (Llewelyn & Mitchell, 1997). McGuirt and Davis (1995) revealed a raised incidence of complications in head and neck cancer patients aged 80 years and above but they also found similar prognosis in terms of survival rate and restoration of function when compared with younger patients. They also noted that age does not appear to have an effect on the sensitivity of the head and neck cancers to radiotherapy. In another retrospective study of patients who had total laryngectomy, old age was not found to be a contributing factor for postoperative complications. Conversely, patients older than 70 have been showed to demonstrate a higher tendency of developing a second primary neoplasm after treatment of laryngeal cancer. Another study that looked at post laryngectomy patients revealed a pronounced decrease in long-term expiratory function in patients over the age of sixty five, (Nilsson, Ekberg, Olsson, & Hindfelt, 1996).

Age is an important predictor for the risk of death attributable to comorbid disease. Therefore, it is logical to combine age and multimorbidity into a prognosticating head and neck cancers staging system as a predictor of survival or mortality. Elderly patients have more overall comorbidities though, there was no improvement in the prognostic capability, when incorporating age variations to the Charlson comorbidity index (CCI). The study thereby suggests that the CCI is an independent predictor of tumor specific survival. Comorbidity may serve as an indicator of the host's immunologic status. This further supports the concept that comorbidity may have an impact on the behavior of head and neck tumors. More studies are needed to confirm the influence of comorbidity on survival rates, and to combine its effects with the Tumor, Nodal and distal Metastasis (TNM) staging system for a more accurate prediction of over patient survival. (Charlson, Pompei, Ales, & MacKenzie, 1987) (Sabin, Rosenfeld, Sundaram, Har-EI, & Lucente, 1999).

CONCLUSION

Aging affects the function of the ears, nose, and throat in varying degrees with greater possibility of exposure to ENT diseases at that older age especially when there are associated multimobidities. Accumulated effects of regular exposure to loud noise, abuse of the voice, various infections in the past and use of hard substances has been implicated. While the principles of management of ENT disorders in the elderly are not so different from what is obtainable for other age groups, it is very important to take note of the specific differences in the pathophysiology of ENT diseases in older age group and apply individualized treatment plan for better outcome and improved quality of life, knowing fully well that some older people are affected more than others. Dose of medications, ability to withstand stress, frailty, performance score, length of surgical operations and other modalities of treatment among other factors are considerable in management of elderly ones. Subtle complaints from elderly patients should not be over looked or managed by unqualified personnel. They should be referred early to specialists in multidiscipline centres for proper management.

REFERENCES

AAO—HNSF. (2006). *Geriatric Care Otolaryngology.*

Adegbiji, W. A., Aremu, S. K., & Aluko, A. A. A. (2019). Geriatric Otorhinolaryngology, Head and Neck Emergency in a Nigerian Teaching Hospital, Ado Ekiti. *International Journal of Otolaryngology and Head & Neck Surgery.*, *8*(3), 81–90.

Albernaz, P. L. M. (2014). Vertigo in elderly patients: A review of 164 cases in Brazil. *Ear, Nose, and Throat Journal*, *93*(8), 322–330.

Alenezi, N. G., Alenazi, A. A., Elboraei, Y. A. E., Alanazi, T. H., Alruwaili, A. K., Alanazi, A. S., ... Alanazi, A. F. (2017). Ear diseases and factors associated with ear infections among the elderly attending hospital in Arar city, Northern Saudi Arabia. *Electronic Physician*, *9*(9), 5304–5309.

Aviv, J. E. (1997). Effects of aging on sensitivity of the pharyngeal and supraglottic areas. *The American Journal of Medicine*, *103*, 74S–76S.

Ayodele, S. O., Olarinoye, J. K., Alabi, B. S., & Ologe, F. E. (2020). Comparison of Nasoendoscopic Findings and Quality of Life between Type II Diabetics and Non-Diabetics with Chronic Rhinosinusitis. *ARC Journal of Diabetes and Endocrinology, 6*(1), 14–21. doi:10.20431/2455-5983.0601003

Balatsouras, D. G., Koukoutsis, G., Fassolis, A., Moukos, A., & Apris, A. (2018). Benign paroxysmal positional vertigo in the elderly: Current insights. *Clinical Interventions in Aging, 13*, 2251–2266.

Boyce, J. M., & Shone, G. R. (2006). Effects of ageing on smell and taste. *Postgraduate Medical Journal, 82*, 239–241.

Charlson, M. E., Pompei, P., Ales, K. L., & MacKenzie, C. R. (1987). A new method of classifying prognostic comorbidity in longitudinal studies: Development and validation. *Journal of Chronic Diseases, 40*, 373–383.

Clegg, A., Young, J., Iliffe, S., Rikkert, M. O., & Rockwood, K. (2013). Frailty in elderly people. *Lancet, 381*(9868), 752–762.

Edelstein, D. R. (1996). Aging of the normal nose in adults. *The Laryngoscope, 106*, 1–25.

Fokkens, W. J., Lund, V. J., Hopkins, C., Hellings, P. W., Kern, R., Reitsma, S., & Zwetsloot, C. P. (2020). European Position Paper on Rhinosinusitis and Nasal Polyps 2020. *Rhinology, 58*(Suppl 29), 1–464.

Higgins, M. B., & Saxman, J. H. (1991). A comparison of selected phonatory behaviors of healthy aged and young adults. *Journal of Speech and Hearing Research, 34*, 1000–1010.

Iwasaki, S., & Yamasoba, T. (2015). Dizziness and Imbalance in the Elderly: Age-related Decline in the Vestibular System. *Aging and Disease, 6*(1), 38–47.

Jiang, R. S., & Hsu, C. Y. (2001). Endoscopic sinus surgery for the treatment of chronic sinusitis in geriatric patients. *Ear, Nose, and Throat Journal, 80*, 230–232.

Kanai, R., Kanemaru, S., Tamura, K. N., Umezawa, N., Yoshida, M., Miwa, T., & Kumazawa, A. (2021). Hearing Outcomes and Complications of Cochlear Implantation in Elderly Patients over 75 Years of Age. *Journal of Clinical Medicine, 10*, 3123.

Kaylie, D. M. (2022). *Effects of Aging on the Ears*. Nose, and Throat.

Knutson, J. W., & Slavin, R. G. (1995). Sinusitis in the Aged. *Drugs & Aging, 7*, 310–316.

Le, G. N., & Marrone, N. (2017). Age-Related Vestibular Disorders: Implications for Older Adult Patients. Arizona.

Llewelyn, J., & Mitchell, R. (1997). Survival of patients who needed salvage surgery for recurrence after radiotherapy for oral carcinoma. *British Journal of Oral & Maxillofacial Surgery, 35*, 424–428.

Lunedo, S. M. C., Sass, S. M. G., Gomes, A. B., Kanashiro, K., & Bortolon, L. (2008). The Prevalence of the Major ENT Symptoms in an Ambulatorial Geriatric Population. *International Archives of Otorhinolaryngology, 12*(1), 95–98.

McGuirt, W. F., & Davis, S. P. (1995). Demographic portrayal and outcome analysis of head and neck cancer surgery in the elderly. *Archives of Otolaryngology—Head & Neck Surgery, 121*, 150–154.

Meador, J. A. (1995). Cerumen impaction in the elderly. *Journal of Gerontological Nursing, 21*(12), 43–45.

Mohammad, A., & Muhammad, S. A. (2017). Audiologic Pattern in Elderly Patients: A Tertiary Care Experience. *International Journal of Open Access Otolaryngology, 1*(1), 1–5.

Nilsson, H., Ekberg, O., Olsson, R., & Hindfelt, B. (1996). Quantitative assessment of oral and pharyngeal function in Parkinson's disease. *Dysphagia, 11*, 144–150.

Ologe, F. E., Segun-Busari, S., Abdulraheem, I. S., & Afolabi, A. O. (2005). Ear Diseases in Elderly Hospital Patients in Nigeria. *The Journals of Gerontology. Series A, Biological Sciences and Medical Sciences, 60A*(3), 404–406.

Orfila, F., Carrasco-Ribelles, L. A., Abellana, R., Roso-Llorach, A., Cegri, F., Reyes, C., & Reyes, F. (2022). Validation of an electronic frailty index with electronic health records: eFRAGICAP index. *BMC Geriatrics, 22*(1), 404.

Oskvig, R. M. (1999). Special Problems in the Elderly. *Chest Journal, 115*(5), 158S–164S.

Roy, N., Kim, J., Courey, M., & Cohen, S. M. (2016). Voice disorders in the elderly: A national database study. *The Laryngoscope, 126*, 421–428.

Roy, N., Stemple, J. C., Merrill, R. M., & Thomas, L. (2007). Epidemiology of voice disorders in the elderly: Preliminary findings. *The Laryngoscope, 117*, 628–633.

Sabin, S. L., Rosenfeld, R. M., Sundaram, K., Har-EI, G., & Lucente, F. E. (1999). The impact of comorbidity and age on survival with laryngeal cancer. *Ear, Nose, and Throat Journal, 78*(8), 578–584.

Sara, H. H., Chowdhury, M. A. B., & Haque, M. A. (2018). Multimorbidity among elderly in Bangladesh. *Aging Medicine*, *1*(3), 267–275.

Shaker, R., Ren, J., Zamir, Z., Sarna, A., Liu, J., & Sui, Z. (1994). Effect of aging, position, and temperature on the threshold volume triggering pharyngeal swallows. *Gastroenterology*, *107*(2), 396–402.

Sogebi, O. A. (2013). Profile of ear diseases among elderly patients in Sagamu, South-Western Nigeria. *Nigerian Journal of Medicine*, *22*(3), 257.

Sogebi, O. A., Ariba, A. J., Otulana, T. O., & Osalusi, B. S. (2014). Vestibular disorders in elderly patients: Characteristics, causes and consequences. *The Pan African Medical Journal*, *19*, 146.

Sreenivas, V., Natashya, H. S., & Sumy, P. (2021). The Role of Comorbidities in Benign Paroxysmal Positional Vertigo. *Ear, Nose, and Throat Journal*, *100*(5), NP225–NP230.

Stachler, R. J., Francis, D. O., Schwartz, S. R., Damask, C. C., Digoy, G. P., Krouse, H. J., & McCoy, S. J. (2018). Clinical Practice Guideline: Hoarseness (Dysphonia) (Update). *Otolaryngology - Head and Neck Surgery*, *00*(0), 1–42.

Tafiadis, D., Chronopoulos, S. K., Helidoni, M. E., Kosma, E. I., Voniati, L., & Papadopoulos, P. … Velegrakis, G. A. (2019). Checking for voice disorders without clinical intervention : The Greek and global VHI thresholds for voice disordered patients. *Scientific Reports, 9*, 1–9. doi:10.1038/s41598-019-45758-z

Tsuji, K., Velázquez-Villaseñor, L., Rauch, S. D., Glynn, R. J., Wall, C., & Merchant, S. N. (2000). Temporal bone studies of the human peripheral vestibular system. Aminoglycoside ototoxicity. *The Annals of Otology, Rhinology & Laryngology. Supplement*, *181*, 20–25.

Winkler, S., Garg, A. K., Mekayarajjananonth, T., Bakaeen, L. G., & Khan, E. (1999). Depressed taste and smell in geriatric patients. *The Journal of the American Dental Association*, *130*(12), 1759–1765.

Woo, P., Casper, J., Colton, R., & Brewer, D. (1992). Dysphonia in the aging: Physiology versus disease. *The Laryngoscope*, *102*, 139–144.

Zhang, Z., Adappa, N. D., Lautenbach, E., Chiu, A. G., Doghramji, L., Howland, T. J., & … . (2014). The effect of diabetes mellitus on chronic rhinosinusitis and sinus surgery outcome. *International Forum of Allergy & Rhinology*, *4*(4), 315–320.

Chapter 9
Stress and Alzheimer's Disease in Elderly Patients

Syed Zafar Sultan Rizvi
Mohammed Ali Jauhar University, India

Mohammad Akram
Aligarh Muslim University, India

Gulfisha Qureshi
Gautam Buddha University, India

Ahmad Sheraz
University of the Punjab, Pakistan

Rimsha Razzaq
University of the Punjab, Pakistan

EXECUTIVE SUMMARY

Stress is one of the main causes of various psychological and physiological changes. Those type of changes cause by excessive secretion of stress hormones like cortisol and adrenaline into the blood stream from adrenal gland in kidney. There is underline neuroendocrine pathways which carries signals from hypothalamus to pituitary gland than secretion of adrenocorticotropic hormone which ultimately stimulates the Adrenal cortex and release the Epinephrine and nor Epinephrine. When the cortisol and adrenaline level increase in blood stream. That causes the physiological changes like elevated level of blood pressure, glucose level, dilation of pupil and immunological response, as soon as, the threat is subsides this level down towards the normal. It is also a leading cause of hospitalization, especially in the elderly population. Elderly people who have comorbidities like Alzheimer's, cardiovascular disorders are more prone to wards minor stressors, it worsens their disease. It is essential to overcome the stress in elderly through various methods e.g., music therapy, social support.

DOI: 10.4018/978-1-6684-2354-7.ch009

INTRODUCTION

Nowadays, people from different age groups are suffering from various kinds of diseases ranging from mild to severe mental health issues which sometimes become the major cause of their death. Among them, due to a very nature of psycho-physiological deterioration, elderly people are always on higher risk of mental health disorder, Immunity disorders or other Neurodegenerative disorders. As per the current researches revealed that, Alzheimer's is one of the most frequently seen disease in elderly patients and it's become more troublesome if it's appears with other co-morbidities like diabetes, hypertension, CAD or other major health disorders in elder patients. Geriatric population are more prone to mental health related issues e.g. Stress disorder, depression, anxiety, Alzheimer's, schizophrenia and dementia etc. while going through this kind of diseases, they become gradually depend on other people for special care and change in life style to prevent these types of complications. Apart from the care from others there are also some protective factors that can be important for the betterment of their life. Further, it has been proven by different research studies that proper sleep, diet, exercise and positive thinking can significantly change the prognosis of disease. A meta-analysis based on the factors related to depression, revealed that it may be responsible and become the cause of probability of hypertension, furthermore, the chances have also been found significantly associated with the development of symptoms of depression at baseline (Meng, et al., 2012). Since long various psychologists have been trying to figure out the major causes of psychological disorders and the factors which are responsible for elimination these disorders. Hence, among all studies variables, recent researches have presented a view that stress related problems are generally appear more in elderly peoples who have some negative factors in their life, and these negative factors are because of many reasons e.g. loneliness, fear of death, over thinking or major diseases that cause pain which may be physiological or psychological in nature.

On the basis of large theoretical work available on stress and its effect on human being, it has been found out that stress is one of the major factors in the development and progression of diseases. Stress is a reaction that occurs in response to a perceived threat or challenge, affecting both physical and psychological aspects of an individual. If not managed, stress can result in various health issues such as anxiety, depression, high blood pressure, heart disease, and weakened immune system function. In the context of palliative care, stress also encompasses the emotional and psychological burden that patients and their caregivers experience when dealing with a terminal illness. The main objective of palliative care is to alleviate suffering and enhance the quality of life for patients and their loved ones, which includes addressing stress and its associated symptoms. Palliative care interventions can take various forms,

173

such as medication, counselling, and support groups, to help manage the physical, emotional, and spiritual aspects of stress and its related co-morbidities.

While considering the role of stress, it is identified that the physiological processes that cause stress have a detrimental negative impact on various psychological aspect such as emotional state of individual, psychological wellbeing, interpersonal relationships, and anxiety, healing, coping, and maintaining a prolonged positive quality of life. Among these entire psychosocial disturbances in people' life, majority of psychological disorders have been thus becoming increasingly pronounced in neurodegenerative diseases. If going through the conceptual framework of neurodegenerative disorders, these have been found responsible to impair mainly brain circuits that regulate stress related responses in addition to causing the tragic loss of cognitive and motor function among people, which is stressful in itself. The disruption of these circuits turns into an abnormal emotional and aggressive behavior that produces a very long-term care particularly in a challenging manner. In addition, high level of stress might make symptoms generally worse and can increases the probably of the occurrence of severe disease. The researchers have introduced that the neuronal and endocrine mechanisms that are engaged by both clinically and experimentally, stress usually interacts with a neurodegenerative illness that is already present.

On the basis of enormous literature studying stress as a causing factor for various psycho-physiological diseases, it has been identified that stress is often a contributing factor to or exacerbating many medical conditions ranging from psoriasis to irritable bowel syndrome, possibly because it leads to impaired immunity. Additionally, stress can also be one of the prominent causes of cardiovascular disturbance among elderly patients. It can particularly produce various causes like minor to major cardiac events among individuals who are above the age of 60 years or suffering from any kind of disease earlier. Generally, cardiac problems are found to be more related with hypertension, coronary artery disease, arrhythmia etc. While having a close observation on the demography of population, the rapidly increasing portion of population who are high in these diseases are the elder people, and by considering the rate of elderly people who are more prone to such disease, it has been estimated that by 2030, around 70 million peoples, or one in every fifth will be older than sixty-five years of age (Mozaffarian et al., 2003). Similar Reports presenting the estimation for the year 2030 that one in every fifth persons in the United States (approximately 35 million people) will be older than age 65 years (Vincent, 2010). If focus should be given on the reasons of death among elderly people, the major cause of death in those who are above the age of 65 years is heart disease that produces a very serious form of challenges in diagnosis and treatment plan for these elderly people (Roger et al., 2011). Further, as per the available data on aging it has been studied that the aging process is found to be quite related with higher probably of anatomic and physiological changes in the cardiovascular system and is responsible to start a kind of manifestation of heart disease in the geriatric population which is quite different from those diseases which are found in younger patients (Wong, et al., 2011). Furthermore, hypertension, coronary heart disease, and diabetes co-morbidities are among the major reasons for the acute level of depression and can insert a serious influence on the treatment and prognosis of disease among people who are in their older age (Zhang, Chen, & Ma, 2018).

Additionally, on the basis of recent evidence, it has been assumed that stress may be involved in accelerating the onset of Alzheimer's disease as well as exacerbating the course of the disease. So, if considering the nature of this disease, stress has been proven as one of the significant factors in the development and progression of any psycho-physiological disease. Humans' capacity to recover from loss, deal with adversity, and keep their spirits up can all be negatively impacted by the physiological mechanisms made possible by stress. Often, stress seems to have a time- and place-varying impact on a variety of brain systems and neural networks. Stress initially activates the hypothalamus and brainstem, and a subsequent action in the amygdala increases dopaminergic and noradrenergic stimulation and alters PFC performance (Arnsten, 2009). So, when the sympathetic nervous system is turned on, the regular production of adrenaline and noradrenaline by the adrenal medulla trains the body for a "fight or flight" response (Suzuki, 2013). The hypothalamic-pituitary-adrenal (HPA) axis is then thought to become activated, a process that takes place within a matter of minutes. Cortisol, the much more important glucocorticoid in humans, is made by the HPA and can be found in saliva in as little as 25 minutes. Cortisol can also usually cross the blood-brain barrier and bind to neural receptors in the hippocampus, the amygdala, and the prefrontal cortex, all of which are important for a healthy stress response (Lupien, et al., 2009; Yaribeygi, et al., 2017). Finally, the body responds to psychological stress by secreting pro-inflammatory cytokines, which may have an immediate effect on brain functioning (Harrison, et al., 2015).

While going through the all literature presented above is about physiological mechanism about stress and its related diseases, however, considering the earlier researches about dementia, it is quite considerable that various researchers have explored dementia awareness among medical learners from distinct nations and concluded that knowledge of dementia was shown to be ordinary throughout medical undergraduates but better among last-year learners than first year (2.5% of first year and 68.0% of final year students) (Nagle, Usita, & Edland, 2013; Sharma et al., 2018). Though Alzheimer disease is gaining immense attention among the healthcare professional, there are quite minimum number of published studies available about estimation of knowledge of Alzheimer's disease among public (Algahtani et al., 2018; Alqahtani et al., 2017).

STRESS AND ALZHEIMER'S DISEASE

While going through the available researches, our knowledge about stress and Alzheimer's comes from a large database of animal studies, because studying and manipulating stress in humans is still requires more subtle empirical studies. The main toxic protein at the heart of Alzheimer's disease patients is beta-amyloid, which forms plaques in the brain and around blood vessels and plays as a key pathological marker of Alzheimer's disease. Further, stress has been shown as an increasing component for production of toxic beta-amyloid in animal models of Alzheimer's disease under acute and chronic stress. This was further found to be related with the rapid cognitive decline in these animal models as compared with those animal models that were diagnosed as without any stress. In addition, early life stress can have long-term and permanent effects on the brains of these animals, with marked increases in brain and cerebrospinal fluid (CSF) amyloid levels.

Dementia refers to a group of conditions characterized by a significant decline in cognitive abilities, to the point where it affects the potential of a person to carry out everyday tasks autonomously. Rather than being a single disease, dementia is best understood as a syndrome. It has been noticed that the elderly people eventually start taking immense worry about Alzheimer's disease when these kinds of symptoms start to appear. It is a neurodegenerative dementia, which means that it is irreversible and results in the loss of brain tissue. Another type of dementia that results from inadequate blood flow to the brain is vascular dementia, which is equally irreversible. However, it has also been identified that Alzheimer's disease-related dementia and vascular dementia can remain in a coexisted manner. Alzheimer's disease is a distinct form of dementia that is identified by the buildup of unusual proteins in the brain. On the other hand, dementia is a general concept that encompasses a reduction in cognitive abilities resulting from various disorders.

Alzheimer's disease (AD) has been diagnosed as a form of quickly increasing, age-independent, progressive brain dysfunction (Nagle et al., 2013; Williams, 2013). Dementia is characterised by memory loss, trouble focusing, and an inability to do even the most basic tasks. The empirical evidence shows that among people with a wide range of clinical dementia symptoms, AD is by far the most prevalent aetiology (Bature, et al., 2017). Also, it is clear that AD is much more common in low- and middle-income nations (Prince et al., 2015).

Alzheimer's Disease and its Continuum

Alzheimer's disease (AD) is the most devastating and dreaded type of dementia that appears late in life and has severe effects on patients as well as society. People suffering from AD mainly experience a deterioration in memory and related intellectual abilities, making it difficult to do things like remembering to eat or take a shower, ultimately leading to complete disability and death. The patient is obviously the primary focus, but it's safe to say that no other condition has such a far-reaching and terrible impact on the patient's loved ones. This is stated that AD is considered as one of the most common form of dementia without a prior cause. Based on its nature and symptoms, AD is an age-related progressive neurodegenerative disorder characterized by multiple cognition related deficiencies, often accompanied by behavioural and mood disorders. It is a kind of devastating disease that leaves a detrimental effect in declining the true self-confidence among the people who suffer from that disease. AD prevalence is usually likely to increase as life expectancy increases for most populations, imposing a significant social and economic burden on societies and health care systems (Shead et al., 2021). It has an insightful impact on patients, families, caregivers, communities and society at large. Current treatments for Alzheimer's are ineffective and have no prospect of cure. Lee et al. (2022) stated that Alzheimer's disease, a progressive decline in mental faculties, is one of the leading causes of disability among the elderly. Short-term memory loss, alterations to personality and temperament, and psychological issues like anger and irritability are among the earliest symptoms of Alzheimer's disease.

According to Irina Skylar-Scott (2021), a clinical assistant professor of neurology and neurological sciences at Stanford University in California stated that only stress may not cause Alzheimer's disease, but if someone has been already going to have Alzheimer's disease, it is certainly one of the prominent elements among several that affects whether the symptoms will appear sooner or later. Patients with high levels of stress may find it more difficult to manage the pathological changes associated with Alzheimer's disease, and their symptoms may be more noticeable.

A research study explained the view that the Alzheimer disease (AD) is the commonest form of dementia that manifests in old age and has severe effects on patients as well as society wherein the patients live and interacted (Mark & Sitskoorn, 2013). Neurodegeneration in the brain typically progresses for years before the ailment is recognised as such. Due to the considerable lag time between the onset of the initial pathophysiological alterations and the onset of clinical manifestations, it is likely that Alzheimer's disease can be divided into several etiological stages. Thus, before the onset of dementia, there is an initial stage known as prodromal, generally can be understood as a mild cognitive impairment (MCI), defined by cognitive decline, yet not to a point where it severely interferes with daily life (Woods, et al., 2012). Moreover, preclinical AD stages have already been described in the preclinical continuum of MCI. Symptoms of subjective cognitive decline (SCD) and the development of brain biomarkers describe this preliminary phase. In a general sense, SCD can be defined as the presence of mild cognitive problems that the patient reports despite actual performance on common intelligence tests

(Jessen et al., 2014). There is widespread agreement, however, that therapeutic approaches are most likely to be beneficial when implemented as early as possible in the AD continuum, despite the fact that this is where the disease typically begins. The next step is to urgently find early markers that can reveal the course of silent neurodegeneration before the onset of clinical indications of dementia. There have been a lot of suggested candidates. Our goal in this publication is to draw attention to stress as a potentially significant contributor to AD risk.

GLOBAL BURDEN AND PREVALENCE OF ALZHEIMER'S DISEASE

Alzheimer's disease killed 24 million people every year, making it the sixth leading cause of death in the world (Nichols et al., 2019). A comprehensive systematic review for the Global Burden of AD in 2016 found that 438 million people around the world have dementia. Dementia affects more women than men (Nichols et al., 2019). Alzheimer's disease International (2015) estimates that by 2050, the number of people living with the disease will reach 131.5 million, with the preponderance of those living in poor and middle-class nations. Researchers have calculated that 6.4% of the population in Saudi Arabia has dementia. A variety of other factors, including age, lack of schooling, hypertension, and coronary disorders, were additionally recognised as major risk variables for cognitive decline (Alkhunizan, Alkhenizan, & Basudan, 2018). However, prior research has revealed that most people and their families dismiss AD's symptoms as inevitable signs of growing older and hence do not pursue any immediate medical treatments (Alkhunizan et al., 2018).

STRESS AND THE TREATMENT OF ALZHEIMER'S DISEASE

When it becomes clearer that stress can negatively affect the development of Alzheimer's disease as well as other neurodegenerative diseases, the issue arises as to whether this knowledge will prove useful in the treatment of AD. It's possible to take several perspectives on this. Animal models of Alzheimer's disease show that stress plays an exacerbating role in the disease's development, suggesting that adopting a healthier lifestyle that reduces sources of stress should be promoted as a means of protecting against dementia. CRFR1 inhibitors and other drugs that specifically lower the amount of stress hormones in the body should also be looked into to see if they can slow the progression of AD in people. In a similar way, the CRFR1 inhibitor R121919 has been shown to reduce amyloid pathology and improve synaptic and mental performance in AD model mice, but it hasn't been tried on people with dementia yet (Zhang et al., 2016).

Hence, so far as the empirical testing of any treatment is concerned, there are few research evidences presented that pharmacological methods that target various parts of the HPA axis have indeed been tried, with varying findings, in individuals with AD. As seen in mice models, therapy with the glucocorticoid receptor inhibitor RU486 reduces AD development (Baglietto-Vargas et al., 2015; Lanté et al., 2015), resulted in a slight but statistically significant increase in cognitive performance in a clinical study (Justice, 2018).

Consequently, the treatment of Alzheimer's disease should take into account the consequences of AD advancement on stress signalling. Abnormal stress reactions, despair, apathy, and hostility are experienced by a subset of people with Alzheimer's disease and other forms of dementia (Amore, et al., 2007). There is a strong temptation to think that each of these groups of symptoms is caused by the breakdown of a different brain circuit. More neuropsychiatric emphasis and possibly pharmaceutical management, especially to ameliorate symptoms, should be given to the subgroups of AD patients that demonstrate depression, severe anxiety, and/or violence. Even though anti-depressants are often well accepted by the elderly, several typical anxiolytics (e.g., benzodiazepines) are contraindicated in instances of dementia due to their negative effects on cognitive efficiency and sharpness (Crocco, et al., 2017; Picton, Marino, & Nealy, 2018).

PALLIATIVE CARE FOR TREATING AD IN ELDERLY PATIENTS

Though it has always been the matter of concern to treat any illness by using pharmaceuticals treatment, new anti-anxiety drugs that don't cause that weird thing to happen would be proven quite helpful in alleviating anxiety sensations in the elderly population suffering from dementia. Numerous researchers have identified that there are various factors prevailing in social system of patients with dementia can play an effective role positively. Such as various nonpharmacologic treatments might play a leading and vital function in the management of AD's associated psychiatric disorders. Clinical experiments with individuals having dementia found that therapeutic touch, which has been shown to relieve stress, lowered anxiety-related speech patterns and pacing and resulted in a modest reduction in salivary Cortisol concentrations (Woods et al., 2012). Dementia sufferers can benefit from music therapy since it reduces their stress and slows their cognitive decline (Baird & Thompson, 2018). People who are living with the patient of dementia can also become a supportive factor for them. Various research studies have identified the role of social support in the treatment of dementia patients. Social Support was found a significant predictor of physical and mental health among elderly people, it thus reduces the deteriorating consequences of stress effectively (Tate, Swift, & Bayomi, 2013). Another study conducted by Thoits (2013) gave the fact that social support is quite capable indirectly helps to reduce stress by effectively bolstering the self-esteem in elderly people who have the symptoms of dementia. It is requiring to successfully defining the social supports and its differential relationship with health outcomes (Grant, Patterson, & Yager, 1988). Furthermore, if the contribution of social support can be recognized in the development of fully functioning human being, Social support is a crucial part of an individual life, as it gives a feeling of security, sense of belonging, and it enhance the self-worth of the patients (Fatima, Rizvi, & Jamal, 2020). Moreover, along with social support, there are many other external factors that should be considered like financial constraints, loneliness, childhood trauma, or pain related disorders. In today's modern time where people are compelled to live far from their family which causes the emergence of psychological disturbance mainly loneliness among people which certainly put a serious negative effect on the mental health of elderly people. Mostly isolated elderly is more prone towards stress related problems in later life, they are unable to share and express their feelings of depression, agony, sadness or anxieties. Those elder who have various modes of communications, or they have a lot of grandchildren's or people who cares them in their old age are most happiness and less likely develop stress related problems. Although the results of these research point to the potential benefits of stress management for Alzheimer's disease individuals, it is not yet known whether this also slows the advancement of the disease.

So as per the various research studies about the physiological functioning behind dementia and its association with stress, it can be summarized in such a manner that stress alone cannot be called as one of the major factors in the onset of Alzheimer's disease; however, it may play an important role for the progression of disease, as well as for the exacerbation of symptoms due to impaired immune responses, which are quite essential in Alzheimer's disease. Additionally, stress can be control through various techniques e.g. music therapy, meditation, pharmaceutical intervention and psychological resilience, social support or availability of various resources that are need at the time of stress dealing such as family, friend, finance etc. While non pharmaceutical treatments should therefore be primary concern, these have no such ill effects and far more benefits then it seems. If stress is uncontrollable then it's not only increase the progression of Alzheimer's disease but it also significant contributor of other health related problems (CAD, diabetes, immunity disorders etc).

SELF-CONTROL REHABILITATION

Apart from various treatments related to neurological functioning of brain of elderly people, various social and personal factors can also be used as an effective treatment for elderly patients suffering from dementia. Since, these kinds of patients are mainly suffering from the problems related to memory, emotion regulation and functioning of various body parts to accomplish different daily task. In that kind of situation, caregivers of these elderly people can give them a helping hand in regulating emotion to some extent. Behavioural techniques can also be used to motivate elderly patient for their daily work however caregivers must provide support to them. Therapies related to communication and self-control can also be given to the dementia patients. Music and stories related to their past experiences can be useful supporting their communication capability. Further, teaching them self-control to the patients, difficult task should be demonstrated in a very easy manner so that they can find themselves capable enough to complete their daily work for personal need at least (Golembiewski & Zeisel, 2022). Though these factors can provide only additional support to the treatment of elderly patients with dementia, it is still in the process of identifying to the very only effective treatment or therapy for the Alzheimer's disease.

Therefore, apart from the neurological and social factors, there are still a lot of variables related to patients' environment and genetic compositions; need to be studied to identify its effective role in dealing the diseases like dementia. Therefore, more work needs to be done on patients before clinical recommendations can be made. It is still need to better understand neurological as well as non-pharmaceutical treatment underpinnings of stress in general and elder populations suffering from Alzheimer disease, and make the updated intervention to reduce these problems. In this sequence, social and psychological therapies can be used to reduce the probability of occurrence of any cognitive degenerative diseases like dementia or Alzheimer's diseases among elderly population. With the average level of understanding of patients' behaviour, caregivers should take the initiate with the help of behavioural scientist to deal the elderly patients suffering from such diseases.

REFERENCES

Alkhunizan, M., Alkhenizan, A., & Basudan, L. (2018). Prevalence of mild cognitive impairment and dementia in Saudi Arabia: A community-based study. *Dementia and Geriatric Cognitive Disorders. Extra*, 8(1), 98–103. doi:10.1159/000487231 PMID:29706986

Alqahtani, A. H., Al Khedair, K., Al-Jeheiman, R., Al-Turki, H. A., & Al Qahtani, N. H. (2018). Anxiety and depression during pregnancy in women attending clinics in a University Hospital in Eastern province of Saudi Arabia: Prevalence and associated factors. *International Journal of Women's Health*, 101–108.

Amore, M., Tagariello, P., Laterza, C., & Savoia, E. (2007). Subtypes of depression in dementia. *Archives of Gerontology and Geriatrics*, *44*, 23–33. doi:10.1016/j.archger.2007.01.004 PMID:17317430

Arnsten, A. (2009). Vías de sinalización de tensións que deterioran a estrutura ea función da cortiza prefrontal. *Nat Rev Neurosci, 10*, 410-2210.1038.

Baglietto-Vargas, D., Chen, Y., Suh, D., Ager, R. R., Rodriguez-Ortiz, C. J., Medeiros, R., Myczek, K., Green, K. N., Baram, T. Z., & LaFerla, F. M. (2015). Short-term modern life-like stress exacerbates Aβ-pathology and synapse loss in 3xTg-AD mice. *Journal of Neurochemistry*, *134*(5), 915–926. doi:10.1111/jnc.13195 PMID:26077803

Baird, A., & Thompson, W. F. (2018). The impact of music on the self in dementia. *Journal of Alzheimer's Disease*, *61*(3), 827–841. doi:10.3233/JAD-170737 PMID:29332051

Bature, F., Guinn, B., Pang, D., & Pappas, Y. (2017). Signs and symptoms preceding the diagnosis of Alzheimer's disease: A systematic scoping review of literature from 1937 to 2016. *BMJ Open*, *7*(8), e015746. doi:10.1136/bmjopen-2016-015746 PMID:28851777

Crocco, E. A., Jaramillo, S., Cruz-Ortiz, C., & Camfield, K. (2017). Pharmacological management of anxiety disorders in the elderly. *Current Treatment Options in Psychiatry*, *4*(1), 33–46. doi:10.100740501-017-0102-4 PMID:28948135

Fatima, S., Rizvi, S. Z. S., & Jamal, S. R. (2020). Social support, health procrastination and flourishing in cancer patients. *IAHRW International Journal of Social Sciences Review*, *8*(7-9), 296–300.

Golembiewski, J. A., & Zeisel, J. (2022). Salutogenic Approaches to Dementia Care. The Handbook of Salutogenesis, 513-532.

Grant, I., Patterson, T. L., & Yager, J. (1988). Social supports in relation to physical health and symptoms of depression in the elderly. *The American Journal of Psychiatry*. PMID:3421347

Harrison, N. A., Cercignani, M., Voon, V., & Critchley, H. D. (2015). Effects of inflammation on hippocampus and substantia nigra responses to novelty in healthy human participants. *Neuropsychopharmacology*, *40*(4), 831–838. doi:10.1038/npp.2014.222 PMID:25154706

Jessen, F., Amariglio, R. E., Van Boxtel, M., Breteler, M., Ceccaldi, M., Chételat, G., & Van Der Flier, W. M. (2014). A conceptual framework for research on subjective cognitive decline in preclinical Alzheimer's disease. *Alzheimer's & Dementia*, *10*(6), 844–852. doi:10.1016/j.jalz.2014.01.001 PMID:24798886

Justice, N. J. (2018). The relationship between stress and Alzheimer's disease. *Neurobiology of Stress*, *8*, 127–133. doi:10.1016/j.ynstr.2018.04.002 PMID:29888308

Lanté, F., Chafai, M., Raymond, E. F., Salgueiro Pereira, A. R., Mouska, X., Kootar, S., Barik, J., Bethus, I., & Marie, H. (2015). Subchronic glucocorticoid receptor inhibition rescues early episodic memory and synaptic plasticity deficits in a mouse model of Alzheimer's disease. *Neuropsychopharmacology*, *40*(7), 1772–1781. doi:10.1038/npp.2015.25 PMID:25622751

Lee, J.-H., Yang, D.-S., Goulbourne, C. N., Im, E., Stavrides, P., Pensalfini, A., ... Berg, M. J. (2022). Faulty autolysosome acidification in Alzheimer's disease mouse models induces autophagic build-up of Aβ in neurons, yielding senile plaques. *Nature Neuroscience*, *25*(6), 688–701. doi:10.103841593-022-01084-8 PMID:35654956

Lupien, S. J., McEwen, B. S., Gunnar, M. R., & Heim, C. (2009). Effects of stress throughout the lifespan on the brain, behaviour and cognition. *Nature Reviews. Neuroscience*, *10*(6), 434–445. doi:10.1038/nrn2639 PMID:19401723

Mark, R. E., & Sitskoorn, M. M. (2013). Are subjective cognitive complaints relevant in preclinical Alzheimer's disease? A review and guidelines for healthcare professionals. *Reviews in Clinical Gerontology*, *23*(1), 61–74. doi:10.1017/S0959259812000172

Meng, L., Chen, D., Yang, Y., Zheng, Y., & Hui, R. (2012). Depression increases the risk of hypertension incidence: A meta-analysis of prospective cohort studies. *Journal of Hypertension*, *30*(5), 842–851. doi:10.1097/HJH.0b013e32835080b7 PMID:22343537

Mozaffarian, D., Kumanyika, S. K., Lemaitre, R. N., Olson, J. L., Burke, G. L., & Siscovick, D. S. (2003). Cereal, fruit, and vegetable fiber intake and the risk of cardiovascular disease in elderly individuals. *Journal of the American Medical Association*, *289*(13), 1659–1666. doi:10.1001/jama.289.13.1659 PMID:12672734

Nagle, B. J., Usita, P. M., & Edland, S. D. (2013). United States medical students' knowledge of Alzheimer disease. *J Educ Eval Health Prof, 10*(4), 10.3352.

Nichols, E., Szoeke, C. E., Vollset, S. E., Abbasi, N., Abd-Allah, F., Abdela, J., ... Asgedom, S. W. (2019). Global, regional, and national burden of Alzheimer's disease and other dementias, 1990–2016: A systematic analysis for the Global Burden of Disease Study 2016. *Lancet Neurology*, *18*(1), 88–106. doi:10.1016/S1474-4422(18)30403-4 PMID:30497964

Picton, J. D., Marino, A. B., & Nealy, K. L. (2018). Benzodiazepine use and cognitive decline in the elderly. *Bulletin - American Society of Hospital Pharmacists*, *75*(1), e6–e12. doi:10.2146/ajhp160381 PMID:29273607

Prince, M. J., Wimo, A., Guerchet, M. M., Ali, G. C., Wu, Y.-T., & Prina, M. (2015). World Alzheimer Report 2015-The Global Impact of Dementia: An analysis of prevalence, incidence, cost and trends.

Roger, V. L., Go, A. S., Lloyd-Jones, D. M., Adams, R. J., Berry, J. D., Brown, T. M., & Ford, E. S. (2011). Executive summary: Heart disease and stroke statistics—2011 update. *Circulation*, *123*(4), 459–463. doi:10.1161/CIR.0b013e3182009701 PMID:21160056

Shead, V. L., Rodriguez, R. L., Dreeben, S. J., McBride, S. A., Byrne, G., & Pachana, N. (2021). Anxiety in older adults across care settings. *Anxiety in older people: Clinical and research perspectives*, 157-172.

Silbersweig, D., Safar, L. T., & Daffner, K. R. (2020). *Neuropsychiatry and Behavioral Neurology*. Principles and Practice. McGraw Hill Professional.

Suzuki, K. (2013). „Garfinkel, S. *N „Critchley, HD, & Se exteroceptive and interoceptive domains modulates ropsychologic1, 5*(13), 2909-2917.

Tate, R. B., Swift, A. U., & Bayomi, D. J. (2013). Older men's lay definitions of successful aging over time: The Manitoba follow-up study. *International Journal of Aging & Human Development*, *76*(4), 297–322. doi:10.2190/AG.76.4.b PMID:23855184

Thoits, P. A. (2013). Self, identity, stress, and mental health. Handbook of the sociology of mental health, 357-377.

Vincent, G. K. (2010). *The next four decades: The older population in the United States: 2010 to 2050*. US Department of Commerce, Economics and Statistics Administration.

Williams, S. C. (2013). Alzheimer's disease: Mapping the brain's decline. *Nature*, *502*(7473), S84–S85. doi:10.1038/502S84a PMID:24187700

Wong, C. Y., Chaudhry, S. I., Desai, M. M., & Krumholz, H. M. (2011). Trends in comorbidity, disability, and polypharmacy in heart failure. *The American Journal of Medicine, 124*(2), 136–143. doi:10.1016/j.amjmed.2010.08.017 PMID:21295193

Woods, B., Aguirre, E., Spector, A. E., & Orrell, M. (2012). Cognitive stimulation to improve cognitive functioning in people with dementia. *Cochrane Database of Systematic Reviews*, 2. doi:10.1002/14651858.CD005562.pub2 PMID:22336813

Yaribeygi, H., Panahi, Y., Sahraei, H., Johnston, T. P., & Sahebkar, A. (2017). The impact of stress on body function: A review. *EXCLI Journal, 16*, 1057. PMID:28900385

Zhang, C., Kuo, C.-C., Moghadam, S. H., Monte, L., Campbell, S. N., Rice, K. C., Sawchenko, P. E., Masliah, E., & Rissman, R. A. (2016). Corticotropin-releasing factor receptor-1 antagonism mitigates beta amyloid pathology and cognitive and synaptic deficits in a mouse model of Alzheimer's disease. *Alzheimer's & Dementia, 12*(5), 527–537. doi:10.1016/j.jalz.2015.09.007 PMID:26555315

Zhang, Y., Chen, Y., & Ma, L. (2018). Depression and cardiovascular disease in elderly: Current understanding. *Journal of Clinical Neuroscience, 47*, 1–5. doi:10.1016/j.jocn.2017.09.022 PMID:29066229

Chapter 10
Cognitive Deficits Leading to Functional Deficits:
An Analytical Perspective

Deoshree Akhouri
Aligarh Muslim University, India

Tabassum Bashir
Aligarh Muslim University, India

Hamza
Aligarh Muslim University, India

Mohammed Reyazuddin
Aligarh Muslim University, India

Zarnish Habib
University of Leeds, UK

EXECUTIVE SUMMARY

This chapter will enlighten you to know about cognitive functions in the elderly and how these functions get affected and lead to downfall progression (neurodegeneration) with aging not only in terms of structural changes but also functional which cause age-associated illnesses. The evidence of cognitive deficit is obvious among the elderly population and needs to be tackled very effectively in keeping the view of maintaining functional independence in their routine activities. Throughout the chapter, different phenomena related to age-associated disorders and comorbidity have highlighted the high frequency of cognitive impairment and we will also be going to know about the role of the COVID-19 pandemic in worsening these symptoms. Neuropsychological assessment at an early stage plays a crucial role in pointing out cognitive deficits earlier which can further lead to decelerating of symptoms through pharmacological and psychosocial rehabilitation.

DOI: 10.4018/978-1-6684-2354-7.ch010

INTRODUCTION

The term cognition can be understood as the process of knowing, including attending, remembering, and reasoning. It can also be defined as the content of these processes, such as concepts and memories (American Psychological Association, 2000). Cognition includes all forms of awareness such as perceiving, remembering, reasoning, judging, imagining, and problem-solving. In the early stages of childhood, this cognition developed through the interaction of genetic or innate capacities, and psychosocial environmental factors but as the age of the individuals increases chances become higher of having a cognitive decline (CD). The CD is more common in the elderly but not every elderly has a CD.

CD is a comprehensive term that involves difficulty in processing thoughts that leads to memory loss, difficulties in decision-making, poor concentration, and learning difficulties. A cross-sectional study in the age ranges from 18 to 60 years suggested that increased age is correlated with lower levels of cognition/cognitive performance (Salthouse, T. A. 2009). CD is inclined to defy Occam's razor, challenging clinicians and nosologists with comorbidity, multiplicity, and unclear boundaries. Such concerns are of utmost true for the elderly, the demographic group most at risk for cognitive disorders. The CD is associated with multimorbidity in the elderly. Older adults are living with multimorbidity with the coexistence of multiple chronic conditions (Goodman, R. A., et al., 2013). Multiple chronic conditions are ongoing causes of substantial ill health and disability that further leads to premature death.

The decline in cognition can range from mild impairment to dementia and this decline further leads to physical impairment. The early stage of decline in cognition is sometimes self-reported by individuals with symptoms of memory problems or confusion, known as the subjective decline in cognition. This self-reported memory problem that has been happening more often or getting worse in the past twelve months becoming common with a prevalence of 11.1% or 1 in 9 adults after the age of 45 years (CDC, 2015-16).

CD represents the complex interface among medicine, neurology, and psychiatry in those neurological or medical circumstances that often lead to cognitive disorders which in return are correlated with behavioral symptoms. According to the Centers for disease control and prevention (CDC), impaired cognition has a profound impact on an individual's overall health and well-being. A severe decline in CD is the major predictor of mortality and has a marked adverse impact on survival (Bassuk, S. S., Wypij, D., & Berkmann, L. F. 2000).

Numerous studies have been provided by the researchers and it was found that age-related illnesses can increase the chance of neural dysfunction, loss of neuronal structure, and loss of synapses among the elderly population which can significantly lead to cognitive deficits and impaired normal functioning (Persson, 2006).

Age-related losses, the number of changes in the brain stem, and in other parts of brain regions can alter normal functioning and lead decline in cognition significantly. Researchers have also provided a number of reasons and protective factors, and lifestyle modifications that can contribute to reducing the early onset of decline (Murman DL, 2015).

The high frequency of cognitive impairment and the COVID-19 pandemic serves as one objective of future studies to be addressed on this topic. A systematic review conducted by Tavares-Júnior, J. W. L. et al., (2022) and they have pointed out several phenomena (impairment in executive functions, attention, and episodic memory) are related to cognitive deficits, functional impairment, and the role of COVID-19 and how these correlated to each other.

COGNITIVE DEFICIT LEADING TO FUNCTIONAL DEFICIT

The term cognitive deficit is an inclusive term used to describe the cognitive impairment. The impairment can be associated to any domains of human cognition. This is essential to recognize what kinds of fluctuations or changes in cognition which could be predictable as an element of normal aging or a change that can be considered or lead to neurocognitive disorders. Functional impairment or deficit is an interchangeable word for disability in mental disorders. The disability is not appropriate to describe all kind of mental disorders in this criterion so for that impairment word instead of disability are used to categories all illness except few. Functional impairment is not new term for the mental health professional, and researchers, but in few cases policy maker used the term disability for mental illness (Park, 2003).

Several consequences are related to aging, cognitive decline, general pathology related cognitive deficits and how normal aging correlate with depression, dementia, and other cognitive disorders (Dhakal and Bobrin, 2022). Cognitive deficit is not a narrow and limited phenomenon to any specific illness or conditions but it could also be the manifestations of an underlying condition. The duration of cognitive deficit can be short or progressive and permanent affecting the person's life (Andreescu and Aizenstein). Neuroimaging (functional MRI and PET imaging) findings reveal that cognitive deficits occur frequently in Parkinson's disease (PD) and provide potential cause for Mild Cognitive Impairment in PD (PD-MCI) that emerged recently in findings. Patients with mild impairment are at risk of developing dementia, and thus it is a topic of growing interest to know more about it (Christopher, L., & Strafella, A. P., 2013). The role of prefrontal cortex (PFC) has been extensively evaluated in numerous studies and it plays a central role in cognitive control functions, and dopamine in the PFC modulates cognitive control, thereby influencing attention, impulse inhibition, prospective memory, and cognitive flexibility and if any discrepancy happened between the systems, leads cognitive impairment in these areas (Natural Medicine, 2020). It was seen that the overlap in brain regions between areas of prefrontal, frontal and dorsolateral region engaged in reflection about oneself and reflection about other people raises the possibility that thinking about other minds involves a sort of simulation of the same processes that are engaged in thinking about oneself and if any damages due to any cause occurred would definitely affect cognitive functions and made them vulnerable to deficits in normal as well as in elderly population (Laureys, 2016).Cognitive deficit affecting person's day to activity and if any region of the brain suffered from any disease such as prions disease, pick disease, Alzheimer's disease, dementia, brain cancer, epilepsy and other seizure disorders, mental disorders, Parkinson's and other movement disorders, stroke and transient ischemic attack (TIA) would leads significant malfunctions that are not limited to only thinking and memory deficits but it also includes disorientation, language deficits, reduce ability to direct, focus, sustain and shift attention and reduce ability in visuoconstructional perpetual ability. Cognitive deficit can occur in any of the cognitive domain such as in attention, executive ability, knowledge and memory, verbal, perceptual activity, and social cognition in elderly population. This can cause significant functional impairment that interferes with previous functioning (Jolles, 2012).

The epidemiology of cognitive decline and deficit can't be predicted among elderly population. The onset of cognitive decline increases with increasing age. The prevalence and incidence of dementia, it's estimated to reach around 20-25 million worldwide. Ongoing as well as already done studies from the past few decades reveals that the growing population towards aging reflects strong association with increased cognitive disorder specially Alzheimer's disease. Alzheimer's disease is the most common type of dementia, and it accounts nearly 50 to 70% cases of dementia worldwide (Prince et al., 2015).

The pathophysiology of cognitive deficits is specifically related to the brain areas that is controlling a certain activity. Brain areas such as hippocampus, amygdale, grey matter, cortex, thalamus, basal ganglia and the white matter are responsible for certain activities and if any damages or diseases occurred in any of the above mentioned areas, lead functional deficit (Okonkwo, Schultz, Oh et al., 2014). Diversity of factors might cause accumulative damage in the brain; age itself can yield cognitive deficits. These factors comprise impairment to the brain causing cerebral ischemia, bran injury and traumatic incidence. Toxins such as alcohol, cannabis, opioids, or other psychoactive substance in a long and chronic use can cause functional deficits in both physical and cognitive level among elderly as well as in other sample population. Other finding related to neurotransmitters, glutamate is the most common excitatory neurotransmitter of our nervous system, and it is also a plentiful neurotransmitter that plays crucial role in cognitive functions like thinking, learning and memory. The prefrontal cortex (PFC) becomes evidently impaired by stress, producing measurable deficits in working memory noted by researchers (Shansky and Lipps, 2013). Chemical substances called hormones regulates the simple as well as complex functions of the human body in order to serve the purpose to maintain various processes, such as growth, emotions and even cognition. Various previous studies have examined the relationship between hormonal effects and cognitive function in almost every age group and progression. An excessive secretion of stress hormones (cortisol) is showed positive correlation in the development, and it also maintained a deteriorating condition of dementia especially Alzheimer's disease (Ali, Begum, & Reza, 2018). Degenerative dementias are the furthermost collective cause of important delayed-life cognitive deterioration, but an amalgamation of influences is shared (Persson et al., 2006). Study findings reveal that more trails, preventive measures, and neurocognitive test are needed to promote awareness and prevent the early onset of mild cognitive impairment as well as dementia (Jongsiriyanyon and Limpawattana, 2018).

From the structural and functional point of view human brain has four different kinds of lobes (frontal lobe, parietal lobe, temporal lobe, occipital lobe) with specific assigned functions respectively and if any damage occurred in parietal lobe, then individual may have inability of get dressed, distortion in space or surrounding, and visuospatial dysfunction. Damage to the frontal lobe lead deficit in planning, abstract understanding and if any damages occurred in temporal lobe leads memory, attention, and executive malfunctioning.

Any underlined physical, neurological, psychological conditions associated with aging and if it became the prominent part of their living would lead marked deficits and functional impairment in term of poor ability of decision making, decrease social interaction, poverty of speech, incoherent thought processes, poor understanding, poor executive functioning (Carvalho, I M, Parimon, Cusack et al., 2014). Mental health professionals, clinician, imaging, medical findings, and research-based study, all of that led their emphasis to understand the illnesses, causes, prognosis, nature, onset, and associated risk factors whether in physical illness or mental illness, lead functional impairment that ultimately minimizes the capability of managing even daily routine. Age associated illness among elderly limits the basic capacity of functioning or limit oneself to be independent. Elderly after certain age (more than 65 of age) would likely to depending on others for normal routine work and if person with underlying illnesses, become more dependent on others on activity comprising facing difficulty in maintaining personal hygiene, cleaning and washing, cooking food, difficulty in initiation and maintaining of social relation and communication, difficulty in normal day to day decision making, marketing and taking part in community and recreational activities, lack of adaptive skills. Restrictions in cognitive abilities can also impact an individual's ability to accomplish efficiently medical regimens. This can result in poor outcomes related comorbidities such as enduring diseases like hypertension, diabetes, and cardio related diseases. The findings suggested that if mental illness has physical comorbidities such as cardiac disease, lungs disease, and respiratory related illnesses and so then it worsens the functioning in the presence of neurocognitive disorders among elderly population (Vannorsdall, 2022). Impairment in every field of social, cognitive, personal, educational, occupational, and family has been studied by researchers to establish a better understanding of independence functioning vs. dependent functioning. Mental health review board, mental health professional and clinician have studied the phenomenon of disability or impairment in terms of outcomes, frequency, and caregiver burden and it's distinct from one to another scientifically, and it was seen that it is still unclear in both the diagnostic criteria of American Psychological Association (APA) and World Health Organization (WHO) about their use in formulating diagnoses of mental disorders (Kennedy, 2009).

COGNITIVE DISORDERS IN ELDERLY

Major Neurocognitive Disorder (Dementia)

The prevalence of dementia is continuing to rise and is predicted to affect more than 130 million people worldwide by 2050 (Alzheimer's Disease International, 2015) another study reported that there is an estimation that 50 million people worldwide in 2018 were living with dementia and this prediction will rise to 152 million by 2050 (Welsh, 2019). The cognitive decline must characterize a change from the patient's prior level of cognitive ability, which is persistent and progressive over time and is not correlated with an episode of delirium exclusively. This decline also creates impairment in the patient's ability to function and perform routine tasks (Emmady, School, Tadi, 2022). The Diagnostic and Statistical Manual- 5 (DSM-5) classifies nine major types of dementia, (1) dementia of the Alzheimer's type, which usually occurs in persons older than 65 years of age and is manifested by progressive intellectual disorientation and dementia, delusions, or depression; (2) vascular dementia, caused by vessel thrombosis or hemorrhage; (3) human immunodeficiency virus (HIV) disease; (4) head trauma; (5) Pick's disease or frontotemporal lobar degeneration; (6) Prion disease such as Creutzfeldt-Jakob disease, which is caused by a slow-growing transmittable virus); (7) substance-induced, caused by toxin or medication (e.g., gasoline fumes, atropine); (8) multiple etiologies; and (9) not specified (if the cause is unknown). It is a neurodegenerative and complex condition in which no two elderly experience similar symptoms or progression (Alzheimer's Society 2020). Dementia is a syndrome, that provides an umbrella term for a cluster of symptoms that can be understood from the combination of biological, psychological, and social perspectives (World Health Organization. (2012).

With cognitive impairment, functional impairment is also common in dementia and is most likely to be associated with the occurrence of depressive features, though the relationship between the severity of cognitive impairment and depressive features is not clear (Payne, J. L., Lyketsos, C. G., Steele, C., Baker, L., Galik, E., Kopunek, S., & Warren, A. 1998). Depression is associated with dementia and is more prevalent in vascular dementia & Alzheimer's types than others (Kuring, J. K., Mathias, J. L., & Ward, L. 2018). Elevated depressive symptoms and anxiety is correlated with multimorbidity and three or more medical conditions deliberated a 2.30-fold increase in elevated anxiety. Thirteen medical triads are associated with depressive symptoms while twenty are associated with anxiety (Gould, C. E., O'Hara, R., Goldstein, M. K., & Beaudreau, S. A. 2016). Multimorbidity has been robustly associated with subsequent dementia when its onset is in midlife rather than late life (Hassen, Fayosse, Landré, Raggi, Bloomberg, Sabia, & Singh-Manoux, 2022). Elderly with multimorbidity have a higher risk of having dementia for a mean of 8.4 years (mean age 75 years) (Grande et al., 2021). Elderly with cardiovascular, neuropsychiatric, and sensory impairment/cancer multimorbidity are at higher risk of developing dementia; concurrent inflammation and genetic predisposition further elevated this risk (Grande et al., 2021).

The prevalence of dementia is higher in elderly women than in elderly men; this might be due to the fact that women have a longer life span (Tonelli et al, 2017). Functional morbidities like fractures and osteoporosis falls are more common in females living with dementia. Dementia is a risk factor for falls and in accumulation, it is also associated with poor recovery, which further intensifies this issue. It is very certain that multimorbidity and functional deficits are more common in the elderly with dementia. The complex relationship of dementia with long-term health conditions leads to a cumulative spiral of increasing risk that leads to an adverse outcome. Dementia also changes the natural course of an extremely prevalent condition such as hypertension. In disparity with the general population, systolic blood pressure (BP) has started falling up to 6 years before the progress of clinically apparent dementia and continues to fall afterward (Stewart et.al, 2009). This detected fall in BP is possibly sufficient to move an individual below the treatment threshold. This collaboration consequently has suggestions for monitoring BP and treatment in people with dementia compared to cognitively intact people. The mortality risk also increased in the presence of dementia, morbidity burden, and depending on age by 1.54 to 6.38 (Tonelli et al, 2017). The elderly living with dementia and cancer has less chances for diagnostic testing or chemotherapy compared to those with cancer but without dementia (Huang, Hsieh, Hsieh, & Wang, 2017). The National Institute of Health and Care Excellence (NICE) guidelines for multimorbidity suggest that the management of multimorbidity is more problematic in the presence of dementia and that cautious attention to any harm or benefits of intervention is required (National Institute for Clinical Excellence. 2016).

Amnestic Disorder

In DSM-5 amnestic disorders are classified as major neurocognitive disorders caused by other medical conditions, toxins, or unknown causes.

The main symptom of the amnestic disorder is the progress of memory disorder that is characterized by impairment in the ability to recall/remember previously remember memories or knowledge (retrograde amnesia), impairment in the ability to acquire new memories or information (anterograde amnesia), loss of memory of events dealing with particular sense such as taste, hearing, etc.(sense-specific amnesia) while sometimes it is the temporary loss of memory and these episodes are sudden and generally do not extend beyond 24 hours (transient amnesia). The impairment is usually found in short-term and recent memory. Sometimes patients lose time or place orientation (the name of the hospital, city), and in some rare cases, even self-orientation is lost in amnestic disorder. These symptoms must result in significant difficulties for patients in their personal, social, or occupational functioning. Gross and subtle changes in personality can go together with the symptoms of memory impairment. Patients with this disorder do not have good insight into their neuropsychiatric conditions; they sometimes even put effort to hide their confusion through confabulatory answers to the questions. Apart from the normal population elderly above 65 years of age have higher chances of developing amnestic disorders and those who are above 75 years have the highest rates of developing it due to traumatic brain injury (TBI).

There are multiple medical conditions that can cause amnestic disorders. Conditions include seizures, head trauma, cerebral tumor, thiamine deficiency, hypoglycemia, brain stroke, hydrocephalus, damage to blood vessels causing ischemia, brain surgery, tumors in the brain, and interrupted oxygen supply to the brain. Amnestic disorders are also caused by certain psychological disorders like schizophrenia, bipolar disorder, and depression (Andreescu and Aizenstein, 2009). The development of amnestic disorder depends upon its etiology, commonly it has a static course with no progression or deterioration but little improvement can be seen over time. The amnestic disorder that is secondary to stroke, infection, and tumor are irreversible, further leading to multimorbidity like holding jobs or occupation, impaired interpersonal relationships, and even inability to care for oneself. TBI and alcohol dependence is associated with a decline in verbal memory. Inhibitory control declined, independence of risk factors, and to a larger extent the mortality for the people who are homeless and precariously housed people (Gicas et al, 2020).

Delirium

Delirium is characterized by a severe deterioration in both the level of consciousness and cognition with impairment in attention particularly. It is a reversible disorder of the central nervous system but it is quite threatening as most of the time it involves perceptual disturbances, sleep cycle impairment, and abnormal psychomotor activity. The impairment in consciousness usually occurs in association with global impairment of cognitive functions that come with disturbance in mood, perception, and behavior. It is also associated with neurological dysfunctions like Tremors, asterixis, nystagmus, incoordination, and urinary incontinence. Delirium is a common disorder with the highest incidence and prevalence the in the elderly population with 1 percent of elderly in the age above 55 years or older and 13% in the age 85 years and older group. Patients with no history of delirium developed it during the time of hospitalization with a prevalence of 5-30%, 10-15% during general surgical patients, 30% of cardiological interventions, 21% of patients with severe burns, 30-40% of patients with AIDS and more than 50% of patients treated for hip fractures alone. The major risk of developing delirium is advanced age. It is estimated that and 30-40% of hospitalized elderly with more than 65% years of age have an episode of delirium another independent risk factor is the male gender. The mortality rate for patients with a single episode of delirium is as high as 50%. The patients who experienced delirium during hospitalization have a 21-75% mortality rate. Chances of delirium doubled as the age becomes 80 years (41.8%) this is due to uncommon predisposing factors in younger age (Marquetand et. al., 2021).

The major predisposing factors for delirium were found to be 65 years with the male gender, frailty, and dementia (Monacelli et al., 2022). and on the cognitive status the individuals who have a history of delirium, depression, and cognitive impairment have higher chances of having delirium. History of falls, low levels of activity, hearing, or a visual impairment, and decreased oral intake are also predisposing factors. Coexisting medical conditions like stroke, chronic renal or hepatic disease, neurological disease, infection with the human immunodeficiency virus, fractures or trauma, and terminal disease make individuals more vulnerable to delirium. Disease interaction and medication use in the multimorbid elderly can precipitate delirium (Savaskan, 2012). Neurosensorial multimorbidity is most prevalent in delirium including in patients with cerebrovascular diseases, sensory impairment, and dementia & at baseline neural connectivity and brain function govern the vulnerability sign for the overall system disruption in the occurrence of acute insults. (Monacelli et al., 2022). In socioeconomically deprived people multimorbidity occurs earlier that inevitably leads to poorer quality of life, and functioning, premature death, and increased healthcare utilization. The primary mechanism for the development of multimorbidity is complex, multilevel, and interrelated but somehow, they are related to the biological mechanism of aging (Skou et al., 2022).

TRENDS OF COVID 19

Corona virus disease 2019 (COVID-19) was announced as Pandemic worldwide by the World Health Organization (WHO) on March 11, 2020. The effect of COVID-19 is not limited to China only but it also spread rapidly at global level with the nature of contamination or communicable across the nations. The rapid outbreak of coronavirus disease was threatening to all level of society causing mortality and morbidity. COVID-19 is an infectious or communicable in nature cause by severe acute respiratory syndrome coronavirus 2 (SARS-CoV-2) by means of substantial mortality and morbidity (Wu et. al., 2020). Covid related protocols, government restrictions, and covid related appropriate measures such as social distancing, home quarantine, lockdown etc. led negative impact on every individual from every sector of society. No single population was left behind of its negative impact including anxiety, depression, insomnia, posttraumatic stress disorders, stress and adjustment related disorders, obsessive compulsive and related disorders, substance use disorders, and so. Elderly those who lived alone or with their spouses during pandemic faced a number of psychological problems and this population are more vulnerable to multiple psychological conditions including problem related to substantial central nervous system (CNS) linking that varieties from acute disorientation (delirium) to meningoencephalitis (Mcloughlin, 2020). Acute and severe symptoms and manifestations indicators have been distinguished by researchers and health professional affecting to the elderly as well as normal healthy population, but long-standing neuropsychiatric and cognitive consequences still not so clear to understand it in detail, (Tavares-Júnior et al., 2022). Roberta Eduarda Grolli et al (2021), conducted a study and found that chronic condition and other medical or psychiatric illness work as precipitating factor for highest risk of comorbidity and mortality during COVID-19. Additionally, it was also found that elderly with previous psychiatric conditions reflects some downfall in neurological and immunological symptoms.

The effect of COVID -19 is not only restricted to physical health related condition but also had a negative impact on extensive series of medical manifestation. Nervous system related indicators of deterioration due to covid-19 were evident among elderly population during pandemic, including cognitive deficits/ impairment including dementia, mild cognitive impairment (MCI), subjective cognitive decline (SCD). During and after COVID-19, clinical evaluation was demonstrated on elderly patient and it found that the neurobiological manifestation being more common (Wu et al., 2020). Outbreak of COVID-19 led to various clinical manifestation including headache, wooziness, faintness, altered sensorium, altered consciousness, stroke, severe episodes of anxiety, panic attacks, insomnia, gastrointestinal disease, and ataxia (Guan et al., 2019). Mao et al. (2022) conducted a study on elderly patient and found that patients those were having severe illness are more to be expected and prone toward progress of nerve related disorder such as disorders of consciousness, acute cerebrovascular disease, and musculoskeletal disease. Among elderly population, functional impairment is seen evidently which significantly goes to put negatively impact of managing daily life independence. Alemanno et al (2021) conducted research study with the help of questionnaire and have applied different assessment tools to ensure the role of COVID-19 on cognitive deficit, using Mini Mental Status Evaluation (MMSE), Montreal Cognitive Assessment (MOAC), Functional Independence Measures (FIM), and Hamilton Rating Scale for Depression (HAM-D). Interestingly 80% of patients have found to have cognitive impairment which in turn can affect the functional outcome of elderly. Moreover Deing et al., (2014), found that the annual progression rate of minor to major mental deficiency among adults over 65 years of age is around 12 to 18%. The prevalence rate and neurological amnestic alteration rate is around 10 to 15% and now it is most prevalent among older adults during pandemic period.

MANAGEMENT

Early detection of cognitive decline is crucial step to be taken into consideration to reduce the global disability and care giver burden among elderly. Non-pharmacological management used to manage core symptoms as well as the root causes. Non-pharmacological management targets on the less productive routine of the elderly and male them less dependent on their caregivers. The core symptoms in elderly are cognitive deficit, functional deficits, and social decline. Therapist, medical social worker, mental health professional can provide personalized approaches to presenting problems for cognitive deficits such as dementia, delirium, amnestic and other neurocognitive disorders. Techniques of cognitive stimulation are a program of memory provoking, problem-solving skills and conversational fluency activities, face naming training. These are very effective techniques for the management of dementia. Reality Orientation Therapy also used to get quick information about the patient's presence of mind. This is done to reorient the person by repetitive orientation to the environment. Maintaining of dairy on daily basis, reading newspaper articles and placing things on their appropriate fix places can reduce the burden of dependency. Caregiver intervention programs are based on comprehensive training to the family caregiver so that effective management can be done, and family burden can be reduced which ultimately going to serve satisfaction. Light therapy, aromatherapy, music therapy, pet therapy, physical activities recreational activities, and multisensory stimulation play a significant role in the management of elderly with deficits. Scheduled toileting and routine prompted voiding for incontinence, graded assistance, and positive reinforcement are very effective to increase functional independence.

Colcombe & Kramer, 2003; Corre-Leite et al., in 2001, analyzed eighteen clinical trials to monitor the impact of physical activities interventions on the cognition of the elderly and reported benefits in managing executive functions, planning, abstraction, selection of relevant sensory information, and other higher level cognitive functioning. Another meta-analysis was published by Kramer et al., 2005, they noticed the positive significant effect of aerobic exercise and strength training on executive functioning and global cognitive improvement. These randomized control trials proved the efficacy of cognitive training in the elderly. The role of cognitive intervention in the management of CD is important and shouldn't be denied.

Kramer et al., 2004, memory training can improve recall, recognition, visuospatial ability, perceptual discrimination, and other related perception. Memory training-based intervention is not only effective for older with significant deficits but also good for healthy individuals as well. Evidence of mnemonic-based memory last in long-term memory and it is also useful for remembering fact-based information. According to McDougall, 2000, memory training is nothing but teaching a new way of storing and retaining information for a long. The memory function of the elderly can improve through self-monitoring, problem-solving, relaxation, and feedback. Memory performance can be enhanced by training. Training includes stress management, learning of coping skill, improvement of self-efficacy, promoting effective health management through proper routine follow-up, one or two-step mathematical calculations, maintaining mindful based daily activity, and a supported environment has also been tested in older adults in a retirement residence (McDougall, 2000). In a Longitudinal study by Schaie et al., 2004, a cognitive training program was demonstrated in older adults with existing cognitive declines. They have identified decline related to inductive reasoning or spatial orientation training programs for 5 hours which were designed to improve skills that are needed to manage day-to-day activities. And in this training program of 7 years follow up after training, 40% improvement was achieved. In this follow-up study, cognitive training was proved to be more effective for this precise cognitive ability (day-to-day activities).

The ACTIVE (Advanced Cognitive Training for Independent and Vital Elderly) can also serve as potential findings in the management of the elderly. Clinical trials of 2000 older adults have randomly divided into three groups and provided them three different training of verbal episodic memory, inductive reasoning, and processing speed 10 sessions. Post-training improvements occurred in specific focused skills that continued for 2 years (Ball et al., 2002). Another study by Wills et al (2006), they have reported significant improvement in 10 sessions of ACTIVE intervention as booster treatment for specific cognitive domains such as memory, reasoning, or processing speed. According to Wolinsky et al., 2006, randomized trials of control versus experimental group found that the participants those who were in the experimental group were less likely to undergo significant deficits in memory as well as health-related quality of life, and these findings leads to the direction for continuing research to test the impact of cognitive interventions on everyday lives of elderly in future.

The role of social intervention also provides evidence of the protective effects of social involvement, social support, and productive activities on cognition in aging. Fried et al., 2004 conducted study on older adults for 15 hours in weekly sessions over one year in school as an add-on treatment of cognitive protective intervention. In this program elderly worked with students in elementary school and played the role of supportive person and an interactive activity was done that involves bodily activity, strength building, effective social support networks, and cognition related activity that positively increases the cognitive ability of elders. This program is serving as a crucial institutive in focusing on societal engagement interventions in order to enhance cognitive ability for older adults and aims to minimize deficits and maximize functioning in every sphere of life. The finding of this study provides support to social theories that claim the role of social support and engagement in the betterment of meaningful functioning, and these played a critical role in "successful aging."

Researchers and health professionals cannot avoid the potential role of nutritional intervention on aging and cognitive decline. A number of clinical trials were carried out and found to be effective in the management of decline whether cognitive, functional, or social. The nutritional effect can serve as a potential intervention to improve cognitive function. In a study in 2005 by Wouter-Wesseling et al., on a small sample of 67 participants of the older adult with minimal or no measurable impairment was taken for 6-months trial testing and at last, it was noted that short and intermediate memory improved after the intervention.

CONCLUSION

It's a very crucial to know and detect early signs and symptoms including frequent forgetting of appointments, social events, loosening of association, difficulty in formulating of thoughts and speech, difficulty in following one to one as well as group conversations and emotional reciprocity, poor understanding of basic instructions, difficulty in making routine decision, poor judgment ability, disorientation, confusions, difficulty in planning, unable to reason and think well, difficulty in problem solving, face difficulty in motor functioning, and trouble in finding locations. Sometimes in some cases it was misdiagnose and there is also treatment gap because family members and other close associates can't distinguish between normal aging symptoms and neurocognitive disorders related to comorbidities and identification of manifestation of abnormalities in brain level functions. Symptoms associated with aging among elderly significantly impacted their life functioning and made them vulnerable to many other psychiatric including depression, anxiety, agitation, paranoia, personality changes, hallucinations, inappropriate behavior, substance use, obstructive sleep apnea, insomnia, obsessive compulsive disorder as well as physical comorbidities including diabetes, obesity, high cholesterol, hypertension, cardiac disease. Aging is a downfall growing stage of multiple comorbidities and its need to be managed effectively. Therefore, keeping all the above-mentioned recent evidence in the field of cognitive deficit and progressive decline with aging, it is very crucial to rule out every possible way to prevent the onset, an initial assessment is needed to be done, management should be planned ahead, and treatment are needed to provide so that the burden of global disability, mortality, morbidity could be reduced.

REFERENCES

Alemanno, F., Houdayer, E., Parma, A., Spina, A., Del Forno, A., Scatolini, A., Angelone, S., Brugliera, L., Tettamanti, A., Beretta, L., & Iannaccone, S. (2021, February 8). COVID-19 cognitive deficits after respiratory assistance in the subacute phase: A COVID-rehabilitation unit experience. *PLoS One, 16*(2), e0246590. doi:10.1371/journal.pone.0246590 PMID:33556127

Ali, S. A., Begum, T., & Reza, F. (2018, July). Hormonal influences on cognitive function. *The Malaysian Journal of Medical Sciences: MJMS, 25*(4), 31–41. doi:10.21315/mjms2018.25.4.3 PMID:30914845

Almeria M, Cejudo JC, Sotoca J, Deus J, Krupinski J. (2020). Cognitive profile following COVID-19 infection: Clinical predictors leading to neuropsychological impairment. *Brain, behavior, & immunity-health.*

Alvarez, M., Trent, E., Goncalves, B. D., Pereira, D. G., Puri, R., Frazier, N. A., Sodhi, K., & Pillai, S. S. (2022). Cognitive dysfunction associated with COVID-19: Prognostic role of circulating biomarkers and microRNAs. *Frontiers in Aging Neuroscience, 14*, 14. doi:10.3389/fnagi.2022.1020092 PMID:36268187

Anderson, D. K., Lord, C., Risi, S., DiLavore, P. S., Shulman, C., Thurm, A., & Pickles, A. American Psychiatric Association. (2013). Diagnostic and statistical manual of mental disorders. The Linguistic and Cognitive Effects of Bilingualism on Children with Autism Spectrum Disorders.

Andreescu, C., & Aizenstein, H. J.*Amnestic Disorders and Mild Cognitive Impairment. Kaplan & Sadock's Comprehensive Textbook of Psychiatry. Baskı* (B. J. Sadock, B. A. Sadock, & P. Ruiz, Eds.).

Ball, K., Berch, D. B., Helmers, K. F., Jobe, J. B., Leveck, M. D., Marsiske, M., Morris, J. N., Rebok, G. W., Smith, D. M., Tennstedt, S. L., Unverzagt, F. W., & Willis, S. L.ACTIVE Study Group. (2002, November 13). Effects of cognitive training interventions with older adults: A randomized controlled trial. *Journal of the American Medical Association, 288*(18), 2271–2281. doi:10.1001/jama.288.18.2271 PMID:12425704

Bassuk, S. S., Wypij, D., & Berkmann, L. F. (2000, April 1). Cognitive impairment and mortality in the community-dwelling elderly. *American Journal of Epidemiology, 151*(7), 676–688. doi:10.1093/oxfordjournals.aje.a010262 PMID:10752795

Carvalho, A., Rea, I. M., Parimon, T., & Cusack, B. J. (2014, April 12). Physical activity and cognitive function in individuals over 60 years of age: A systematic review. *Clinical Interventions in Aging*, 661–682. PMID:24748784

Castaño, E. (2020, April). Discourse analysis as a tool for uncovering the lived experience of dementia: Metaphor framing and well-being in early-onset dementia narratives. *Discourse & Communication, 14*(2), 115–132. doi:10.1177/1750481319890385

Chehrehnegar, N., Nejati, V., Shati, M., Rashedi, V., Lotfi, M., Adelirad, F., & Foroughan, M. (2020, March). Early detection of cognitive disturbances in mild cognitive impairment: A systematic review of observational studies. *Psychogeriatrics, 20*(2), 212–228. doi:10.1111/psyg.12484 PMID:31808989

Christopher, L., & Strafella, A. P. (2013, September). Neuroimaging of brain changes associated with cognitive impairment in Parkinson's disease. *Journal of Neuropsychology, 7*(2), 225–240. doi:10.1111/jnp.12015 PMID:23551844

Crivelli, L., Palmer, K., Calandri, I., Guekht, A., Beghi, E., Carroll, W., Frontera, J., García-Azorín, D., Westenberg, E., Winkler, A. S., Mangialasche, F., Allegri, R. F., & Kivipelto, M. (2022, May). Changes in cognitive functioning after COVID-19: A systematic review and meta-analysis. *Alzheimer's & Dementia, 18*(5), 1047–1066. doi:10.1002/alz.12644 PMID:35297561

Darley, D. R., Dore, G. J., Cysique, L., Wilhelm, K. A., Andresen, D., Tonga, K., Stone, E., Byrne, A., Plit, M., Masters, J., Tang, H., Brew, B., Cunningham, P., Kelleher, A., & Matthews, G. V. (2021, April 1). Persistent symptoms up to four months after community and hospital-managed SARS-CoV-2 infection. *The Medical Journal of Australia*, *214*(6), 279–280. doi:10.5694/mja2.50963 PMID:33657671

Dhakal, A., & Bobrin, B. D. (2022). Cognitive Deficits. Treasure Island (FL): StatPearls Publishing.

Ding, D., Zhao, Q., Guo, Q., Meng, H., Wang, B., Luo, J., Mortimer, J. A., Borenstein, A. R., & Hong, Z. (2015, March 1). Prevalence of mild cognitive impairment in an urban community in China: A cross-sectional analysis of the Shanghai Aging Study. *Alzheimer's & Dementia*, *11*(3), 300–309. doi:10.1016/j.jalz.2013.11.002 PMID:24613707

Emmady, P. D., Schoo, C., & Tadi, P. (2022). Major Neurocognitive Disorder (Dementia). In StatPearls [Internet]. Treasure Island (FL): StatPearls Publishing.

Gicas, K. M., Jones, A. A., Thornton, A. E., Petersson, A., Livingston, E., Waclawik, K., Panenka, W. J., Barr, A. M., Lang, D. J., Vila-Rodriguez, F., Leonova, O., Procyshyn, R. M., Buchanan, T., MacEwan, G. W., & Honer, W. G. (2020, March). Cognitive decline, and mortality in a community-based sample of homeless and precariously housed adults: 9-year prospective study. *BJPsych Open*, *6*(2), e21. doi:10.1192/bjo.2020.3 PMID:32043436

Goodman, R. A., Posner, S. F., Huang, E. S., Parekh, A. K., & Koh, H. K. (2013). Peer reviewed: defining and measuring chronic conditions: imperatives for research, policy, program, and practice. *Preventing Chronic Disease*, 10.

Gould, C. E., O'Hara, R., Goldstein, M. K., & Beaudreau, S. A. (2016, October). Multimorbidity is associated with anxiety in older adults in the Health and Retirement Study. *International Journal of Geriatric Psychiatry*, *31*(10), 1105–1115. doi:10.1002/gps.4532 PMID:27441851

Grande, G., Marengoni, A., Vetrano, D. L., Roso-Llorach, A., Rizzuto, D., Zucchelli, A., Qiu, C., Fratiglioni, L., & Calderón-Larrañaga, A. (2021, May). Multimorbidity burden and dementia risk in older adults: The role of inflammation and genetics. *Alzheimer's & Dementia*, *17*(5), 768–776. doi:10.1002/alz.12237 PMID:33403740

Grolli, R. E., Mingoti, M. E., Bertollo, A. G., Luzardo, A. R., Quevedo, J., Réus, G. Z., & Ignacio, Z. M. (2021, May). Impact of COVID-19 in the mental health in elderly: Psychological and biological updates. *Molecular Neurobiology*, *58*(5), 1905–1916. doi:10.100712035-020-02249-x PMID:33404981

Ho, F. F., Xu, S., Kwong, T. M., Li, A. S., Ha, E. H., Hua, H., Liong, C., Leung, K. C., Leung, T. H., Lin, Z., Wong, S. Y., Pan, F., & Chung, V. C. H. (2023, January 19). Prevalence, Patterns, and Clinical Severity of Long COVID among Chinese Medicine Telemedicine Service Users: Preliminary Results from a Cross-Sectional Study. *International Journal of Environmental Research and Public Health*, *20*(3), 1827. doi:10.3390/ijerph20031827 PMID:36767195

Huang, H. K., Hsieh, J. G., Hsieh, C. J., & Wang, Y. W. (2017, September 9). Do cancer patients with dementia receive less aggressive treatment in end-of-life care? A nationwide population-based cohort study. *Oncotarget*, *8*(38), 63596–63604. doi:10.18632/oncotarget.18867 PMID:28969014

Jolles, J., Verhey, F. R., Riedel, W. J., & Houx, P. J. (1995, December). Cognitive impairment in elderly people: Predisposing factors and implications for experimental drug studies. *Drugs & Aging*, *7*(6), 459–479. doi:10.2165/00002512-199507060-00006 PMID:8601053

Jongsiriyanyong, S., & Limpawattana, P. (2018, December). Mild cognitive impairment in clinical practice: A review article. *American Journal of Alzheimer's Disease and Other Dementias*, *33*(8), 500–507. doi:10.1177/1533317518791401 PMID:30068225

Kurdoğlu, Z. (2021). Do the COVID-19 vaccines cause menstrual irregularities. *International Journal of Women's Health and Reproduction Sciences*, *9*(3), 158–159. doi:10.15296/ijwhr.2021.29

Kuring, J. K., Mathias, J. L., & Ward, L. (2018, December 15). Prevalence of depression, anxiety, and PTSD in people with dementia: A systematic review and meta-analysis. *Neuropsychology Review*, *28*(4), 393–416. doi:10.100711065-018-9396-2 PMID:30536144

Langa, K. M., Larson, E. B., Karlawish, J. H., Cutler, D. M., Kabeto, M. U., Kim, S. Y., & Rosen, A. B. (2008, March 1). Trends in the prevalence and mortality of cognitive impairment in the United States: Is there evidence of a compression of cognitive morbidity? *Alzheimer's & Dementia*, *4*(2), 134–144. doi:10.1016/j.jalz.2008.01.001 PMID:18631957

Laureys, S., Gosseries, O., & Tononi, G. (Eds.). (2015 Aug 12). *The neurology of consciousness: cognitive neuroscience and neuropathology*. Academic Press.

Lee, J. K., & Jeong, H. W. (2021, January). Wearing face masks regardless of symptoms is crucial for preventing the spread of COVID-19 in hospitals. *Infection Control and Hospital Epidemiology*, *42*(1), 115–116. doi:10.1017/ice.2020.202 PMID:32372736

Marquetand, J., Bode, L., Fuchs, S., Ernst, J., von Känel, R., & Boettger, S. (2021). Predisposing, and precipitating factors for delirium in the very old (≥ 80 years): A prospective cohort study of 3,076 patients. *Gerontology, 67*(5), 599–607. doi:10.1159/000514298 PMID:33789299

Mcloughlin, B. C., Miles, A., Webb, T. E., Knopp, P., Eyres, C., Fabbri, A., Humphries, F., & Davis, D. (2020, October). Functional and cognitive outcomes after COVID-19 delirium. *European Geriatric Medicine, 11*(5), 857–862. doi:10.100741999-020-00353-8 PMID:32666303

Miyawaki, C. E., Bouldin, E. D., Taylor, C. A., & McGuire, L. C. (2020, August 13). Baby boomers as caregivers: Results from the Behavioral Risk Factor Surveillance System in 44 states, the District of Columbia, and Puerto Rico, 2015–2017. *Preventing Chronic Disease, 17*, E80. doi:10.5888/pcd17.200010 PMID:32790608

Monacelli, F., Signori, A., Marengoni, A., Di Santo, S., Rossi, E., Valsecchi, M. G., Morandi, A., & Bellelli, G. (2022, May 1). of Delirium IS. Delirium and clusters of older patients affected by multimorbidity in acute hospitals. *Journal of the American Medical Directors Association, 23*(5), 885–888. doi:10.1016/j.jamda.2021.10.004 PMID:34798007

Monacelli, F., Signori, A., Marengoni, A., Di Santo, S., Rossi, E., Valsecchi, M. G., Morandi, A., & Bellelli, G. (2022, May 1). of Delirium IS. Delirium and clusters of older patients affected by multimorbidity in acute hospitals. *Journal of the American Medical Directors Association, 23*(5), 885–888. doi:10.1016/j.jamda.2021.10.004 PMID:34798007

Murman, D. L. The impact of age on cognition. In Seminars in hearing 2015 Aug (Vol. 36, No. 03, pp. 111-121). Thieme Medical Publishers. doi:10.1055-0035-1555115

Park, H. L., O'Connell, J. E., & Thomson, R. G. (2003, December). A systematic review of cognitive decline in the general elderly population. *International Journal of Geriatric Psychiatry, 18*(12), 1121–1134. doi:10.1002/gps.1023 PMID:14677145

Payne, J. L., Lyketsos, C. G., Steele, C., Baker, L., Galik, E., Kopunek, S., Steinberg, M., & Warren, A. (1998, November). Relationship of cognitive and functional impairment to depressive features in Alzheimer's disease and other dementias. *The Journal of Neuropsychiatry and Clinical Neurosciences, 10*(4), 440–447. doi:10.1176/jnp.10.4.440 PMID:9813790

Persson, J., Nyberg, L., Lind, J., Larsson, A., Nilsson, L. G., Ingvar, M., & Buckner, R. L. (2006, July 1). Structure–function correlates of cognitive decline in aging. *Cerebral Cortex (New York, N.Y.), 16*(7), 907–915. doi:10.1093/cercor/bhj036 PMID:16162855

Pilotto, A., Cristillo, V., Cotti Piccinelli, S., Zoppi, N., Bonzi, G., Sattin, D., Schiavolin, S., Raggi, A., Canale, A., Gipponi, S., Libri, I., Frigerio, M., Bezzi, M., Leonardi, M., & Padovani, A. (2021, December). Long-term neurological manifestations of COVID-19: Prevalence and predictive factors. *Neurological Sciences*, *42*(12), 4903–4907. doi:10.100710072-021-05586-4 PMID:34523082

Prince, M., Ali, G. C., Guerchet, M., Prina, A. M., Albanese, E., & Wu, Y. T. (2016, December). Recent global trends in the prevalence and incidence of dementia, and survival with dementia. *Alzheimer's Research & Therapy*, *8*(1), 1–3. doi:10.118613195-016-0188-8 PMID:27473681

Prince, M. J., Wimo, A., Guerchet, M. M., Ali, G. C., Wu, Y. T., & Prina, M. (2015). *World Alzheimer Report 2015-The Global Impact of Dementia: An analysis of prevalence, incidence, cost, and trends*. WAA.

Renzi, A., Verrusio, W., Messina, M., & Gaj, F. (2020, November). Psychological intervention with elderly people during the COVID-19 pandemic: The experience of a nursing home in Italy. *Psychogeriatrics*, *20*(6), 918–919. doi:10.1111/psyg.12594 PMID:32770596

Salthouse, T. A. (2009, April 1). When does age-related cognitive decline begin? *Neurobiology of Aging*, *30*(4), 507–514. doi:10.1016/j.neurobiolaging.2008.09.023 PMID:19231028

Savaskan, E. (2012, December 1). Delirium and multimorbidity in the elderly. *Praxis (Bern)*, *101*(25), 1633–1636. doi:10.1024/1661-8157/a001147 PMID:23233102

Stewart, R., Xue, Q. L., Masaki, K., Petrovitch, H., Ross, G. W., White, L. R., & Launer, L. J. (2009, August 1). Change in blood pressure and incident dementia: A 32-year prospective study. *Hypertension*, *54*(2), 233–240. doi:10.1161/HYPERTENSIONAHA.109.128744 PMID:19564551

Tavares-Júnior, J. W., de Souza, A. C., Borges, J. W., Oliveira, D. N., Siqueira-Neto, J. I., Sobreira-Neto, M. A., & Braga-Neto, P. (2022, April 18). COVID-19 associated cognitive impairment: A systematic review. *Cortex*, *152*, 77–97. doi:10.1016/j.cortex.2022.04.006 PMID:35537236

Tonelli, M., Wiebe, N., Straus, S., Fortin, M., Guthrie, B., James, M. T., Klarenbach, S. W., Tam-Tham, H., Lewanczuk, R., Manns, B. J., & Quan, H. (2017, August 14). Multimorbidity, dementia and health care in older people: A population-based cohort study. *Canadian Medical Association Open Access Journal.*, *5*(3), E623–E631. PMID:28811281

Üstün, B., & Kennedy, C. (2009, June 1). What is "functional impairment"? Disentangling disability from clinical significance. *World Psychiatry; Official Journal of the World Psychiatric Association (WPA), 8*(2), 82–85. doi:10.1002/j.2051-5545.2009.tb00219.x PMID:19516924

Vannorsdall, T. D., Brigham, E., Fawzy, A., Raju, S., Gorgone, A., Pletnikova, A., Lyketsos, C. G., Parker, A. M., & Oh, E. S. (2022, March 1). Cognitive dysfunction, psychiatric distress, and functional decline after COVID-19. *Journal of the Academy of Consultation-liaison Psychiatry, 63*(2), 133–143. doi:10.1016/j.jaclp.2021.10.006 PMID:34793996

Welsh, T. J. (2019). Multimorbidity in people living with dementia. *Case Reports in Women's Health*, (Jul), 23. PMID:31193805

Williams, K. N., & Kemper, S. (2010, May 1). Interventions to reduce cognitive decline in aging. *Journal of Psychosocial Nursing and Mental Health Services, 48*(5), 42–51. doi:10.3928/02793695-20100331-03 PMID:20415290

Woo MS, Malsy J, Pöttgen J, Seddiq Zai S, Ufer F, Hadjilaou A, Schmiedel S, Addo MM, Gerloff C, Heesen C, Schulze Zur Wiesch J. (2020). Frequent neurocognitive deficits after recovery from mild COVID-19. *Brain communications, 2*(2).

World Health Organization. (2004). International Statistical Classification of Diseases and related health problems: Alphabetical index (Vol. 1, 2, 3). World Health Organization.

Wu, Y., Xu, X., Chen, Z., Duan, J., Hashimoto, K., Yang, L., Liu, C., & Yang, C. (2020, July 1). Nervous system involvement after infection with COVID-19 and other coronaviruses. *Brain, Behavior, and Immunity, 87*, 18–22. doi:10.1016/j.bbi.2020.03.031 PMID:32240762

Zhang, L., Shooshtari, S., St. John, P., & Menec, V. H. (2022, November 10). Multimorbidity and depressive symptoms in older adults and the role of social support: Evidence using Canadian Longitudinal Study on Aging (CLSA) data. *PLoS One, 17*(11), e0276279. doi:10.1371/journal.pone.0276279 PMID:36355773

Zhou, H., Lu, S., Chen, J., Wei, N., Wang, D., Lyu, H., Shi, C., & Hu, S. (2020, October 1). The landscape of cognitive function in recovered COVID-19 patients. *Journal of Psychiatric Research, 129*, 98–102. doi:10.1016/j.jpsychires.2020.06.022 PMID:32912598

Chapter 11
Of Multimorbidity:
Case Histories in Care Planning

Aisha Ansari
iD https://orcid.org/0000-0002-1512-8504
Capella University, USA

EXECUTIVE SUMMARY

An argument is made that multi-morbidity can be distinguished between three categories: male, female, and elderly. Another identifier linked to multi-morbidity is military service and veterans. Managed care and care planning are offered as common solutions when managing elder care. The topics of hypoxia, palliative care, abdominal distention, and pharmacology are examined to show their effects on elder care and multi-morbidity. For multi-morbidity, the role of chronic illnesses as a public health stressor must also be examined. Cases, solutions, and other outcomes in this chapter will discuss the overall diagnosis in some patients. Financial management in healthcare gains nominal attention because of its importance in our society, culture, and human behaviors.

INTRODUCTION

Social, Cultural, And Behavioral Disparities in Multi-Morbidity

History displays a wide array of hospitalizations and caring for the wounded, sick, elderly and mentally ill. Often when visualizing care and hospitalization we view wounded soldiers and their rehabilitation and re-entry into society as being a model in managing care. As adults receiving our first diagnosis and prescription, we move along our life journey without heeding these prescribed precautions. Subsequently,

DOI: 10.4018/978-1-6684-2354-7.ch011

we accumulate more illnesses, diagnosis, and prescriptions. This is the foundation of multi-morbidity. Lack of mobility carries a plethora of concerns which include hypoxia, palliative care, abdominal weight gain, and weight loss. Accepting frailty as a part of growing old and old age does not necessarily affect all individuals. This chapter attempts to link multi-morbidities with age and chronic illnesses. Examples of co-morbidities and defining it are embedded within this chapter contexts of each patient and their environments. The World Health Organization (WHO) describes co-morbidities as being 65 years and older with a combined diagnosis of diabetes, heart disease, mental illness, and immobility. In real world scenarios co-morbidities are simply more than one disease found within the same person. The target audience which includes medical professionals and family members who are care givers will find examples and definitions throughout this chapter with cases in care planning examples. This chapter reiterates the importance of healthy heart and brain stem messaging which communicates vital life instructions throughout our life cycles. Definitions and examples of co-morbidities and the need for proper medical care guidelines are illustrated throughout this chapter through our literature reviewed case studies.

The first hospital dates to the 4th century in Persia and the 6th century in Syria. Persian Academy of Gondishapur was established for medical training in 529 A.D. Al Wahid Bimarstan was the first Islamic hospital and built in Syria between 706 and 707 A.D. Spanish hospitals are the forerunners dates from 1503 in the Americas with Hospital St. Nicolas de Bari in Dominican Republic. The first hospital in the United States was founded in Philadelphia in 1751, Philadelphia Hospital, under the leadership of Dr. Thomas Bond and Benjamin Franklin. Philadelphia Hospital mission was to care for the sick, insane, poor, and homeless. Care at the first hospital in Philadelphia distinguished between the sick, insane, poor, and homeless under the same roof with specific care plans. Over 140 years ago in 1881, Clara Barton is credited with the American Red Cross, serving the wounded and poor, with an emphasis at that time for American soldiers. A Congressional Charter in the 1900's set a path of charitable personal and emergency disaster relief in the United States. All these cases in caring for the sick, injured, mentally challenged, and the homeless are the basis for of the research done in healthcare treatment and outcomes.

Distinguishing between the different environments found in patients with multi-morbidity stems from gender, and the conditions which will be reiterated throughout this paper. These conditions being gender, social and economic descriptive, medical treatment and prescriptions will be targeted as common denominators when possible, reducing the extensive burden in diagnosis and treatment. Cases in managed care facilities often see disparities in diagnosis and treatment based on the patient's ability to pay. Despite being housed in the same location, segmented care plans are put into place to manage each society demands in healthcare accountability. Recount the early days of mid-wife visits and caring for the sick, all done within the privacy of our homes. Today many palliative care patients choose to remain under the care of a physician while staying at home with the nursing care of family members. Personal contacts and observations while visiting the elderly and those residents receiving managed and palliative care, over a seven-year period, offered cases linked in life cycles, cultural, social and economic factors which contribute to multi-morbidity.

When charting the first palliative care case, one patient in 1948 started the movement, and the first planned care facility in 1967. Palliative care evolved from the London boroughs with families meeting and planning care for their dying family members and spread to more than 1.5 million homes (Saunders, 2000). Saunders described the first patient, being a male Jew from Warsaw Poland, and died from rectal cancer (Saunders, 2000). However, the author Dame Cicely Saunders and St. Christophers are credited with started the palliative care movement. Ms. Saunders died at St. Christophers in 2006. The author is known for her work in "total pain". As with opioids in our society today, people in the 1940's were convinced that narcotic relief would free patients of pain and discomfort, which Saunders refer to as myths (2000). In 1970's a double-blind study was done with morphine and diamorphine, and with findings that there is no difference between the two drugs.

Alcohol and substance abuse in our society crosses all boundaries in social, cultural, and human behaviors. When associating alcohol with multiple chronic illnesses there is little delineation between social and economic effects in diagnosis. Sexual transmitted diseases are another common denominator found in chronic diseases, often attributed to mobility and morbidity. Greenstein et al., relate the case of a 75-year-old veteran with complex comorbidities and is an alcoholic with his estranged wife as primary caregiver (2021). Patient has been admitted to the VA Medical Center over 150 times with injuries from alcoholism and mental illness (Greenstein et. al, 2021). Suffering from Vietnam War trauma, the patient has been diagnosed with chronic liver disease, mental illness, post-traumatic stress disorder (PTSD), aging, and alcoholism. With personal care and hygiene lagging, the patient has a risk of cardiovascular disease due to his cognitive ability and non-adherence to the medical team care planning (Greenstein et al., 2021). Therefore, the VA medical care team relies on interdisciplinary care because of the complexities found, this patient is an example of comorbidities.

Collaborations between the state and local governments with the VA at the federal level offer financial solutions when caring for veterans' complex needs. The Veterans Administration, VA, touts a budget of sixty-eight billion dollars for 9 million veterans (Kaufman et al., 2022). The VA per capita budget is three times the local efforts found in veteran agencies and medical centers. The case of the local tribe members in Alaska and Indian community, The Indian Health Services, IHS, which offers their veterans 4,078 dollars per capita, significantly less that US prisoners at 10, 742 dollars in 2017 (Kaufman et al., 2022). Most veterans combine local and federal dollars to cover their medical expenses. This study found that only 45 percent of all veterans utilized the system of funding medical expenses using both local and federal dollars. Veterans in this study when distinguishing between the male veterans and female veterans found that females were slightly younger in age. Female veterans sixty-five and older were 10 percent, while male veterans were 41.3 percent (Kaufman et al., 2022). Recently the Department of Defense, DOD, acknowledged the service of the United States LGBT, lesbian, gay, black, and transgender, community. Missing demographic data in this military population challenges the VA medical mission and administration when delivering medical services (Watkins, 2022). Service members are often asked to identify themselves as veterans without respect to lifestyles and sexual preferences.

Recent concerns with chronic obstructive pulmonary disease, (COPD) and healthy hearts; linking the two maladies, COPD, and coronary heart disease, (CHD) seem appropriate for the case of comorbidities and aging. Aging men and women experience a decline in the desire to interact sexually. Steptoe reported in a recent study that age and morbidities were used as continuous variables in people over 50 years of age diagnosed with CHD, analyzing marital status and partnerships, and excluding participants with diabetes (2016). Findings show that the number of comorbidities were higher in patients with CHD and a confidence level of p=>0.001, that 94.7 percent women and 93.6 percent men were considered heterosexual throughout their lifetimes (Steptoe, 2016). This large data set involved 2979 men and 3711 women, which did not include diabetes as a covariate but did consider arthritis and any form of cancer accompanied by their detailed prescription records within the last four years (Steptoe, 2016). Because with COPD the lungs and the heart are dependent on each other, and without adequate purified oxygen the mind and body fail to respond appropriately in most situations including sexual activity.

So often as in most instances disparity in healthcare is brought on by race, cultural identity, and socio-economic well-being. Perhaps revisiting the Critical Race Theory is not advised; however, many experts suggest that the theory holds reflective wins in connecting with our respective race and heritage. Corona virus disease, COVID-19, in 2019 globally affected the vulnerable and underlined public health disparities.

The National Library of Medicine reports that racially diverse mature adults with psychiatric needs experience hardships during the pandemic and COVID 19. Characteristics found in this vulnerable population during the pandemic include isolated individuals with psychiatric needs, posing complications in co-morbidities such as diabetes, SARS and other respiratory infections, and hypertension (Diaz et al., 2021). Diaz et al. reported that in the United Kingdom minorities, for example, Bangladeshi, Pakistani, and Indian were reported as experiencing far more mental distress than their White British counterparts. Blacks in the United Kingdom also measured with more distress than their White British counterparts. Areas around the globe with more access to the Internet experienced less mental health and distress, with Asian and Hispanics reporting spikes in hospitalization and contemplated suicide (Diaz et al., 2021). During the pandemic, India reported increased agitation between Muslims and their religious majority, using social media to spread virus phobias and discriminate comments (Diaz et al., 2021). The elderly experienced social isolation during the pandemic and COVID 19 was in North Africa, Middle East, including the Sub-Sahara countries due to lack of Internet access for in-home health appointments. Because of COVID 19 isolation and lack of Internet use, elderly patients could not utilize telehealth. Managing health visits and health management strategies were limited with an increase in depression and trauma (Diaz et al., 2021). Quality of life measures seek to eliminate pain and suffering gained from being diagnosed with a terminal illness.

VULNERABLE POPULATIONS IN MULTI-MORBIDITY: THE ELDERLY, HOMELESS, AND MENTAL ILLNESS

When examining the vulnerability found in multiple morbidities, Herrman et al. (2022) reminds us that a healthy brain as our stem, plays a key role in maintaining health throughout our complete life cycle. Herman gives evidence that depression is heterogenous, and that the trajectory of mental illness does not change despite environment and context of the morbidity. The authors also relate that depression is experienced during our lifetime, and reactions and responses are different clinicians and caregivers are challenged with care planning. Evidence-based research supports that the physical health is intricately linked to mental health. During this discussion we will refer to depression as being ongoing with diagnosis thresholds varying because of depression sparse data. Researchers found underlying depression in both male and female patients, young and old, and across all social and economic barriers. Herrmann et al., (2022) linked comorbidities and chronic illnesses including cardiovascular disease, cancer, and diabetes to depression and mental health.

The elderly, when compared to other vulnerable populations with multiple morbidities, require multidisciplinary care planning. McCarthy links sleeping disorders in the elderly to co-morbidity (2021). With a multidisciplinary and multi-faceted care plan adults 65 years of age and older suffering from depression require holistic care and medical treatment. Because of the complexity of depression and sleeping disorders in the elderly when coupled with other chronic illnesses, present care givers with the need for transparency and early diagnosis. By the time a patient reaches sixty-five with comorbidities, McCarthy offers a strategy and care planning which is systematic and multidomain.

Qassem et al. and in a recent survey of elderly patients with depression and co-morbidity, Adult Psychiatric Morbidity Survey, found that age and social environments played major roles (2021). In a sample of 7325 English participants, 3163 men and 4162 women, the probability of, post-traumatic stress disorder (PTSD), was present in 7112 participants (Qassem et al., 2021). Most prevalent in the findings were depression, social phobias, and anxieties. Substance abuse in the elderly was minimal with race and cultural backgrounds more prominent variables (Qassem et al., 2021). Because of temporal and overlooked underlying cases in depression, PTSD, there were differences in outcomes linking depression and co-morbidity. However, results were conclusive enough to suggest that there is an overlap and strong association in depression and co-morbidity. Continued care in the elderly populations always advises care and patience. Coupling old age, depression, and co-morbidity need age old remedies in holistic care which do not rely solely on care planning and pharmacology.

Multi-Morbidity Cases: Frailty, Hypoxia, And Pharmacology

Multi-morbidity acts as a vector for hypoxia being complex and requiring multiple illnesses and diseases. Infections obstructing the airways for breathing in recent COVID-19 elderly patients. However, not without the array of overlapping concerns in cognitive abilities, sleep disorders, heart and stroke complications, depression, and anxiety. Respiratory syndrome and corona virus, these infections affect HDL functions and cause chronic inflammation in elderly patients (AbdelHafez, 2022). Hypoxia in the elderly should not be confused with prescription side effects, but the euphoria of light headedness without adequate oxygen in their environments.

Centers for Disease Control and Prevention report in Emerging Infectious Diseases, 2017, a case of an elderly patient and his death during a blood transfusion in New York, USA. The patient died from septic shock two weeks following a perioperative blood transfusion and transmission of anaplasmosis (Goel et al., 2017). The seventy-eight-year-old patient suffered from anemia, received 14 transfusions, and had a long history of chronic illness, including coronary heart and kidney disease, and diabetes (Goel et al., 2017). An investigation and autopsy concluded that the donated blood used in the transfusion was from a patient with Lyme disease. The donated blood, after 90 days, was now considered compromised with human granulocytic ehrlichiosis, HGA, tick-borne disease and is normally asymptomatic in healthy humans (Goel et al, 2017). In this case of the seventy-eight-year-old patient, with the transmitted HGA blood, septic shock and respiratory complications were fatal. After this investigation a call for judicious protocols in blood transfusions and regulated guidelines. Currently the Food and Drug Administration does not have standards in place for donated blood (Goel et al., 2017). Hypoxia linked to breathing and respiratory malfunction, occurs during sepsis and toxic shock. Most cases of sepsis originate in the healthcare facility environment and are a fatal trajectory in older and chronically ill patients. Sepsis is one of the World Health Organization sustainable goals in healthy 2030. The WHO passed Resolution WHA70.7 in response to emerging threats and early clinical management of Sepsis.

Revisiting our argument that elderly patients and co-morbidity often accompany mental fatigue and mental disorders. Sleep apnea and anxiety require medical treatment to allow the elderly proper and sufficient sleep and healthy hearts. Elderly patients experiencing multiple health conditions and the use of multiple drug therapies. Experts found that the interaction between drugs analysis for the effects and common illnesses most patients experience while on various drug therapies.

Frailty in older patients stems from an intestinal infection. Nivet et al. describe the possible cause of intestinal infection as clostridium difficile, CDI, and affects adults over eighty years old with co-morbidities (2022). However, a recent study in France used participants ages 18 – 79 as a control group and found that fecal microbiota transplant therapy works as a deterrent in CDI infections (Nivet et al., 2022). The survival rate in patients 80 years of age and older at 52 weeks when using this intervention of FMT. Overall survival rate and recurrence free rates between the two groups did not vary, 78.9 versus 89.7 percent respectively (Nivet et al., 2022). The same for re-occurrence free between the two groups at 86.9 and 94.3 percent (Nivet et al, 2022). While FMT is not a world-wide recommendation in patients, frailty in elderly patients does not prove to be a significant factor in actual outcomes. Authors offer a conclusion that FMT limits a loss of motor skills in older patients, improves quality of life, and care settings do not affect patient outcome (Nivet et al, 2022).

Dawood and McNamara, (2022), quote Khalil Gibran about the value of having elderly people in our lives, with "Seek ye the counsel……. hardened to the voices of life". "Even if their counsel……. pay heed to them," Khalil Gibran. Elderly people provide us with countless benefits in wisdom and life lessons. Dawood and McNamara remind us of that global public health has seen a cross section of same diseases and suffering during this last decade (2022). The authors recommend having clarity in communicating quality of life treatments in elderly care from the emergency room back to their homes.

Ribarič (2022) argues that physical exercise, PE, is an alternative to pharmacology in patients with Alzheimer's and cardiovascular diagnosis. Benefits of physical exercise include increased cardio muscle strength, increased oxygen, and blood capillary network. Physical exercise, a non-pharmacological intervention, enhanced with proper nutrition, improves Alzheimer's and cognitive functions in adults >65 years of age (Ribarič, 2022). Aging is associated with systemic chronic infection, SCI, and continues degrading and damaging body tissues. When SCI spreads to the patient's gut, brain, liver, and kidney may lead to diabetes and cancer (Ribarič, 2022). Key factors triggering systemic chronic infection are diet, social and cultural lifestyle changes, and existing chronic infections which lead to inhibited metabolic function in aging (Ribarič, 2022). Experts suggest that practitioners do not fully understand SCI and need ongoing research. Patients with SCI should avoid highly processed foods and cognitive decline.

FOCUS: MANAGING MULTI-MORBIDITY AND PALLIATIVE CARE

Palliative care requires pain management and holistic care when the patient no longer responds to other methods of care including spiritual healing and prayer. The concept of palliative care, PC, adopted in definition by the World Health Organization, WHO in 1990. According to Llop-Medina et al. the European Association for Palliative Care, EAPC, expanded the treatment of patients with life-threatening and end stages of diseases, to include management of spiritual, social, and psychological care (2022). Palliative Care, PC, focused on improving the patient and their family quality life, easily gains attention in elderly care and co-morbidity. Reuters, 2011 charted 6162 records and five studies which revealed that elderly patients with multi-morbidities care needs most often involved emotionally caring individuals as caregivers. This study done in a care-giving setting and used cohort professionals. Again, most patients required holistic care because of their depression and anxiety. The need for spiritual care reported because of the study setting, and patients felt that staffing and resources did not reflect their religious values (Llop-Medina et al., 2022).

Moving past initial palliative care planning, and pandemic palliative care, Crawford et al. link palliative care and legal care during these end-of-life decisions in advance care (2021). Recollecting that the care plan becomes a part of the patient's medical records and can be subpoenaed by legal professionals in legal proceedings caring for the elderly and end-of-life patients. The palliative care team initiates advance care and document planning and resuscitation as found in the Advance Care Directive, ACD, a legislative and common law instrument (Crawford et al., 2021). However, with stress and human behavior adherence to a protocol in communication and clarity between patient, team members, and family members remain barriers in palliative care. This observance was documented by hospital care team in Australia using a 7 Step Pathway and prepared by its clinicians and communicated to patient, staff and family members (Crawford et al., 2021). The South Australia hospital utilized eight focus groups in quality data collection. The patient's case in acute oncology required a care team consisting of nurses both regular and emergency room, medical interns, specialists, and social workers (Crawford et al., 2021). Documentation and activities were not transmitted across the spectrum of the care team, causing the end-of-life wishes to be undermined (Crawford et al., 2021).

Multidisciplinary care approaches seek to reduce the hospital length of stay and readmissions. Palliative care considered as a solution to long hospital stay. Since decision-making is a vital component of palliative care, adequate care giving, and support are catalysts in progressive treatment and release from long term care. A team of physicians and social workers in a one thousand bed teaching hospital offered routine multi-disciplinary recommendations twice weekly (Hagiwara & Yuya, 2022). Out 13, 941 patients, 5644 patients were 65 years of age and older. Using a linear regression model, the length of stay decreased by mean=0.36, while readmissions were unchanged at -1.17% (Hagiwara & Yuya, 2022). Managing multi-morbidity and palliative care requires a multidisciplinary approach as seen in a care plan.

There are several types of care plans. For this discussion we will concern ourselves with a care plan for the elderly. Managed care and nursing home long term care utilize care plans which are broken down into categories starting with assessment, diagnosis, objective, intervention, rationale, and evaluation. The fact that care plans are subject to the Health Insurance Portability and Accountability Act, HIPPA, and are part of the individual and patient medical record, reflects the need for patient information privacy and protection. Each care plan is specifically designed for the individual patient and supports staffing, care, and insurance reimbursement and is subject to privacy in health information guidelines and regulations.

Nursing care plans are prescribed and prepared for the patient by registered nurses, approved by the family physician and passed on to family members and the nursing facility staff. When viewing a recent care plan all the environment and contexts of the patient and background affect care planning outcomes. The care plan starts with the subjective and objective. When interviewing the patient, the health professional finds that there is an expression of fatigue and anxiety. Targeting loss of sleep, the care plan progresses to manage the objective with a short-term diagnosis. After diagnosis, a nursing intervention is recommended, a rationale given for actions taken, and evaluations given after the care planning.

The National Institute of Nursing offers information and resources in palliative care. According to the Institute, palliative includes a multidisciplinary team. Palliative care teams may include doctors, nurses, social workers, therapists, spiritual advisers, nutritionists, pharmacists, and other counselors including legal attorneys. The Journal of Nurse Practitioners explains that in palliative care, end-of-life decisions are discussed. Some observations in palliative care are that the age spectrum varies, while most are elderly there are individuals in palliative care < 65 years of age. Therefore end-of-life discussions require sound mental health and stability, since individuals in palliative care are concerned with support and pain management.

Table 1. Nursing care plan

Subjective: Patient reports loss of sleep and fatigue	Diagnosis: Imbalance and activity intolerance	Objective: Short term objectives include	Intervention: Assess patient and ADL	Rationale: Choices in activities influenced	Evaluation Care plan intervened with Increased activity
Objective: Recommend sleep and elevated bed rest	Problem with oxygen supply and delivery	Increase tolerance in ADL after nursing intervention	Note any changes in gait/muscle weakness	Nutrition and diet changes in B_{12} targeting falls and bone density	Psychological tolerance in social settings returned to a normal range per laboratory data
Check vital statistics in blood pressure and respiratory functions	Low oxygen for lower body requirements	Long term objectives after nursing intervention increased muscle strength	Advise more activity with assistance, quiet atmosphere, elevated bed pillows	Increase rest, improving heart and oxygen supply	Demonstrated more independent activity

The cost of palliative care is covered by most insurances just as Medicare and Medicaid may participate in some palliative care. The Journal of Nurse Practitioners relates that there are three areas of concern in palliative care. Coordination of care involves collaboration between all members of the palliative team to ensure clarity and communication for referrals and transitions during care planning. Palliative care requires education and resources in elder care and support. The Journal of Nurse Practitioners also reported that when the term support care was used instead of palliative care, referral increased 41 percent (2022). Palliative care also suffers from patient and family member's misconceptions. Patients' negative feelings are exposed during palliative care because of end-stage life and decision making. One third of the adults in the United States receiving palliative care require a family member for cognitive and sound decision-making. This person of authority and power of attorney, in most cases, needs the trust of the patient and the palliative care team.

COVID-19 offered more challenges to patients and their families with the environment of uncertainty. The Journal of Nurse Practitioners report that communications skills across the multidisciplinary teams lacked support and resources in competent palliative care planning (2022). In Africa, only eight countries were prepared to respond to the COVID 19 pandemic. WHO 2020 readiness assessment found 62 percent of African countries were adequately prepared for the pandemic, with 34 countries participating. African countries witnessed the universal experience with COVID 19 and their elderly and vulnerable patients with co-morbidities. The 2005 International Health Regulations Survey was mailed to 166 African Palliative

Care Association members and partners. Using a descriptive analysis of COVID 19 preparedness, 21 countries responded (Boufkhed et al., 2020). The survey reported triage conditions and patients complained of breathlessness and psychological distress (Boufkhed et al., 2020). COVID 19 patients referred to palliative care complained of fever, cough, spiritual, existential threats, and resources supporting end-of-life decision-making (Boufkhed et al., 2020).

Of the respondents, there were 17 physicians, 12 nurses, 1 psychosocial professional, and 46 front-line managers. Staff members reported anxiety about contracting the COVID 19 virus and the stigma of caring for the pandemic victims (Boufkhed et al., 2020). Staff members also reported socio-economic concerns in employment, training additional staff, and personal protective equipment resources (Boufkhed et al., 2020). During the pandemic staff members utilized mobile phone applications to monitor, instruct, and communicate COVID 19 measures and outcomes. Fifty-two percent of the respondents were prepared with palliative protocols, while 42 percent reported scarcity in resources to train staff during the pandemic (Boufkhed et al., 2020). COVID 19 pandemic measures were found adequate in the 34 African nations responding to the WHO International Health Regulations Survey, however resources mainly monetary, remain a challenge.

McAteer and Wellbery offer in an editorial with American Family Physician, that the World Health Organization and its sustainable goals for all nations support improved palliative care (2013). Statistics on elderly deaths reflect a need for improvement in palliative care. McAteer and Wellbery estimate that one million deaths with 45 percent in the United States hospices, could have been avoided (2013). With protocols in multidisciplinary teams and documented activities in care, palliative care still reported upward trends in deaths including discharges and readmissions (2013). With some variances between hospice care and palliative care, the common concern is quality of life there are positives in the case of palliative care, especially in the hospices that the patient feels a sense of improved quality of life, caring, support, and management of end-of life- and life-threatening illness.

The World Health Organization, WHO, reports that seventy-eight percent of adults living in low to moderate income countries need palliative care. The WHO has taken the initiative and included palliative care as part of their Sustainable Development Goal, SDG, making it an integral part of healthcare delivery. A campaign for insurance coverage and palliative care inclusion in technical advancement, measurement and assessment tools. WHO, with a strategy in palliative care will focus on elder frailty, end-stage chronic illnesses, cardiovascular disease, and cancer? Strategies also include social and spiritual development goals for patients throughout palliative care.

BARRIERS TO PALLIATIVE CARE

The Eastern Mediterranean has seen recent emerging non-communicable diseases. The World Health Organization, WHO, with resources and resolutions seek to tackle disparities in access to palliative care. Since many patients are diagnosed with late-stage cancer and life-threatening illnesses, palliative care is needed as an integral part of their primary care and support. Fadhil et al, (2017) report that palliative care is available in this region of the world, but care is sporadic and inconsistent. Author's report that based on income Saudi Arabia scored lower than Egypt and Morocco. Saudi Arabia ranked 60 out of 80 high income countries in palliative care at 30.8 percent. However, Saudi Arabia has implemented through their National Cancer Centre and Saudi Health Council and intensive care and pain management plan for palliative patients (Osman & Yamout, 2022). Palliative care in its early stages in Saudi Arabia and Jordan with evidence starting in the 1990's. Saudi Arabia, Jordan, and Egypt have the largest number palliative care programs, with Jordan and Saudi Arabia recognizing palliative care as a specialty (Osman & Yamout, 2022). Saudi Health Council in 2018 adopted their Saudi Palliative Care National Clinical Guideline for Oncology, which offers quality standards in pain management, and life-threatening patient assessments throughout the caring period. These qualitative standards are guidelines found in National Cancer Centre is evidenced based and scalable to most palliative patients, including patients with diverse backgrounds, religions including Islam and eastern cultures. The full 2018 report can be accessed at Saudi Health Council government Internet site. Morocco and Egypt considered amongst the low-income countries scored 33.8 and 32.9 percent respectively (Fadhil et al., 2017). Iraq, in the middle-income group, had the lowest Quality of Life ranking at 12.5 percent. This report forecast improvement and development of palliative care using psychological resources (Fadhil et al., 2017). When considering global palliative care quality reports, most nations do not have policies in place governing palliative care, but in this case Kuwait and Tunisia a standalone plan is implemented (Fadhil et al., 2017). This World Health Organization, WHO, NCD, non-communicable disease country report list Saudi Arabia and Syria with home-based palliative care, with Lebanon having palliative care that is non-governmental agencies (Fadhil et al., 2017). Concerns that when palliative care is available in Eastern Mediterranean countries, it's in the developmental stages of delivery, however like most palliative care globally offering quality end stage life support in pain management, social and spiritual activities in decision-making.

In 2014, the World Health Organization, WHO, established primary care inclusion goals in palliative care. The objective of this World Health Assembly Resolution 76.19 recognized palliative care as an integral part of universal health and well-being, and to improve palliative care globally. In the Eastern Mediterranean region an estimated forty million people need palliative care. WHO explains palliative barriers and non-communicable diseases access to service as?

- Palliative care is not considered as a global health policy and agenda
- Improved and non-existent training is needed for healthcare and allied health professionals in palliative care
- Social and cultural misconceptions and the lack of community awareness about palliative care its benefits and accessibility.
- Misconceptions, and the need for education and public awareness in the international conventions about opioid benefits and substance abuse

Barriers in palliative care for women with gynecological cancers are experienced globally. The stigma of female gynecological cancer resonates globally, in a world the perhaps expectations in the female gender are being a mother, friend, beautiful, and healthy. Western policies in palliative care for patients seeking home care have developed to represent dignity and family care. However, women make-up the bulk of palliative caregivers and require professional representation in the workforce. Low- and middle-income countries are now reporting an increase in female gynecological cancers. Policy and resource barriers continue to challenge caregivers, patients and their families in caring for palliative patients diagnosed with life-threatening conditions. Authors Cain and Denny argue that the cost of medications and opioids in palliative care continues to be a barrier (2018). Palliative care calls for complete integration in primary care as soon as the patient is diagnosed with a life-threatening illness.

Low- and middle-income countries in this section of our discussion will refer to Latin America. The spectrum in access and support in palliative care in Latin America for women diagnosed with oncological cancers see the highest rates in Costa Rica. The gap in service based on population is 16.06 palliative care units per 1 million inhabitants' population (Cain & Denny, 2018). Costa Rica if followed by Honduras with 0.24 units per inhabitants. With these disparities in palliative care, Mexico ranks the highest country in palliative training a course integration in medical curricula (Cain & Denny, 2018). Palliative care calls for multi-disciplinary care globally, and most often it starts with family and the community. Lack of access and resources, palliative care often sees the community as the front-line managers, and family members as caregivers. Community and family members are indispensable in palliative care with a wealth of experience in the patient's psychosocial, spiritual, medical, pain and comfort management. Palliative care management timing and intervention are critical to the patient's quality of life. Treating bowel and constipation irritabilities in women with terminal cancer diagnosis has proven effective in continuity of care (Cain & Denny, 2018). Other methods of treatment and care include surgeries with stents and reduce hospital stays. In cervical cancer patients, and ovarian cancers bowel motility is of importance, and palliation care must be individually implemented for optimum outcomes (Cain & Denny, 2018). Pulmonary, breast, and ovarian cancers are managed with hyperthermic chemotherapy, radiation, and talc powders. Long term care has promise in pulmonary issues with opioids and morphine (Cain & Denny, 2018). Women often experience barriers in palliative care because of resources, accessibility, and policies governing care. Open communication and planned strategies that put the patient first are needed to relieve the main services in palliative care, pain management and support. Reassurance that terminal illnesses are understood and that family, community, the care-giving team are committed to extending and improving suffering works across cultures, and diseases. Because most caregivers are women, palliative care education and training can improve how the world view women and palliative care.

Blumberg, 2015, reports that the United Kingdom tops the list of countries with palliative care and credits this outcome to their incorporation with the National Health Service. Australia and New Zealand follow next, and these statistics were linked to healthcare funding in the respective countries for palliative care. Countries were scored based on quality weights of healthcare environments and contexts, training and staffing of health professionals, affordability of palliative care, quality of care, and community engagement (Blumberg, 2015). Environment, human resources and training of palliative care professionals, and affordability weighed in at 20 per cent. Quality of care at 30 per cent, and community engagement at 10 per cent. Changing views about the benefits and challenges in substance abuse and opioids was seen as an opportunity to improve palliative care. Community engagement and partnerships in care involving families, patients, and healthcare professionals are needed to strengthen palliative care awareness.

A WORD FORWARD: SOLUTIONS AND RECOMMENDATIONS

Care planning acts as the best model and best practice solution in elderly and palliative care. In this chapter the various cultures and demographics were examined and determined that co-morbidities require multi-discipline and emphatic caring. Health solutions which address end-stage disease progression, patient decision-making empowers, and strengthens the care in care planning for the patient. With palliative care, barriers to care, the need for trained professionals as care givers echo concern and sparse resources. Since the patient has been given life threatening circumstances to navigate presumably for a short period of time, a focus on the patient and their overall well-being are key to successful outcomes.

Since caregivers and multi-disciplinary teams work together for maximum results in patient outcomes, sharing of best practices are required globally as care planning becomes the accepted practice in elderly care. Our preceding discussions in palliative care recommended that care planning strategies should put the patient and their needs first. This empowerment allows for sound decision making during stress and uncertainty. Care planning and palliative care should be incorporated within the health care delivery and not as a stand alone in elderly care. This healthcare incorporates cost and availability when implementing care planning and palliative care, ensuring a certain level of inclusion and equitable access. This call for prescriptions and pharmacies suitable for public, men, and women, economically challenged continues to challenge world health systems.

Visioning post corona virus diseases and elderly palliative care, support and technology seek to aid sustainable life trends. Research is needed in telemedicine and the prospect of the elderly finding this technology user- friendly and supportive. Technologies including the computer and cellphone would allow the patient privacy while gaining empowerment in decision-making situations.

CONCLUSION: FORECASTING MULTI-MORBIDITY AND FUTURE DISCUSSIONS

Forecasting and future care planning discussions, focus-groups in multi – morbidity cases are expected to assist the patients and their families with care and support. Multi-morbidity, hypoxia, pharmacology, fragility, dementia, and mental wellness require caregivers who are empathetic to growing old and with multiple chronic illnesses. Care planning across the spectrum of disciplines addresses the individual patient preferences and is flexible in change and quality of life measures.

Care planning works best when the care plan is available and understood by the patient, and their family members. With support from all team members both medical and patient linked, a research action approach can be applied to recovery and quality of life. Palliative care strives in a supportive environment for decision making, which are often social and psychosomatic. Therefore, having a trusting team of care givers allows the patient to reflect and make important end of life decisions. Global advocacy in palliative caring is needed along with our existing world of primary care.

Women and men both require care planning and palliative care, however because female caregivers outnumber male caregivers; women often make up much of the managed care workforce. Innovative approaches and break through therapies merging male and female care planning may improve outcomes. Without regards to social demographics, improved outcomes and lower mortality rates offer chances for better health communication strategies in elderly care.

REFERENCES

AbdelHafez, M. A. (2022). Protective and therapeutic potentials of HDL and ApoA1 in COVID-19 elderly and chronic illness patients. *Bulletin of the National Research Center*, *46*(1), 222. doi:10.118642269-022-00886-x PMID:35915785

Blumberg, A. (2015). 10 Countries with the Best Care for the Dying. *Huffington Post*.

Boufkhed, S., Namisango, E., Luyirika, E., Sleeman, K. E., Costantini, M., Peruselli, C., Normand, C., Higginson, I. J., & Harding, R. (2020). Preparedness of African Palliative Care Services to Respond to the COVID-19 Pandemic: A Rapid Assessment. *Journal of Pain and Symptom Management*, *60*(6), e10–e26. doi:10.1016/j.jpainsymman.2020.09.018 PMID:32949761

Cain, J. M., & Denny, L. (2018, October). Palliative care in women's cancer care: Global challenges and advances. *International Journal of Gynaecology and Obstetrics: the Official Organ of the International Federation of Gynaecology and Obstetrics*, *143*(Suppl 2), 153–158. doi:10.1002/ijgo.12624 PMID:30306578

Crawford, G. B., Hodgetts, K., Burgess, T., & Eliott, J. (2021). Documenting plans for care: Advance care directives and the 7-step pathway in the acute care context. *BMC Palliative Care*, *20*(1), 1–9. doi:10.118612904-021-00838-8 PMID:34503479

Dawood, M., & McNamara, R. (2022). Do no harm. *Emergency Medicine Journal: EMJ*.

Diaz, A., Baweja, R., Bonatakis, J. K., & Baweja, R. (2021, April 19). Global health disparities in vulnerable populations of psychiatric patients during the COVID-19 pandemic. *World Journal of Psychiatry*, *11*(4), 94–108. doi:10.5498/wjp.v11.i4.94 PMID:33889535

Early palliative care initiation: Role of the primary care clinician. (2022). *The Journal for Nurse Practitioners, 18*(5), 493-495.

Fadhil, I., Lyons, G., & Payne, S. (2017, March). Barriers to, and opportunities for, palliative care development in the Eastern Mediterranean Region. *The Lancet. Oncology*, *18*(3), e176–e184. doi:10.1016/S1470-2045(17)30101-8 PMID:28271872

Fancourt, D., & Steptoe, A. (2019). Comparison of physical and social risk-reducing factors for the development of disability in older adults: A population-based cohort study. *Journal of Epidemiology and Community Health, 73*(10), 906–912. doi:10.1136/jech-2019-212372 PMID:31243046

Goel, R., Westblade, L. F., Kessler, D. A., Sfeir, M., Slavinski, S., Backenson, B., & Cushing, M. M. (2018). Death from Transfusion-Transmitted Anaplasmosis, New York, USA, 2017. *Emerging Infectious Diseases, 24*(8), 1548–1550. doi:10.3201/eid2408.172048 PMID:30016241

Greenstein, A. P., Solomon, H. V., & Funk, M. C. (2021). Caring for aging veterans with alcohol use disorder and multiple morbidities. *Generations Journal, 44*(4), 1–6.

Hackett, R. A., & Steptoe, A. (2016, October). Psychosocial Factors in Diabetes and Cardiovascular Risk. *Current Cardiology Reports, 18*(10), 95. doi:10.100711886-016-0771-4 PMID:27566328

Hagiwara, Yuya, M.D., M.A.C.M. (2022). Interprofessional geriatric and palliative care intervention associated with fewer hospital days. *Journal of Pain and Symptom Management, 63*(4), 629.

Herrman, H., Patel, V., Kieling, C., Berk, M., Buchweitz, C., Cuijpers, P., & Wolpert, M. (2022). Time for united action on depression: A lancet –World psychiatric association commission. *Lancet, 399*(10328), 957–1022. doi:10.1016/S0140-6736(21)02141-3 PMID:35180424

Kaufman, C. E., Grau, L., Begay, R., Reid, M., Goss, C. W., Hicken, B., Shore, J. H., & O'Connell, J. (2022). American indian and alaska native veterans in the indian health service: Health status, utilization, and cost. *PLoS One, 17*(4), e0266378. doi:10.1371/journal.pone.0266378 PMID:35363822

Llop-Medina, L., Fu, Y., Garcés-Ferrer, J., & Doñate-Martínez, A. (2022). Palliative care in older people with multimorbidities: A scoping review on the palliative care needs of patients, carers, and health professionals. *International Journal of Environmental Research and Public Health, 19*(6), 3195. doi:10.3390/ijerph19063195 PMID:35328881

McAteer, R., & Wellbery, C. (2013, December 15). Palliative care: Benefits, barriers, and best practices. *American Family Physician, 88*(12), 807–813. PMID:24364543

McCarthy, C. E. (2021). Sleep disturbance, sleep disorders and co-morbidities in the care of the older person. *Medical Science, 9*(2), 31. PMID:34063838

Nivet, C., Duhalde, V., Beaurain, M., Delobel, P., Quelven, I., & Laurent, A. (2022). Fecal microbiota transplantation for refractory clostridioides difficile infection is effective and well tolerated even in very old subjects: A real-life study. *The Journal of Nutrition, Health & Aging*, *26*(3), 290–296. doi:10.100712603-022-1756-1 PMID:35297473

Oladimeji, M., Asiyanbi, G., Fadeyi, A., Belle, O., Olanipekun, S., & Adekola, O. (2019). ESICM LIVES 2019.

Osman, H., & Yamout, R. (2022). Palliative Care in the Arab World. In H. O. Al-Shamsi, I. H. Abu-Gheida, F. Iqbal, & A. Al-Wadhi (Eds.), *Cancer in the Arab World*. Springer. doi:10.1007/978-981-16-7945-2_24

Qassem, T., Aly-ElGabry, D., Alzarouni, A., Abdel-Aziz, K., & Danilo, A. (2021). Psychiatric comorbidities in post-traumatic stress disorder: Detailed findings from the adult psychiatric morbidity survey in the english population. *The Psychiatric Quarterly*, *92*(1), 321–330. doi:10.100711126-020-09797-4 PMID:32705407

Resolution WHA67. (2014). *19. Strengthening of palliative care as a component of comprehensive care throughout the life course*. Sixty-seventh World Health Assembly.

Ribarič, S. (2022). Physical exercise, a potential non-pharmacological intervention for attenuating neuroinflammation and cognitive decline in Alzheimer's disease patients. *International Journal of Molecular Sciences*, *23*(6), 3245. doi:10.3390/ijms23063245 PMID:35328666

Salari, P., O'Mahony, C., Henrard, S., Welsing, P., Bhadhuri, A., Schur, N., Roumet, M., Beglinger, S., Beck, T., Jungo, K. T., Byrne, S., Hossmann, S., Knol, W., O'Mahony, D., Spinewine, A., Rodondi, N., & Schwenkglenks, M. (2022). Cost-effectiveness of a structured medication review approach for multimorbid older adults: Within-trial analysis of the OPERAM study. *PLoS One*, *17*(4), e0265507. doi:10.1371/journal.pone.0265507 PMID:35404990

Saudi Palliative Care National Clinical Guideline for Oncology. (n.d.). SHC. shc.gov.sa/ar/NCC/Documents/Saudi%20Palliative%20Care%20National%20Clinical%20Guideline%20for%20Oncology.pdf

Saunders, C. (2000). The evolution of palliative care. *Patient Education and Counseling*, *41*(1), 7–13. doi:10.1016/S0738-3991(00)00110-5 PMID:10900362

Steptoe, A., Jackson, S. E., & Wardle, J. (2016). Sexual activity and concerns in people with coronary heart disease from a population-based study. *Heart (British Cardiac Society)*, *102*(14), 1095–1099. doi:10.1136/heartjnl-2015-308993 PMID:27126394

World Health Organization. (2018). *Integrating palliative care and symptom relief into primary health care: a WHO guide for planners, implementers, and managers.* WHO.

KEY TERMS AND DEFINITIONS

Chronic Diseases: People with chronic illnesses are prone to other infections and maladies because of underlying and existing disease. For example, diabetes, heart, and kidney diseases, which are concurrent with any emerging illnesses. Most patients began therapy for an illness such as heart disease and continue until clinicians see improvement to release the patient from the diagnosed regime. Since the patient is still being considered under physician care, any other illnesses become multiple conditions in health care and medical statistics. Chronic ill patients sometimes are part of a group of behavioral linked and diagnosed individuals due to symptoms and outcomes. The Center for Disease Control, CDC, define chronic disease as any condition by which an individual is treated for more than 1 year and currently undergoing treatment. The CDC also offers risk factors such as alcohol and tobacco use, nutrition and diet, exercise, and physical activities.

Elderly: The Agency for Healthcare Research and Quality, AHRQ, define elderly in the United States as people aged sixty-five and older and having one or more chronic illnesses or comorbidities. Often the elderly requires specialized care which is managed by family members. The AHRQ estimates that by 2030 the elderly will comprise 20 percent of the US population.

Homeless: The National Institute of Health, NIH, and their National Library of Medicine definition of homeless stems from the Stuart B. McKinney Assistance Act in 1987, which gives several conditions to be considered homeless. First, the individual does not have a stable or fixed address during the nighttime. An individual has a nighttime address which is a shelter, or hotel temporary housing, transit or rotational housing for the mentally ill. Sleeping or being housed in a private or public place not intended for humans and is applicable to individuals and families.

Hypoxia: The Cleveland Clinic describes hypoxia as being delirium based on the lack of oxygen in human body tissues. Symptoms include bluish skin, rapid heartbeat, confusion, and often accompanied by heart and lung disease.

Mentally Ill: Mental illness is described at the National Alliance on Mental Illness, NAMI, as a disorder that can cause varying amounts of psychological and behavioral impairment in individuals. NAMI also offers several types of mental illness, 1) anxiety, 2) psychosis, 3) schizophrenia, 4) bipolar disorder, 5) major depression disorder, 6) panic attack, 7) adjustment disorder, 8) post-traumatic stress disorder, PTSD, 9) borderline personality disorder, and 10) intellectual disability.

Multi-Morbidity: Adults over the age of sixty-five, living with both physical and mental ailments are classified by the World Health Organization, WHO, as having multi-morbidities. Since individuals with multi-morbidities are at a higher risk of injuries, such as falls, the WHO has devoted much attention to safer elderly primary care. Multi-morbidity conditions include diabetes, heart disease, HIV/AIDS, and mental illness.

Pharmacology: The study of medicines and how they work interacting with the human body, is the definition offered by the British Pharmacological Society. Pharmacology comes from the Latin word "pharmakon" meaning drug, and "logia" meaning knowledge of.

Palliative Care: Evidenced-based quality care for families and practitioners about palliative care and serious illnesses can be found at the National Institute of Nursing. The National Institute of Nursing define palliative care as treatment received concurrently with the illness but being concerned with pain management. Palliative care help to relieve constipation, shortness of breath, loss of appetite, fatigue, loss of sleep, and medical treatment side effects.

Compilation of References

AAO—HNSF. (2006). *Geriatric Care Otolaryngology.*

AbdelHafez, M. A. (2022). Protective and therapeutic potentials of HDL and ApoA1 in COVID-19 elderly and chronic illness patients. *Bulletin of the National Research Center, 46*(1), 222. doi:10.118642269-022-00886-x PMID:35915785

Ackermans, L. L., Rabou, J., Basrai, M., Schweinlin, A., Bischoff, S. C., Cussenot, O., Cancel-Tassin, G., Renken, R. J., Gómez, E., Sánchez-González, P., Rainoldi, A., Boccia, G., Reisinger, K. W., Ten Bosch, J. A., & Blokhuis, T. J. (2022). Screening, diagnosis and monitoring of sarcopenia: When to use which tool? *Clinical Nutrition ESPEN, 48*, 36–44. doi:10.1016/j.clnesp.2022.01.027 PMID:35331514

Adegbiji, W. A., Aremu, S. K., & Aluko, A. A. A. (2019). Geriatric Otorhinolaryngology, Head and Neck Emergency in a Nigerian Teaching Hospital, Ado Ekiti. *International Journal of Otolaryngology and Head & Neck Surgery., 8*(3), 81–90.

Ahmad, T., Pencina, M. J., Schulte, P. J., O'Brien, E., Whellan, D. J., Piña, I. L., Kitzman, D. W., Lee, K. L., O'Connor, C. M., & Felker, G. M. (2014). Clinical implications of chronic heart failure phenotypes defined by cluster analysis. *Journal of the American College of Cardiology, 64*(17), 1765–1774. doi:10.1016/j.jacc.2014.07.979 PMID:25443696

Ahmed, N., Mandel, R., & Fain, M. J. (2007). Frailty: An emerging geriatric syndrome. *The American Journal of Medicine, 120*(9), 748–753. doi:10.1016/j.amjmed.2006.10.018 PMID:17765039

Ai, A. L., & Carrigan, L. T. (2007). Social-strata-related cardiovascular health disparity and comorbidity in an aging society: Implications for professional care. *Health & Social Work, 32*(2), 97–105. doi:10.1093/hsw/32.2.97 PMID:17571643

Albano, C., Cupello, A., Mainardi, P., Scarrone, S., & Favale, E. (2006). Successful treatment of epilepsy with serotonin reuptake inhibitors: Proposed mechanism. *Neurochemical Research, 31*(4), 509–514. doi:10.100711064-006-9045-7 PMID:16758359

Albernaz, P. L. M. (2014). Vertigo in elderly patients: A review of 164 cases in Brazil. *Ear, Nose, and Throat Journal, 93*(8), 322–330.

Alcañiz, M., & Solé-Auró, A. (2018). Feeling good in old age: Factors explaining health-related quality of life. *Health and Quality of Life Outcomes*, *16*(1), 48. doi:10.118612955-018-0877-z PMID:29534708

Alemanno, F., Houdayer, E., Parma, A., Spina, A., Del Forno, A., Scatolini, A., Angelone, S., Brugliera, L., Tettamanti, A., Beretta, L., & Iannaccone, S. (2021, February 8). COVID-19 cognitive deficits after respiratory assistance in the subacute phase: A COVID-rehabilitation unit experience. *PLoS One*, *16*(2), e0246590. doi:10.1371/journal.pone.0246590 PMID:33556127

Alenezi, N. G., Alenazi, A. A., Elboraei, Y. A. E., Alanazi, T. H., Alruwaili, A. K., Alanazi, A. S., ... Alanazi, A. F. (2017). Ear diseases and factors associated with ear infections among the elderly attending hospital in Arar city, Northern Saudi Arabia. *Electronic Physician*, *9*(9), 5304–5309.

Alford, S., Patel, D., Perakakis, N., & Mantzoros, C. S. (2018). Obesity as a risk factor for Alzheimer's disease: Weighing the evidence. *Obesity Reviews*, *19*(2), 269–280. doi:10.1111/obr.12629 PMID:29024348

Alhabib, M. Y., Alhazmi, T. S., Alsaad, S. M., AlQahtani, A. S., & Alnafisah, A. A. (2022). Medication adherence among geriatric patients with chronic diseases in Riyadh, Saudi Arabia. *Patient Preference and Adherence*, *16*, 2021–2030. doi:10.2147/PPA.S363082 PMID:35966222

Ali, S. A., Begum, T., & Reza, F. (2018, July). Hormonal influences on cognitive function. *The Malaysian Journal of Medical Sciences: MJMS*, *25*(4), 31–41. doi:10.21315/mjms2018.25.4.3 PMID:30914845

Alkhunizan, M., Alkhenizan, A., & Basudan, L. (2018). Prevalence of mild cognitive impairment and dementia in Saudi Arabia: A community-based study. *Dementia and Geriatric Cognitive Disorders. Extra*, *8*(1), 98–103. doi:10.1159/000487231 PMID:29706986

Almeria M, Cejudo JC, Sotoca J, Deus J, Krupinski J. (2020). Cognitive profile following COVID-19 infection: Clinical predictors leading to neuropsychological impairment. *Brain, behavior, & immunity-health*.

Alqahtani, A. H., Al Khedair, K., Al-Jeheiman, R., Al-Turki, H. A., & Al Qahtani, N. H. (2018). Anxiety and depression during pregnancy in women attending clinics in a University Hospital in Eastern province of Saudi Arabia: Prevalence and associated factors. *International Journal of Women's Health*, 101–108.

Altonen, B. L., Arreglado, T. M., Leroux, O., Murray-Ramcharan, M., & Engdahl, R. (2020). Characteristics, comorbidities and survival analysis of young adults hospitalized with COVID-19 in New York City. *PLoS One*, *15*(12), e0243343. doi:10.1371/journal.pone.0243343 PMID:33315929

Alvarez, M., Trent, E., Goncalves, B. D., Pereira, D. G., Puri, R., Frazier, N. A., Sodhi, K., & Pillai, S. S. (2022). Cognitive dysfunction associated with COVID-19: Prognostic role of circulating biomarkers and microRNAs. *Frontiers in Aging Neuroscience*, *14*, 14. doi:10.3389/fnagi.2022.1020092 PMID:36268187

Alzheimer's Association. (2022a). *Facts and Figures*. Alzheimer's Association. https://www.alz. org/alzheimers-dementia/facts-figures

Alzheimer's Association. (2022b). *Parkinson's Disease Dementia*. Alzheimer's Association. https://www.alz.org/alzheimers-dementia/what-is-dementia/types-of-dementia/parkinson-s-disease-dementia

Amarya, S., Singh, K., & Sabharwal, M. (2014). Health consequences of obesity in the elderly. *Journal of Clinical Gerontology and Geriatrics*, *5*(3), 63–67. doi:10.1016/j.jcgg.2014.01.004

American Medical Association. (2022). *Patient-physician relationships*. AMA. https://www. ama-assn.org/delivering-care/ethics/patient-physician-relationships

American Psychiatric Association. (2022). Diagnostic and Statistical Manual of Mental Disorders (DSM-5-TRTM) (Fifth Edit). APA

Aminian, A., Brethauer, S. A., Kirwan, J. P., Kashyap, S. R., Burguera, B., & Schauer, P. R. (2015). How safe is metabolic/diabetes surgery? *Diabetes, Obesity & Metabolism*, *17*(2), 198–201. doi:10.1111/dom.12405 PMID:25352176

Amore, M., Tagariello, P., Laterza, C., & Savoia, E. (2007). Subtypes of depression in dementia. *Archives of Gerontology and Geriatrics*, *44*, 23–33. doi:10.1016/j.archger.2007.01.004 PMID:17317430

Anderson, D. K., Lord, C., Risi, S., DiLavore, P. S., Shulman, C., Thurm, A., & Pickles, A. American Psychiatric Association. (2013). Diagnostic and statistical manual of mental disorders. The Linguistic and Cognitive Effects of Bilingualism on Children with Autism Spectrum Disorders.

Anderson, L. M., Scrimshaw, S. C., Fullilove, M. T., Fielding, J. E., Normand, J., & Services, T. F. (2003). Culturally competent healthcare systems: A systematic review. *American Journal of Preventive Medicine*, *24*(3), 68–79. doi:10.1016/S0749-3797(02)00657-8 PMID:12668199

Andreescu, C., & Aizenstein, H. J. *Amnestic Disorders and Mild Cognitive Impairment. Kaplan & Sadock's Comprehensive Textbook of Psychiatry. Baskı* (B. J. Sadock, B. A. Sadock, & P. Ruiz, Eds.).

Andreyeva, T., Sturm, R., & Ringel, J. S. (2004). Moderate and severe obesity have large differences in health care costs. *Obesity Research*, *12*(12), 1936–1943. doi:10.1038/oby.2004.243 PMID:15687394

Angelidi, A. M., Belanger, M. J., Kokkinos, A., Koliaki, C. C., & Mantzoros, C. S. (2022). Novel noninvasive approaches to the treatment of obesity: From pharmacotherapy to gene therapy. *Endocrine Reviews*, *43*(3), 507–557. doi:10.1210/endrev/bnab034 PMID:35552683

Araiza-Garaygordobil, D., Gopar-Nieto, R., Martinez-Amezcua, P., Cabello-López, A., Alanis-Estrada, G., Luna-Herbert, A., González-Pacheco, H., Paredes-Paucar, C. P., Sierra-Lara, M. D., Briseño-De la Cruz, J. L., Rodriguez-Zanella, H., Martinez-Rios, M. A., & Arias-Mendoza, A. (2020). A randomized controlled trial of lung ultrasound-guided therapy in heart failure (CLUSTER-HF study). *American Heart Journal, 227*, 31–39. doi:10.1016/j.ahj.2020.06.003 PMID:32668323

Aramrat, C., Choksomngam, Y., Jiraporncharoen, W., Wiwatkunupakarn, N., Pinyopornpanish, K., Mallinson, P. A. C., Kinra, S., & Angkurawaranon, C. (2022). Advancing multimorbidity management in primary care: A narrative review. *Primary Health Care Research and Development, 23*, e36. doi:10.1017/S1463423622000238 PMID:35775363

Argyropoulou, D., Geladas, N. D., Nomikos, T., & Paschalis, V. (2022). Exercise and Nutrition Strategies for Combating Sarcopenia and Type 2 Diabetes Mellitus in Older Adults. *Journal of Functional Morphology and Kinesiology, 7*(2), 48. doi:10.3390/jfmk7020048 PMID:35736019

Arnsten, A. (2009). Vías de sinalización de tensións que deterioran a estrutura ea función da cortiza prefrontal. *Nat Rev Neurosci, 10*, 410-2210.1038.

Aspray, T. J., & Hill, T. R. (2019). Osteoporosis and the ageing skeleton. *Biochemistry and cell biology of ageing: Part II clinical science*, 453-476.

Aviv, J. E. (1997). Effects of aging on sensitivity of the pharyngeal and supraglottic areas. *The American Journal of Medicine, 103*, 74S–76S.

Ayodele, S. O., Olarinoye, J. K., Alabi, B. S., & Ologe, F. E. (2020). Comparison of Nasoendoscopic Findings and Quality of Life between Type II Diabetics and Non-Diabetics with Chronic Rhinosinusitis. *ARC Journal of Diabetes and Endocrinology, 6*(1), 14–21. doi:10.20431/2455-5983.0601003

Baglietto-Vargas, D., Chen, Y., Suh, D., Ager, R. R., Rodriguez-Ortiz, C. J., Medeiros, R., Myczek, K., Green, K. N., Baram, T. Z., & LaFerla, F. M. (2015). Short-term modern life-like stress exacerbates Aβ-pathology and synapse loss in 3xTg-AD mice. *Journal of Neurochemistry, 134*(5), 915–926. doi:10.1111/jnc.13195 PMID:26077803

Bah, S., Hussain, M., AlHotheyfa, R., AlNujaidi, H. Y., Al-Qahtani, M., AlAnsary, N., & Albagmi, F. M. (2022). *Multimorbidity Prevalence and Contributing Factors in Saudi Arabia*. Academic Press.

Bai, A., Xu, W., Sun, J., Liu, J., Deng, X., Wu, L., Zou, X., Zuo, J., Zou, L., Liu, Y., Xie, H., Zhang, X., Fan, L., & Hu, Y. (2021). Associations of sarcopenia and its defining components with cognitive function in community-dwelling oldest old. *BMC Geriatrics, 21*(1), 292. doi:10.118612877-021-02190-1 PMID:33957882

Baird, A., & Thompson, W. F. (2018). The impact of music on the self in dementia. *Journal of Alzheimer's Disease, 61*(3), 827–841. doi:10.3233/JAD-170737 PMID:29332051

Baker, N. R., & Blakely, K. K. (2017). Gastrointestinal disturbances in the elderly. *Nursing Clinics*, *52*(3), 419–431. PMID:28779823

Balatsouras, D. G., Koukoutsis, G., Fassolis, A., Moukos, A., & Apris, A. (2018). Benign paroxysmal positional vertigo in the elderly: Current insights. *Clinical Interventions in Aging*, *13*, 2251–2266.

Ball, K., Berch, D. B., Helmers, K. F., Jobe, J. B., Leveck, M. D., Marsiske, M., Morris, J. N., Rebok, G. W., Smith, D. M., Tennstedt, S. L., Unverzagt, F. W., & Willis, S. L.ACTIVE Study Group. (2002, November 13). Effects of cognitive training interventions with older adults: A randomized controlled trial. *Journal of the American Medical Association*, *288*(18), 2271–2281. doi:10.1001/jama.288.18.2271 PMID:12425704

Baracos, V. E., & Arribas, L. (2018). Sarcopenic obesity: Hidden muscle wasting and its impact for survival and complications of cancer therapy. *Annals of Oncology: Official Journal of the European Society for Medical Oncology*, *29*, ii1–ii9. doi:10.1093/annonc/mdx810

Barbato, A., D'Avanzo, B., Cinquini, M., Fittipaldo, A. V., Nobili, A., Amato, L., Vecchi, S., & Onder, G. (2022). Effects of goal-oriented care for adults with multimorbidity: A systematic review and meta-analysis. *Journal of Evaluation in Clinical Practice*, *28*(3), 371–381. doi:10.1111/jep.13674 PMID:35355381

Barb, D., Pazaitou-Panayiotou, K., & Mantzoros, C. S. (2006). Adiponectin: A link between obesity and cancer. *Expert Opinion on Investigational Drugs*, *15*(8), 917–931. doi:10.1517/13543784.15.8.917 PMID:16859394

Barnett, K., Mercer, S. W., Norbury, M., Watt, G., Wyke, S., & Guthrie, B. (2012). Epidemiology of multimorbidity and implications for health care, research, and medical education: A cross-sectional study. *Lancet*, *380*(9836), 37–43. doi:10.1016/S0140-6736(12)60240-2 PMID:22579043

Bartosch, P. S., Kristensson, J., McGuigan, F. E., & Akesson, K. E. (2020). Frailty and prediction of recurrent falls over 10 years in a community cohort of 75-year-old women. *Aging Clinical and Experimental Research*, *32*(11), 1–10. doi:10.100740520-019-01467-1 PMID:31939201

Bassuk, S. S., Wypij, D., & Berkmann, L. F. (2000, April 1). Cognitive impairment and mortality in the community-dwelling elderly. *American Journal of Epidemiology*, *151*(7), 676–688. doi:10.1093/oxfordjournals.aje.a010262 PMID:10752795

Bastani, P., Bikineh, P., Mehralian, G., Sadeghkhani, O., Rezaee, R., Kavosi, Z., & Ravangard, R. (2021). Medication adherence among the elderly: Applying grounded theory approach in a developing country. *Journal of Pharmaceutical Policy and Practice*, *14*(1), 1–8. doi:10.118640545-021-00340-9 PMID:34193278

Batsis, J. A., & Dolkart, K. M. (2015). Evaluation of older adults with obesity for bariatric surgery: Geriatricians' perspective. *Journal of Clinical Gerontology and Geriatrics*, *6*(2), 45–53. doi:10.1016/j.jcgg.2015.01.001

Bature, F., Guinn, B., Pang, D., & Pappas, Y. (2017). Signs and symptoms preceding the diagnosis of Alzheimer's disease: A systematic scoping review of literature from 1937 to 2016. *BMJ Open*, *7*(8), e015746. doi:10.1136/bmjopen-2016-015746 PMID:28851777

Baumann, D., Ruch, W., Margelisch, K., Gander, F., & Wagner, L. (2020). Character strengths and life satisfaction in later life: An analysis of different living conditions. *Applied Research in Quality of Life*, *15*(2), 329–347. doi:10.100711482-018-9689-x

Bazargan, M., Smith, J., Yazdanshenas, H., Movassaghi, M., Martins, D., & Orum, G. (2017). Non-adherence to medication regimens among older African American adults. *BMC Geriatrics*, *17*(1), 1–12. doi:10.118612877-017-0558-5 PMID:28743244

Beer, C., Hyde, Z., Almeida, O. P., Norman, P., Hankey, G. J., Yeap, B. B., & Flicker, L. (2011). Quality use of medicines and health outcomes among a cohort of community dwelling older men: An observational study. *British Journal of Clinical Pharmacology*, *71*(4), 592–599. doi:10.1111/j.1365-2125.2010.03875.x PMID:21395652

Bernabeu-Wittel, M., Gómez-Díaz, R., González-Molina, Á., Vidal-Serrano, S., Díez-Manglano, J., Salgado, F., Soto-Martín, M., & Ollero-Baturone, M. (2020). Oxidative stress, telomere shortening, and apoptosis associated to sarcopenia and frailty in patients with multimorbidity. *Journal of Clinical Medicine*, *9*(8), 2669. doi:10.3390/jcm9082669 PMID:32824789

Bertrand, K., Raymond, M. H., Miller, W. C., Ginis, K. A. M., & Demers, L. (2017). Walking aids for enabling activity and participation: A systematic review. *American Journal of Physical Medicine & Rehabilitation*, *96*(12), 894–903. doi:10.1097/PHM.0000000000000836 PMID:29176406

Bezerra de Souza, D. L., Oliveras-Fabregas, A., Espelt, A., Bosque-Prous, M., de Camargo Cancela, M., Teixidó-Compañó, E., & Jerez-Roig, J. (2021). Multimorbidity and its associated factors among adults aged 50 and over: A cross-sectional study in 17 European countries. *PLoS One*, *16*(2), e0246623. doi:10.1371/journal.pone.0246623 PMID:33571285

Biegus, J., Niewinski, P., Josiak, K., Kulej, K., Ponikowska, B., Nowak, K., Zymlinski, R., & Ponikowski, P. (2021). Pathophysiology of Advanced Heart Failure: What Knowledge Is Needed for Clinical Management? *Heart Failure Clinics*, *17*(4), 519–531. doi:10.1016/j.hfc.2021.06.001 PMID:34511202

Bijlsma, A. Y., Meskers, C. G. M., Ling, C. H. Y., Narici, M., Kurrle, S. E., Cameron, I. D., Westendorp, R. G. J., & Maier, A. B. (2013). Defining sarcopenia: The impact of different diagnostic criteria on the prevalence of sarcopenia in a large middle-aged cohort. *Age (Dordrecht, Netherlands)*, *35*(3), 871–881. doi:10.100711357-012-9384-z PMID:22314402

Bisdorff, A., Bosser, G., Gueguen, R., & Perrin, P. (2013). The epidemiology of vertigo, dizziness, and unsteadiness and its links to co-morbidities. *Frontiers in Neurology*, *4*, 29. doi:10.3389/fneur.2013.00029 PMID:23526567

Blach, A., Pangle, A., Azhar, G., & Wei, J. (2022). Disparity and multimorbidity in heart failure patients over the age of 80. *Gerontology & Geriatric Medicine*, *8*, 23337214221098901. doi:10.1177/23337214221098901 PMID:35591952

Blázquez-Bermejo, Z., Farré, N., Llagostera, M., Caravaca Perez, P., Morán-Fernández, L., Fort, A., De-Juan, J., Ruiz, S., & Delgado, J. F. (2020). The development of chronic diuretic resistance can be predicted during a heart-failure hospitalization. Results from the REDIHF registry. *PLoS One*, *15*(10), e0240098. doi:10.1371/journal.pone.0240098 PMID:33007024

Blumberg, A. (2015). 10 Countries with the Best Care for the Dying. *Huffington Post*.

Bof de Andrade, F., Thumé, E., Facchini, L. A., Torres, J. L., & Nunes, B. P. (2022). Education and income-related inequalities in multimorbidity among older Brazilian adults. *PLoS One*, *17*(10), e0275985. doi:10.1371/journal.pone.0275985 PMID:36227899

Boirie, Y. (2009). Physiopathological mechanism of sarcopenia. *JNHA-. The Journal of Nutrition, Health & Aging*, *13*(8), 717–723. doi:10.100712603-009-0203-x PMID:19657556

Borack, M. S., & Volpi, E. (2016). Efficacy and safety of leucine supplementation in the elderly. *The Journal of Nutrition*, *146*(12), 2625S–2629S. doi:10.3945/jn.116.230771 PMID:27934654

Borghammer, P., Knudsen, K., Fedorova, T. D., & Brooks, D. J. (2017). Imaging Parkinson's disease below the neck. *NPJ Parkinson's Disease*, *3*(1), 1–10. doi:10.103841531-017-0017-1 PMID:28649615

Borson, S., & Chodosh, J. (2014). Developing dementia-capable health care systems: A 12-step program. *Clinics in Geriatric Medicine*, *30*(3), 395–420. doi:10.1016/j.cger.2014.05.001 PMID:25037288

Borzuola, R., Giombini, A., Torre, G., Campi, S., Albo, E., Bravi, M., Borrione, P., Fossati, C., & Macaluso, A. (2020). Central and Peripheral Neuromuscular Adaptations to Ageing. *Journal of Clinical Medicine*, *9*(3), 741. doi:10.3390/jcm9030741 PMID:32182904

Bos, C., Gaudichon, C., & Tomé, D. (2000). Nutritional and physiological criteria in the assessment of milk protein quality for humans. *Journal of the American College of Nutrition*, *19*(sup2), 191S-205S.

Bouchard, D. R., Soucy, L., Sénéchal, M., Dionne, I. J., & Brochu, M. (2009). Impact of resistance training with or without caloric restriction on physical capacity in obese older women. *Menopause (New York, N.Y.)*, *16*(1), 66–72. doi:10.1097/gme.0b013e31817dacf7 PMID:18779759

Boufkhed, S., Namisango, E., Luyirika, E., Sleeman, K. E., Costantini, M., Peruselli, C., Normand, C., Higginson, I. J., & Harding, R. (2020). Preparedness of African Palliative Care Services to Respond to the COVID-19 Pandemic: A Rapid Assessment. *Journal of Pain and Symptom Management*, *60*(6), e10–e26. doi:10.1016/j.jpainsymman.2020.09.018 PMID:32949761

Boyce, J. M., & Shone, G. R. (2006). Effects of ageing on smell and taste. *Postgraduate Medical Journal*, *82*, 239–241.

Boyd, C., Smith, C. D., Masoudi, F. A., Blaum, C. S., Dodson, J. A., Green, A. R., & Rich, M. W. (2019). Decision making for older adults with multiple chronic conditions: Executive summary for the American Geriatrics Society guiding principles on the care of older adults with multimorbidity. *Journal of the American Geriatrics Society*, *67*(4), 665–673. doi:10.1111/jgs.15809 PMID:30663782

Boyes, N. G., Marciniuk, D. D., Haddad, H., & Tomczak, C. R. (2022). Autonomic cardiovascular reflex control of hemodynamics during exercise in heart failure with reduced ejection fraction and the effects of exercise training. *Reviews in Cardiovascular Medicine*, *23*(2), 72. doi:10.31083/j.rcm2302072 PMID:35229563

Bradley, T. D., & Floras, J. S. (2003). Sleep apnea and heart failure: Part I: obstructive sleep apnea. *Circulation*, *107*(12), 1671–1678. doi:10.1161/01.CIR.0000061757.12581.15 PMID:12668504

Brännström, J., Lövheim, H., Gustafson, Y., & Nordström, P. (2019). Association between antidepressant drug use and hip fracture in older people before and after treatment initiation. *JAMA Psychiatry*, *76*(2), 172–179. doi:10.1001/jamapsychiatry.2018.3679 PMID:30601883

Bray, G. A., Frühbeck, G., Ryan, D. H., & Wilding, J. P. (2016). Management of obesity. *Lancet*, *387*(10031), 1947–1956. doi:10.1016/S0140-6736(16)00271-3 PMID:26868660

Bray, G. A., Kim, K. K., & Wilding, J. P. H. (2017). Obesity: A chronic relapsing progressive disease process. A position statement of the World Obesity Federation. *Obesity Reviews*, *18*(7), 715–723. doi:10.1111/obr.12551 PMID:28489290

Breen, R., & Müller, W. (2020). *Education and intergenerational social mobility in Europe and the United States*. Stanford University Press.

Brewis, A., SturtzSreetharan, C., & Wutich, A. (2018). Obesity stigma as a globalizing health challenge. *Globalization and Health*, *14*(1), 1–6. doi:10.118612992-018-0337-x PMID:29439728

Briggs, R., Kennelly, S. P., & Kenny, R. A. (2018). Does baseline depression increase the risk of unexplained and accidental falls in a cohort of community-dwelling older people? Data from The Irish Longitudinal Study on Ageing (TILDA). *International Journal of Geriatric Psychiatry*, *33*(2), e205–e211. doi:10.1002/gps.4770 PMID:28766755

Brown, P., McNeill, R., Leung, W., Radwan, E., & Willingale, J. (2011). Current and future economic burden of osteoporosis in New Zealand. *Applied Health Economics and Health Policy*, *9*(2), 111–123. doi:10.2165/11531500-000000000-00000 PMID:21271750

Burnes, D., Sheppard, C., Henderson, C. R. Jr, Wassel, M., Cope, R., Barber, C., & Pillemer, K. (2019). Interventions to reduce ageism against older adults: A systematic review and meta-analysis. *American Journal of Public Health*, *109*(8), e1–e9. doi:10.2105/AJPH.2019.305123 PMID:31219720

Buttigieg, S. C., Ilinca, S., de Sao Jose, J. M., & Larsson, A. T. (2018). Researching ageism in health-care and long term care. In *Contemporary perspectives on ageism* (pp. 493–515). Springer. doi:10.1007/978-3-319-73820-8_29

Cain, J. M., & Denny, L. (2018, October). Palliative care in women's cancer care: Global challenges and advances. *International Journal of Gynaecology and Obstetrics: the Official Organ of the International Federation of Gynaecology and Obstetrics, 143*(Suppl 2), 153–158. doi:10.1002/ijgo.12624 PMID:30306578

Calderón-Larrañaga, A., Vetrano, D. L., Ferrucci, L., Mercer, S., Marengoni, A., Onder, G., Eriksdotter, M., & Fratiglioni, L. (2019). Multimorbidity and functional impairment–bidirectional interplay, synergistic effects and common pathways. *Journal of Internal Medicine, 285*(3), 255–271. doi:10.1111/joim.12843 PMID:30357990

Canada, B., Stephan, Y., Sutin, A. R., & Terracciano, A. (2020). Personality and falls among older adults: Evidence from a longitudinal cohort. *The Journals of Gerontology: Series B, 75*(9), 1905–1910. doi:10.1093/geronb/gbz040 PMID:30945733

Canadian Coalition for Seniors' Mental Health. (2006). National guidelines for seniors' mental health: The assessment and treatment of depression. Toronto, ON: Canadian Coalition for Seniors'. *Mental Health*.

Caramelli, P., & Castro, L. H. M. (2005). Dementia associated with epilepsy. *International Psychogeriatrics, 17*(s1), S195–S206. doi:10.1017/S1041610205002024 PMID:16240490

Carrasco-Ribelles, L. A., Roso-Llorach, A., Cabrera-Bean, M., Costa-Garrido, A., Zabaleta-del-Olmo, E., Toran-Monserrat, P., Orfila Pernas, F., & Violan, C. (2022). Dynamics of multimorbidity and frailty, and their contribution to mortality, nursing home and home care need: A primary care cohort of 1 456 052 ageing people. *EClinicalMedicine, 52*, 101610. doi:10.1016/j.eclinm.2022.101610 PMID:36034409

Carvalho, A., Rea, I. M., Parimon, T., & Cusack, B. J. (2014, April 12). Physical activity and cognitive function in individuals over 60 years of age: A systematic review. *Clinical Interventions in Aging*, 661–682. PMID:24748784

Castaño, E. (2020, April). Discourse analysis as a tool for uncovering the lived experience of dementia: Metaphor framing and well-being in early-onset dementia narratives. *Discourse & Communication, 14*(2), 115–132. doi:10.1177/1750481319890385

Cendes, F., Theodore, W. H., Brinkmann, B. H., Sulc, V., & Cascino, G. D. (2016). Neuroimaging of epilepsy. *Handbook of Clinical Neurology, 136*, 985–1014. doi:10.1016/B978-0-444-53486-6.00051-X PMID:27430454

Centers for Disease Control and Prevention. (2010). *Defining Childhood Overweight and Obesity*. CDC. https://www.cdc.gov/obesity/childhood/defining.html

Charlson, M. E., Pompei, P., Ales, K. L., & MacKenzie, C. R. (1987). A new method of classifying prognostic comorbidity in longitudinal studies: Development and validation. *Journal of Chronic Diseases, 40*, 373–383.

Charokopos, A., Griffin, M., Rao, V. S., Inker, L., Sury, K., Asher, J., Turner, J., Mahoney, D., Cox, Z. L., Wilson, F. P., & Testani, J. M. (2019). Serum and urine albumin and response to loop diuretics in heart failure. *Clinical Journal of the American Society of Nephrology; CJASN*, *14*(5), 712–718. doi:10.2215/CJN.11600918 PMID:31010938

Chehrehnegar, N., Nejati, V., Shati, M., Rashedi, V., Lotfi, M., Adelirad, F., & Foroughan, M. (2020, March). Early detection of cognitive disturbances in mild cognitive impairment: A systematic review of observational studies. *Psychogeriatrics*, *20*(2), 212–228. doi:10.1111/psyg.12484 PMID:31808989

Chen, L. K., Woo, J., Assantachai, P., Auyeung, T. W., Chou, M. Y., Iijima, K., Jang, H. C., Kang, L., Kim, M., Kim, S., Kojima, T., Kuzuya, M., Lee, J. S. W., Lee, S. Y., Lee, W.-J., Lee, Y., Liang, C.-K., Lim, J.-Y., Lim, W. S., ... Arai, H. (2020). Asian Working Group for Sarcopenia: 2019 consensus update on sarcopenia diagnosis and treatment. *Journal of the American Medical Directors Association*, *21*(3), 300–307. doi:10.1016/j.jamda.2019.12.012 PMID:32033882

Cheung, A. K., Chang, T. I., Cushman, W. C., Furth, S. L., Hou, F. F., Ix, J. H., Knoll, G. A., Muntner, P., Pecoits-Filho, R., Sarnak, M. J., Tobe, S. W., Tomson, C. R. V., & Mann, J. F. E. (2021). KDIGO 2021 clinical practice guideline for the management of blood pressure in chronic kidney disease. *Kidney International*, *99*(3), S1–S87. doi:10.1016/j.kint.2020.11.003 PMID:33637192

Cho, B. Y., Seo, D. C., Lin, H. C., Lohrmann, D. K., & Chomistek, A. K. (2018). BMI and central obesity with falls among community-dwelling older adults. *American Journal of Preventive Medicine*, *54*(4), e59–e66. doi:10.1016/j.amepre.2017.12.020 PMID:29433954

Chooi, Y. C., Ding, C., & Magkos, F. (2019). The epidemiology of obesity. *Metabolism: Clinical and Experimental*, *92*, 6–10. doi:10.1016/j.metabol.2018.09.005 PMID:30253139

Christopher, L., & Strafella, A. P. (2013, September). Neuroimaging of brain changes associated with cognitive impairment in Parkinson's disease. *Journal of Neuropsychology*, *7*(2), 225–240. doi:10.1111/jnp.12015 PMID:23551844

Clegg, A., Young, J., Iliffe, S., Rikkert, M. O., & Rockwood, K. (2013). Frailty in elderly people. *Lancet*, *381*(9868), 752–762. doi:10.1016/S0140-6736(12)62167-9 PMID:23395245

Clyne, B., Cooper, J. A., Boland, F., Hughes, C. M., Fahey, T., & Smith, S. M. (2017). Beliefs about prescribed medication among older patients with polypharmacy: A mixed methods study in primary care. *The British Journal of General Practice*, *67*(660), e507–e518. doi:10.3399/bjgp17X691073 PMID:28533200

Cohen, M. (2016). *Technical Series on Safer Primary Care: Multimorbidity*. World Health Organization.

Cohen, R. A., Poppas, A., Forman, D. E., Hoth, K. F., Haley, A. P., Gunstad, J., Jefferson, A. L., Tate, D. F., Paul, R. H., Sweet, L. H., Ono, M., Jerskey, B. A., & Gerhard-Herman, M. (2009). Vascular and cognitive functions associated with cardiovascular disease in the elderly. *Journal of Clinical and Experimental Neuropsychology*, *31*(1), 96–110. doi:10.1080/13803390802014594 PMID:18608677

Coker, R. H., & Wolfe, R. R. (2018). Weight loss strategies in the elderly: A clinical conundrum. *Obesity (Silver Spring, Md.)*, *26*(1), 22–28. doi:10.1002/oby.21961 PMID:29265771

Combes, A., Price, S., Slutsky, A. S., & Brodie, D. (2020). Temporary circulatory support for cardiogenic shock. *Lancet*, *396*(10245), 199–212. doi:10.1016/S0140-6736(20)31047-3 PMID:32682486

Contreras, J. E., Santander, C., Court, I., & Bravo, J. (2013). Correlation between age and weight loss after bariatric surgery. *Obesity Surgery*, *23*(8), 1286–1289. doi:10.100711695-013-0905-3 PMID:23462862

Covey, H. C. (1992). The definitions of the beginning of old age in history. *International Journal of Aging & Human Development*, *34*(4), 325–337. doi:10.2190/GBXB-BE1F-1BU1-7FKK PMID:1607219

Crawford, G. B., Hodgetts, K., Burgess, T., & Eliott, J. (2021). Documenting plans for care: Advance care directives and the 7-step pathway in the acute care context. *BMC Palliative Care*, *20*(1), 1–9. doi:10.118612904-021-00838-8 PMID:34503479

Crespo-Leiro, M. G., Metra, M., Lund, L. H., Milicic, D., Costanzo, M. R., Filippatos, G., Gustafsson, F., Tsui, S., Barge-Caballero, E., De Jonge, N., Frigerio, M., Hamdan, R., Hasin, T., Hülsmann, M., Nalbantgil, S., Potena, L., Bauersachs, J., Gkouziouta, A., Ruhparwar, A., & Ruschitzka, F. (2018). Advanced heart failure: A position statement of the Heart Failure Association of the European Society of Cardiology. *European Journal of Heart Failure*, *20*(11), 1505–1535. doi:10.1002/ejhf.1236 PMID:29806100

Crivelli, L., Palmer, K., Calandri, I., Guekht, A., Beghi, E., Carroll, W., Frontera, J., García-Azorín, D., Westenberg, E., Winkler, A. S., Mangialasche, F., Allegri, R. F., & Kivipelto, M. (2022, May). Changes in cognitive functioning after COVID-19: A systematic review and meta-analysis. *Alzheimer's & Dementia*, *18*(5), 1047–1066. doi:10.1002/alz.12644 PMID:35297561

Crocco, E. A., Jaramillo, S., Cruz-Ortiz, C., & Camfield, K. (2017). Pharmacological management of anxiety disorders in the elderly. *Current Treatment Options in Psychiatry*, *4*(1), 33–46. doi:10.100740501-017-0102-4 PMID:28948135

Cruz-Jentoft, A. J., Bahat, G., Bauer, J., Boirie, Y., Bruyère, O., Cederholm, T., ... Zamboni, M. (2019). Sarcopenia: Revised European consensus on definition and diagnosis. *Age and Ageing*, *48*(1), 16–31. doi:10.1093/ageing/afy169 PMID:30312372

Cruz-Jentoft, A. J., & Sayer, A. A. (2019). Sarcopenia. *Lancet*, *393*(10191), 2636–2646. doi:10.1016/S0140-6736(19)31138-9 PMID:31171417

Curcio, F., Testa, G., Liguori, I., Papillo, M., Flocco, V., Panicara, V., Galizia, G., Della-Morte, D., Gargiulo, G., Cacciatore, F., Bonaduce, D., Landi, F., & Abete, P. (2020). Sarcopenia and heart failure. *Nutrients*, *12*(1), 211. doi:10.3390/nu12010211 PMID:31947528

Cutler, R. L., Fernandez-Llimos, F., Frommer, M., Benrimoj, C., & Garcia-Cardenas, V. (2018). Economic impact of medication non-adherence by disease groups: A systematic review. *BMJ Open*, *8*(1), e016982. doi:10.1136/bmjopen-2017-016982 PMID:29358417

Damarell, R. A., Morgan, D. D., & Tieman, J. J. (2020). General practitioner strategies for managing patients with multimorbidity: A systematic review and thematic synthesis of qualitative research. *BMC Family Practice*, *21*(1), 1–23. doi:10.118612875-020-01197-8 PMID:32611391

Darley, D. R., Dore, G. J., Cysique, L., Wilhelm, K. A., Andresen, D., Tonga, K., Stone, E., Byrne, A., Plit, M., Masters, J., Tang, H., Brew, B., Cunningham, P., Kelleher, A., & Matthews, G. V. (2021, April 1). Persistent symptoms up to four months after community and hospital-managed SARS-CoV-2 infection. *The Medical Journal of Australia*, *214*(6), 279–280. doi:10.5694/mja2.50963 PMID:33657671

Dawood, M., & McNamara, R. (2022). Do no harm. *Emergency Medicine Journal: EMJ*.

de Almeida, L. L., Ilha, T. A., de Carvalho, J. A., Stein, C., Caeran, G., Comim, F. V., Moresco, R. N., Haygert, C. J. P., Compston, J. E., & Premaor, M. O. (2020). Sarcopenia and its association with vertebral fractures in people living with HIV. *Calcified Tissue International*, *107*(3), 249–256. doi:10.100700223-020-00718-y PMID:32683475

De Francesco, E. M., Vella, V., & Belfiore, A. (2020). COVID-19 and diabetes: The importance of controlling RAGE. *Frontiers in Endocrinology*, *11*, 526. doi:10.3389/fendo.2020.00526 PMID:32760352

de Pablo-Fernández, E., Courtney, R., Rockliffe, A., Gentleman, S., Holton, J. L., & Warner, T. T. (2021). Faster disease progression in Parkinson's disease with type 2 diabetes is not associated with increased α-synuclein, tau, amyloid-β or vascular pathology. *Neuropathology and Applied Neurobiology*, *47*(7), 1080–1091. doi:10.1111/nan.12728 PMID:33969516

de Roos, A., van der Grond, J., Mitchell, G., & Westenberg, J. (2017). Magnetic resonance imaging of cardiovascular function and the brain: Is dementia a cardiovascular-driven disease? *Circulation*, *135*(22), 2178–2195. doi:10.1161/CIRCULATIONAHA.116.021978 PMID:28559496

DeCarli, C. (2001). The role of neuroimaging in dementia. *Clinics in Geriatric Medicine*, *17*(2), 255–279. doi:10.1016/S0749-0690(05)70068-9 PMID:11375135

DeCarli, C., Kaye, J. A., Horwitz, B., & Rapoport, S. I. (1990). Critical analysis of the use of computer-assisted transverse axial tomography to study human brain in aging and dementia of the Alzheimer type. *Neurology*, *40*(6), 872–883. doi:10.1212/WNL.40.6.872 PMID:2189080

Delgado, J., Bowman, K., & Clare, L. (2020). Potentially inappropriate prescribing in dementia: A state-of-the-art review since 2007. *BMJ Open*, *10*(1), e029172. doi:10.1136/bmjopen-2019-029172 PMID:31900263

Delgado, J., Jones, L., Bradley, M. C., Allan, L. M., Ballard, C., Clare, L., ... Melzer, D. (2020). Potentially inappropriate prescribing in dementia, multi-morbidity and incidence of adverse health outcomes. *Age and Ageing.* PMID:32946561

Demirkan, H. (2013). A smart healthcare systems framework. *IT Professional, 15*(5), 38–45. doi:10.1109/MITP.2013.35

Dennison, E. M., Sayer, A. A., & Cooper, C. (2017). Epidemiology of sarcopenia and insight into possible therapeutic targets. *Nature Reviews. Rheumatology, 13*(6), 340–347. doi:10.1038/nrrheum.2017.60 PMID:28469267

Derrick, C. D., Shridharani, S. M., & Broyles, J. M. (2015). The safety and efficacy of cryolipolysis: A systematic review of available literature. *Aesthetic Surgery Journal, 35*(7), 830–836. doi:10.1093/asj/v039 PMID:26038367

Devinsky, O. (2004). Diagnosis and treatment of temporal lobe epilepsy. *Reviews in Neurological Diseases, 1*(1), 2–9. PMID:16397445

Dhakal, A., & Bobrin, B. D. (2022). Cognitive Deficits. Treasure Island (FL): StatPearls Publishing.

Di Angelantonio, E., Kaptoge, S., Wormser, D., Willeit, P., Butterworth, A. S., Bansal, N., & Burgess, S. (2015). Association of cardiometabolic multimorbidity with mortality. *Journal of the American Medical Association, 314*(1), 52–60. doi:10.1001/jama.2015.7008 PMID:26151266

Diaz, A., Baweja, R., Bonatakis, J. K., & Baweja, R. (2021, April 19). Global health disparities in vulnerable populations of psychiatric patients during the COVID-19 pandemic. *World Journal of Psychiatry, 11*(4), 94–108. doi:10.5498/wjp.v11.i4.94 PMID:33889535

DiMatteo, M. R., Giordani, P. J., Lepper, H. S., & Croghan, T. W. (2002). Patient adherence and medical treatment outcomes a meta-analysis. *Medical Care, 40*(9), 794–811. doi:10.1097/00005650-200209000-00009 PMID:12218770

Ding, D., Zhao, Q., Guo, Q., Meng, H., Wang, B., Luo, J., Mortimer, J. A., Borenstein, A. R., & Hong, Z. (2015, March 1). Prevalence of mild cognitive impairment in an urban community in China: A cross-sectional analysis of the Shanghai Aging Study. *Alzheimer's & Dementia, 11*(3), 300–309. doi:10.1016/j.jalz.2013.11.002 PMID:24613707

Dinh, T. S., Brueckle, M.-S., González-González, A. I., Fessler, J., Marschall, U., Schubert-Zsilavesz, M., & Schubert, I. (2022). Evidence-Based Decision Support for a Structured Care Program on Polypharmacy in Multimorbidity: A Guideline Upgrade Based on a Realist Synthesis. *Journal of Personalized Medicine, 12*(1), 69. doi:10.3390/jpm12010069 PMID:35055383

Divo, M. J., Martinez, C. H., & Mannino, D. M. (2014). Ageing and the epidemiology of multimorbidity. *The European Respiratory Journal, 44*(4), 1055–1068. doi:10.1183/09031936.00059814 PMID:25142482

Do Cetin, D. C., & Nasr, G. (2014). Obesity in the elderly: More complicated than you think. *Cleveland Clinic Journal of Medicine, 81*(1), 51–61. doi:10.3949/ccjm.81a.12165 PMID:24391107

Dodds, R. M., Granic, A., Robinson, S. M., & Sayer, A. A. (2020). Sarcopenia, long-term conditions, and multimorbidity: Findings from UK Biobank participants. *Journal of Cachexia, Sarcopenia and Muscle*, *11*(1), 62–68. doi:10.1002/jcsm.12503 PMID:31886632

Dodig, S., Čepelak, I., & Pavić, I. (2019). Hallmarks of senescence and aging. *Biochemia medica. Biochemia Medica*, *29*(3), 483–497. doi:10.11613/BM.2019.030501 PMID:31379458

Donaldson, P. J., Grey, A. C., Heilman, B. M., Lim, J. C., & Vaghefi, E. (2017). The physiological optics of the lens. *Progress in Retinal and Eye Research*, *56*, e1–e24. doi:10.1016/j.preteyeres.2016.09.002 PMID:27639549

Dorman, R. B., Abraham, A. A., Al-Refaie, W. B., Parsons, H. M., Ikramuddin, S., & Habermann, E. B. (2012). Bariatric surgery outcomes in the elderly: An ACS NSQIP study. *Journal of Gastrointestinal Surgery*, *16*(1), 35–44. doi:10.100711605-011-1749-6 PMID:22038414

Dozio, E., Vettoretti, S., Lungarella, G., Messa, P., & Corsi Romanelli, M. M. (2021). Sarcopenia in chronic kidney disease: Focus on advanced glycation end products as mediators and markers of oxidative stress. *Biomedicines*, *9*(4), 405. doi:10.3390/biomedicines9040405 PMID:33918767

Drake, S. A., Conway, S. H., Yang, Y., Cheatham, L. S., Wolf, D. A., Adams, S. D., Wade, C. E., & Holcomb, J. B. (2021). When falls become fatal—Clinical care sequence. *PLoS One*, *16*(1), e0244862. doi:10.1371/journal.pone.0244862 PMID:33406164

Drenth-van Maanen, A. C., Wilting, I., & Jansen, P. A. (2020). Prescribing medicines to older people—How to consider the impact of ageing on human organ and body functions. *British Journal of Clinical Pharmacology*, *86*(10), 1921–1930. doi:10.1111/bcp.14094 PMID:31425638

Dudeja, V., Misra, A., Pandey, R. M., Devina, G., Kumar, G., & Vikram, N. K. (2001). BMI does not accurately predict overweight in Asian Indians in northern India. *British Journal of Nutrition*, *86*(1), 105–112. doi:10.1079/BJN2001382 PMID:11432771

Dumbreck, S., Flynn, A., Nairn, M., Wilson, M., Treweek, S., Mercer, S. W., & Guthrie, B. (2015). Drug-disease and drug-drug interactions: Systematic examination of recommendations in 12 UK national clinical guidelines. *BMJ, 350.*

Early palliative care initiation: Role of the primary care clinician. (2022). *The Journal for Nurse Practitioners, 18*(5), 493-495.

Edelstein, D. R. (1996). Aging of the normal nose in adults. *The Laryngoscope*, *106*, 1–25.

Eggenberger, E., Heimerl, K., & Bennett, M. I. (2013). Communication skills training in dementia care: A systematic review of effectiveness, training content, and didactic methods in different care settings. *International Psychogeriatrics*, *25*(3), 345–358. doi:10.1017/S1041610212001664 PMID:23116547

Ekiz, T., Kara, M., Özcan, F., Ricci, V., & Özçakar, L. (2020). Sarcopenia and COVID-19: a manifold insight on hypertension and the renin angiotensin system. *American journal of physical medicine & rehabilitation*.

Ekiz, T., Kara, M., & Özçakar, L. (2020). Fighting against frailty and sarcopenia–As well as COVID-19? *Medical Hypotheses*, *144*, 109911. doi:10.1016/j.mehy.2020.109911 PMID:32505075

Elbahrawy, A., Bougie, A., Loiselle, S. E., Demyttenaere, S., Court, O., & Andalib, A. (2018). Medium to long-term outcomes of bariatric surgery in older adults with super obesity. *Surgery for Obesity and Related Diseases*, *14*(4), 470–476. doi:10.1016/j.soard.2017.11.008 PMID:29249586

Ellison, D. H., & Felker, G. M. (2017). Diuretic treatment in heart failure. *The New England Journal of Medicine*, *377*(20), 1964–1975. doi:10.1056/NEJMra1703100 PMID:29141174

Emmady, P. D., Schoo, C., & Tadi, P. (2022). Major Neurocognitive Disorder (Dementia). In StatPearls [Internet]. Treasure Island (FL): StatPearls Publishing.

Esposito, M., Bader, Y., Pedicini, R., Breton, C., Mullin, A., & Kapur, N. K. (2017). The role of acute circulatory support in ST-segment elevation myocardial infarction complicated by cardiogenic shock. *Indian Heart Journal*, *69*(5), 668–674. doi:10.1016/j.ihj.2017.05.011 PMID:29054200

Etgen, T., Sander, D., Huntgeburth, U., Poppert, H., Förstl, H., & Bickel, H. (2010). Physical activity and incident cognitive impairment in elderly persons: The INVADE study. *Archives of Internal Medicine*, *170*(2), 186–193. doi:10.1001/archinternmed.2009.498 PMID:20101014

Everett, J. A. (2013). The 12 item social and economic conservatism scale (SECS). *PLoS One*, *8*(12), e82131. doi:10.1371/journal.pone.0082131 PMID:24349200

Fadhil, I., Lyons, G., & Payne, S. (2017, March). Barriers to, and opportunities for, palliative care development in the Eastern Mediterranean Region. *The Lancet. Oncology*, *18*(3), e176–e184. doi:10.1016/S1470-2045(17)30101-8 PMID:28271872

Fancourt, D., & Steptoe, A. (2019). Comparison of physical and social risk-reducing factors for the development of disability in older adults: A population-based cohort study. *Journal of Epidemiology and Community Health*, *73*(10), 906–912. doi:10.1136/jech-2019-212372 PMID:31243046

Faragher, R. G., McArdle, A., Willows, A., & Ostler, E. L. (2017). Senescence in the aging process. *F1000 Research*, 6. PMID:28781767

Fatima, S., Rizvi, S. Z. S., & Jamal, S. R. (2020). Social support, health procrastination and flourishing in cancer patients. *IAHRW International Journal of Social Sciences Review*, *8*(7-9), 296–300.

Fattirolli, F., & Pratesi, A. (2015). Cardiovascular prevention and rehabilitation in the elderly: Evidence for cardiac rehabilitation after myocardial infarction or chronic heart failure. *Monaldi Archives for Chest Disease*, *84*(1-2). Advance online publication. doi:10.4081/monaldi.2015.731 PMID:27374045

Feinstein, A. R. (1970). The pre-therapeutic classification of co-morbidity in chronic disease. *Journal of Chronic Diseases*, *23*(7), 455–468. doi:10.1016/0021-9681(70)90054-8 PMID:26309916

Félix, I. B., & Henriques, A. (2021, October). Medication adherence and related determinants in older people with multimorbidity: A cross-sectional study. *Nursing Forum*, *56*(4), 834–843. doi:10.1111/nuf.12619 PMID:34076260

Feng, X., Kelly, M., & Sarma, H. (2021). The association between educational level and multimorbidity among adults in Southeast Asia: A systematic review. *PLoS One*, *16*(12), e0261584. doi:10.1371/journal.pone.0261584 PMID:34929020

Fiuzat, M., Ezekowitz, J., Alemayehu, W., Westerhout, C. M., Sbolli, M., Cani, D., Whellan, D. J., Ahmad, T., Adams, K., Piña, I. L., Patel, C. B., Anstrom, K. J., Cooper, L. S., Mark, D., Leifer, E. S., Felker, G. M., Januzzi, J. L., & O'Connor, C. M. (2020). Assessment of limitations to optimization of guideline-directed medical therapy in heart failure from the GUIDE-IT trial: A secondary analysis of a randomized clinical trial. *JAMA Cardiology*, *5*(7), 757–764. doi:10.1001/jamacardio.2020.0640 PMID:32319999

Foccillo, G. (2020). The Infections Causing Acute Respiratory Failure in Elderly Patients. In *Ventilatory Support and Oxygen Therapy in Elder, Palliative and End-of-Life Care Patients* (pp. 35–45). Springer. doi:10.1007/978-3-030-26664-6_5

Fokkens, W. J., Lund, V. J., Hopkins, C., Hellings, P. W., Kern, R., Reitsma, S., & Zwetsloot, C. P. (2020). European Position Paper on Rhinosinusitis and Nasal Polyps 2020. *Rhinology*, *58*(Suppl 29), 1–464.

Fortin, M., Soubhi, H., Hudon, C., Bayliss, E. A., & Van den Akker, M. (2007). *Multimorbidity's many challenges* (Vol. 334). British Medical Journal Publishing Group.

Frølich, A., Ghith, N., Schiøtz, M., Jacobsen, R., & Stockmarr, A. (2019). Multimorbidity, healthcare utilization and socioeconomic status: A register-based study in Denmark. *PLoS One*, *14*(8), e0214183. doi:10.1371/journal.pone.0214183 PMID:31369580

Fudim, M., Hernandez, A. F., & Felker, G. M. (2017). Role of volume redistribution in the congestion of heart failure. *Journal of the American Heart Association*, *6*(8), e006817. doi:10.1161/JAHA.117.006817 PMID:28862947

Gadelha, A. B., Neri, S. G. R., Bottaro, M., & Lima, R. M. (2018). The relationship between muscle quality and incidence of falls in older community-dwelling women: An 18-month follow-up study. *Experimental Gerontology*, *110*, 241–246. doi:10.1016/j.exger.2018.06.018 PMID:29935953

Ganesan, R., & Vijaya Chamundeeswari, V. (2020). Composite algorithm for pervasive healthcare system–a solution to find optimized route for closest available health care facilities. *Multimedia Tools and Applications*, *79*(7), 5125–5148. doi:10.100711042-018-6136-9

Garin, N., Koyanagi, A., Chatterji, S., Tyrovolas, S., Olaya, B., Leonardi, M., & Ayuso-Mateos, J. L. (2016). Global multimorbidity patterns: A cross-sectional, population-based, multi-country study. *Journals of Gerontology Series A: Biomedical Sciences and Medical Sciences*, *71*(2), 205–214. doi:10.1093/gerona/glv128 PMID:26419978

Gazibara, T., Kurtagic, I., Kisic-Tepavcevic, D., Nurkovic, S., Kovacevic, N., Gazibara, T., & Pekmezovic, T. (2017). Falls, risk factors and fear of falling among persons older than 65 years of age. *Psychogeriatrics*, *17*(4), 215–223. doi:10.1111/psyg.12217 PMID:28130862

Gicas, K. M., Jones, A. A., Thornton, A. E., Petersson, A., Livingston, E., Waclawik, K., Panenka, W. J., Barr, A. M., Lang, D. J., Vila-Rodriguez, F., Leonova, O., Procyshyn, R. M., Buchanan, T., MacEwan, G. W., & Honer, W. G. (2020, March). Cognitive decline, and mortality in a community-based sample of homeless and precariously housed adults: 9-year prospective study. *BJPsych Open*, *6*(2), e21. doi:10.1192/bjo.2020.3 PMID:32043436

Gimeno-Miguel, A., Gutiérrez, A. G., Poblador-Plou, B., Coscollar-Santaliestra, C., Pérez-Calvo, J. I., Divo, M. J., & Ruiz-Laiglesia, F. J. (2019). Multimorbidity patterns in patients with heart failure: An observational Spanish study based on electronic health records. *BMJ Open*, *9*(12), e033174. doi:10.1136/bmjopen-2019-033174 PMID:31874886

Goel, R., Westblade, L. F., Kessler, D. A., Sfeir, M., Slavinski, S., Backenson, B., & Cushing, M. M. (2018). Death from Transfusion-Transmitted Anaplasmosis, New York, USA, 2017. *Emerging Infectious Diseases*, *24*(8), 1548–1550. doi:10.3201/eid2408.172048 PMID:30016241

Gold, D. T., & McClung, B. (2006). Approaches to patient education: Emphasizing the long-term value of compliance and persistence. *The American Journal of Medicine*, *119*(4), S32–S37. doi:10.1016/j.amjmed.2005.12.021 PMID:16563940

Golembiewski, J. A., & Zeisel, J. (2022). Salutogenic Approaches to Dementia Care. The Handbook of Salutogenesis, 513-532.

Gomes, R. S., Barbosa, A. R., Meneghini, V., Confortin, S. C., d'Orsi, E., & Rech, C. R. (2020). Association between chronic diseases, multimorbidity and insufficient physical activity among older adults in southern Brazil: A cross-sectional study. *Sao Paulo Medical Journal*, *138*(6), 545–553. doi:10.1590/1516-3180.2020.0282.r1.15092020 PMID:33331604

Goodman, R. A., Posner, S. F., Huang, E. S., Parekh, A. K., & Koh, H. K. (2013). Peer reviewed: defining and measuring chronic conditions: imperatives for research, policy, program, and practice. *Preventing Chronic Disease*, 10.

Gould, C. E., O'Hara, R., Goldstein, M. K., & Beaudreau, S. A. (2016, October). Multimorbidity is associated with anxiety in older adults in the Health and Retirement Study. *International Journal of Geriatric Psychiatry*, *31*(10), 1105–1115. doi:10.1002/gps.4532 PMID:27441851

Grande, G., Marengoni, A., Vetrano, D. L., Roso-Llorach, A., Rizzuto, D., Zucchelli, A., Qiu, C., Fratiglioni, L., & Calderón-Larrañaga, A. (2021, May). Multimorbidity burden and dementia risk in older adults: The role of inflammation and genetics. *Alzheimer's & Dementia*, *17*(5), 768–776. doi:10.1002/alz.12237 PMID:33403740

Grant, I., Patterson, T. L., & Yager, J. (1988). Social supports in relation to physical health and symptoms of depression in the elderly. *The American Journal of Psychiatry*. PMID:3421347

Gravell, R. (1988). *Communication problems in elderly people: practical approaches to management*. Croom Helm.

Greene, S. J., Butler, J., Albert, N. M., DeVore, A. D., Sharma, P. P., Duffy, C. I., Hill, C. L., McCague, K., Mi, X., Patterson, J. H., Spertus, J. A., Thomas, L., Williams, F. B., Hernandez, A. F., & Fonarow, G. C. (2018). Medical therapy for heart failure with reduced ejection fraction: The CHAMP-HF registry. *Journal of the American College of Cardiology, 72*(4), 351–366. doi:10.1016/j.jacc.2018.04.070 PMID:30025570

Greene, S. J., Fonarow, G. C., DeVore, A. D., Sharma, P. P., Vaduganathan, M., Albert, N. M., Duffy, C. I., Hill, C. L., McCague, K., Patterson, J. H., Spertus, J. A., Thomas, L., Williams, F. B., Hernandez, A. F., & Butler, J. (2019). Titration of medical therapy for heart failure with reduced ejection fraction. *Journal of the American College of Cardiology, 73*(19), 2365–2383. doi:10.1016/j.jacc.2019.02.015 PMID:30844480

Greenstein, A. P., Solomon, H. V., & Funk, M. C. (2021). Caring for aging veterans with alcohol use disorder and multiple morbidities. *Generations Journal, 44*(4), 1–6.

Grolli, R. E., Mingoti, M. E., Bertollo, A. G., Luzardo, A. R., Quevedo, J., Réus, G. Z., & Ignacio, Z. M. (2021, May). Impact of COVID-19 in the mental health in elderly: Psychological and biological updates. *Molecular Neurobiology, 58*(5), 1905–1916. doi:10.100712035-020-02249-x PMID:33404981

Guisado-Clavero, M., Roso-Llorach, A., López-Jimenez, T., Pons-Vigués, M., Foguet-Boreu, Q., Muñoz, M. A., & Violán, C. (2018). Multimorbidity patterns in the elderly: A prospective cohort study with cluster analysis. *BMC Geriatrics, 18*(1), 1–11. doi:10.118612877-018-0705-7 PMID:29338690

Hackett, R. A., & Steptoe, A. (2016, October). Psychosocial Factors in Diabetes and Cardiovascular Risk. *Current Cardiology Reports, 18*(10), 95. doi:10.100711886-016-0771-4 PMID:27566328

Hagiwara, Yuya, M.D., M.A.C.M. (2022). Interprofessional geriatric and palliative care intervention associated with fewer hospital days. *Journal of Pain and Symptom Management, 63*(4), 629.

Halfon, M., Phan, O., & Teta, D. (2015). Vitamin D: A review on its effects on muscle strength, the risk of fall, and frailty. *BioMed Research International, 2015*, 2015. doi:10.1155/2015/953241 PMID:26000306

Hamerman, D. (1999). Toward an understanding of frailty. *Annals of Internal Medicine, 130*(11), 945–950. doi:10.7326/0003-4819-130-11-199906010-00022 PMID:10375351

Hamilton, B. (2010). Vitamin D and human skeletal muscle. *Scandinavian Journal of Medicine & Science in Sports, 20*(2), 182–190. PMID:19807897

Hanna, A., & Frangogiannis, N. G. (2020). Inflammatory cytokines and chemokines as therapeutic targets in heart failure. *Cardiovascular Drugs and Therapy, 34*(6), 849–863. doi:10.100710557-020-07071-0 PMID:32902739

Harrison, N. A., Cercignani, M., Voon, V., & Critchley, H. D. (2015). Effects of inflammation on hippocampus and substantia nigra responses to novelty in healthy human participants. *Neuropsychopharmacology*, *40*(4), 831–838. doi:10.1038/npp.2014.222 PMID:25154706

Haug, N., Deischinger, C., Gyimesi, M., Kautzky-Willer, A., Thurner, S., & Klimek, P. (2020). High-risk multimorbidity patterns on the road to cardiovascular mortality. *BMC Medicine*, *18*(1), 1–12. doi:10.118612916-020-1508-1 PMID:32151252

Hébert, R., & Brayne, C. (1995). Epidemiology of vascular dementia. *Neuroepidemiology*, *14*(5), 240–257. doi:10.1159/000109800 PMID:7477666

Hedman, S., Nydahl, M., & Faxén-Irving, G. (2016). Individually prescribed diet is fundamental to optimize nutritional treatment in geriatric patients. *Clinical Nutrition (Edinburgh, Lothian)*, *35*(3), 692–698. doi:10.1016/j.clnu.2015.04.018 PMID:25998583

Heidenreich, P. A., Bozkurt, B., Aguilar, D., Allen, L. A., Byun, J. J., Colvin, M. M., Deswal, A., Drazner, M. H., Dunlay, S. M., Evers, L. R., Fang, J. C., Fedson, S. E., Fonarow, G. C., Hayek, S. S., Hernandez, A. F., Khazanie, P., Kittleson, M. M., Lee, C. S., Link, M. S., & Yancy, C. W. (2022a). 2022 AHA/ACC/HFSA guideline for the management of heart failure: A report of the American College of Cardiology/American Heart Association Joint Committee on Clinical Practice Guidelines. *Journal of the American College of Cardiology*, *79*(17), e263–e421. doi:10.1016/j.jacc.2021.12.012 PMID:35379503

Heidenreich, P. A., Bozkurt, B., Aguilar, D., Allen, L. A., Byun, J. J., Colvin, M. M., Deswal, A., Drazner, M. H., Dunlay, S. M., Evers, L. R., Fang, J. C., Fedson, S. E., Fonarow, G. C., Hayek, S. S., Hernandez, A. F., Khazanie, P., Kittleson, M. M., Lee, C. S., Link, M. S., & Yancy, C. W. (2022b). 2022 AHA/ACC/HFSA guideline for the management of heart failure: executive summary: a report of the American College of Cardiology/American Heart Association Joint Committee on Clinical Practice Guidelines. *Journal of the American College of Cardiology*, *79*(17), 1757–1780. doi:10.1016/j.jacc.2021.12.011 PMID:35379504

Heiestad, H., Gjestvang, C., & Haakstad, L. A. (2020). Investigating self-perceived health and quality of life: A longitudinal prospective study among beginner recreational exercisers in a fitness club setting. *BMJ Open*, *10*(6), e036250. doi:10.1136/bmjopen-2019-036250 PMID:32513890

Hendrie, H. C., Lindgren, D., Hay, D. P., Lane, K. A., Gao, S., Purnell, C., Munger, S., Smith, F., Dickens, J., Boustani, M. A., & Callahan, C. M. (2013). Comorbidity profile and healthcare utilization in elderly patients with serious mental illnesses. *The American Journal of Geriatric Psychiatry : Official Journal of the American Association for Geriatric Psychiatry*, *21*(12), 1267–1276. doi:10.1016/j.jagp.2013.01.056 PMID:24206938

Hengartner, M. P., & Plöderl, M. (2018). False beliefs in academic psychiatry: The case of antidepressant drugs. *Ethical Human Psychology and Psychiatry*, *20*(1), 6–16. doi:10.1891/1559-4343.20.1.6

Herranz, N., & Gil, J. (2018). Mechanisms and functions of cellular senescence. *The Journal of Clinical Investigation*, *128*(4), 1238–1246. doi:10.1172/JCI95148 PMID:29608137

Herrman, H., Patel, V., Kieling, C., Berk, M., Buchweitz, C., Cuijpers, P., & Wolpert, M. (2022). Time for united action on depression: A lancet –World psychiatric association commission. *Lancet*, *399*(10328), 957–1022. doi:10.1016/S0140-6736(21)02141-3 PMID:35180424

Hetzer, R., Müller, J. H., Weng, Y. G., Loebe, M., & Wallukat, G. (2000). Midterm follow-up of patients who underwent removal of a left ventricular assist device after cardiac recovery from end-stage dilated cardiomyopathy. *The Journal of Thoracic and Cardiovascular Surgery*, *120*(5), 843–855. doi:10.1067/mtc.2000.108931 PMID:11044309

Higgins, M. B., & Saxman, J. H. (1991). A comparison of selected phonatory behaviors of healthy aged and young adults. *Journal of Speech and Hearing Research*, *34*, 1000–1010.

Hoerbst, A., & Ammenwerth, E. (2010). Electronic health records. *Methods of Information in Medicine*, *49*(04), 320–336. doi:10.3414/ME10-01-0038 PMID:20603687

Ho, F. F., Xu, S., Kwong, T. M., Li, A. S., Ha, E. H., Hua, H., Liong, C., Leung, K. C., Leung, T. H., Lin, Z., Wong, S. Y., Pan, F., & Chung, V. C. H. (2023, January 19). Prevalence, Patterns, and Clinical Severity of Long COVID among Chinese Medicine Telemedicine Service Users: Preliminary Results from a Cross-Sectional Study. *International Journal of Environmental Research and Public Health*, *20*(3), 1827. doi:10.3390/ijerph20031827 PMID:36767195

Ho, J. E., Redfield, M. M., Lewis, G. D., Paulus, W. J., & Lam, C. S. (2020). Deliberating the diagnostic dilemma of heart failure with preserved ejection fraction. *Circulation*, *142*(18), 1770–1780. doi:10.1161/CIRCULATIONAHA.119.041818 PMID:33136513

Hollingworth, T. W., Oke, S. M., Patel, H., & Smith, T. R. (2021). Getting to grips with sarcopenia: Recent advances and practical management for the gastroenterologist. *Frontline Gastroenterology*, *12*(1), 53–61. doi:10.1136/flgastro-2019-101348 PMID:33489069

Holmes, G. L. (2015). Cognitive impairment in epilepsy: The role of network abnormalities. *Epileptic Disorders*, *17*(2), 101–116. doi:10.1684/epd.2015.0739 PMID:25905906

Hommet, C., Mondon, K., Camus, V., De Toffol, B., & Constans, T. (2008). Epilepsy and dementia in the elderly. *Dementia and Geriatric Cognitive Disorders*, *25*(4), 293–300. doi:10.1159/000119103 PMID:18311076

Horiuchi, Y., Tanimoto, S., Latif, A. M., Urayama, K. Y., Aoki, J., Yahagi, K., Okuno, T., Sato, Y., Tanaka, T., Koseki, K., Komiyama, K., Nakajima, H., Hara, K., & Tanabe, K. (2018). Identifying novel phenotypes of acute heart failure using cluster analysis of clinical variables. *International Journal of Cardiology*, *262*, 57–63. doi:10.1016/j.ijcard.2018.03.098 PMID:29622508

Horne, R., Chapman, S. C., Parham, R., Freemantle, N., Forbes, A., & Cooper, V. (2013). Understanding patients' adherence-related beliefs about medicines prescribed for long-term conditions: A meta-analytic review of the Necessity-Concerns Framework. *PLoS One*, *8*(12), e80633. doi:10.1371/journal.pone.0080633 PMID:24312488

Horváth, A., Szűcs, A., Hidasi, Z., Csukly, G., Barcs, G., & Kamondi, A. (2018). Prevalence, semiology, and risk factors of epilepsy in Alzheimer's disease: An ambulatory EEG study. *Journal of Alzheimer's Disease*, *63*(3), 1045–1054. doi:10.3233/JAD-170925 PMID:29710705

Huang, A. R., & Mallet, L. (2013). Prescribing opioids in older people. *Maturitas*, *74*(2), 123–129. doi:10.1016/j.maturitas.2012.11.002 PMID:23201325

Huang, H. K., Hsieh, J. G., Hsieh, C. J., & Wang, Y. W. (2017, September 9). Do cancer patients with dementia receive less aggressive treatment in end-of-life care? A nationwide population-based cohort study. *Oncotarget*, *8*(38), 63596–63604. doi:10.18632/oncotarget.18867 PMID:28969014

Ibrahim, N. A., Edis, Z., & Al-Owais, K. S. (2020). Adherence of geriatric patients and their beliefs toward their medicines in the United Arab Emirates. *Journal of Pharmacy & Bioallied Sciences*, *12*(1), 22. doi:10.4103/jpbs.JPBS_93_19 PMID:32801597

Idler, E. L., & Benyamini, Y. (1997). Self-rated health and mortality: A review of twenty-seven community studies. *Journal of Health and Social Behavior*, *38*(1), 21–37. doi:10.2307/2955359 PMID:9097506

Institute of Health Metrics and Evaluation. (2019). Global Health Data Exchange (GHDx). http://ghdx.healthdata.org/gbd-results-tool?params=gbd-api-2019-permalink/d780dffbe8a381b25e1416884959e88b

Itkin, G. P., & Itkin, M. G. (2021). Lymph circulation and heart failure. *Journal of Transplantology and Artificial Organs*, *23*(3), 186–191. doi:10.15825/1995-1191-2021-3-186-191

Itkin, M., Rockson, S. G., & Burkhoff, D. (2021). Pathophysiology of the lymphatic system in patients with heart failure: JACC state-of-the-art review. *Journal of the American College of Cardiology*, *78*(3), 278–290. doi:10.1016/j.jacc.2021.05.021 PMID:34266581

Iwasaki, S., & Yamasoba, T. (2015). Dizziness and Imbalance in the Elderly: Age-related Decline in the Vestibular System. *Aging and Disease*, *6*(1), 38–47.

Jackson Leach, R., Powis, J., Baur, L. A., Caterson, I. D., Dietz, W., Logue, J., & Lobstein, T. (2020). Clinical care for obesity: A preliminary survey of sixty-eight countries. *Clinical Obesity*, *10*(2), e12357. doi:10.1111/cob.12357 PMID:32128994

Jackson, C. F., & Wenger, N. K. (2011). Cardiovascular disease in the elderly. *Revista Española de Cardiología (English Ed.)*, *64*(8), 697–712. doi:10.1016/j.rec.2011.05.003 PMID:21723657

Jackson, M. J. (2009). Strategies for reducing oxidative damage in ageing skeletal muscle. *Advanced Drug Delivery Reviews*, *61*(14), 1363–1368. doi:10.1016/j.addr.2009.07.018 PMID:19737589

Jahng, K. H., Martin, L. R., Golin, C. E., & DiMatteo, M. R. (2005). Preferences for medical collaboration: Patient–physician congruence and patient outcomes. *Patient Education and Counseling*, *57*(3), 308–314. doi:10.1016/j.pec.2004.08.006 PMID:15893213

Jaski, B. E., Ha, J., Denys, B. G., Lamba, S., Trupp, R. J., & Abraham, W. T. (2003). Peripherally inserted veno-venous ultrafiltration for rapid treatment of volume overloaded patients. *Journal of Cardiac Failure*, *9*(3), 227–231. doi:10.1054/jcaf.2003.28 PMID:12815573

Jeffery, C. A., Shum, D. W., & Hubbard, R. E. (2013). Emerging drug therapies for frailty. *Maturitas*, *74*(1), 21–25. doi:10.1016/j.maturitas.2012.10.010 PMID:23141547

Jensen, G. L., & Hsiao, P. Y. (2010). Obesity in older adults: Relationship to functional limitation. *Current Opinion in Clinical Nutrition and Metabolic Care*, *13*(1), 46–51. doi:10.1097/MCO.0b013e32833309cf PMID:19841579

Jessen, F., Amariglio, R. E., Van Boxtel, M., Breteler, M., Ceccaldi, M., Chételat, G., & Van Der Flier, W. M. (2014). A conceptual framework for research on subjective cognitive decline in preclinical Alzheimer's disease. *Alzheimer's & Dementia*, *10*(6), 844–852. doi:10.1016/j.jalz.2014.01.001 PMID:24798886

Jiang, R. S., & Hsu, C. Y. (2001). Endoscopic sinus surgery for the treatment of chronic sinusitis in geriatric patients. *Ear, Nose, and Throat Journal*, *80*, 230–232.

Jimmy, B., & Jose, J. (2011). Patient medication adherence: Measures in daily practice. *Oman Medical Journal*, *26*(3), 155–159. doi:10.5001/omj.2011.38 PMID:22043406

Jin, H., Kim, Y., & Rhie, S. J. (2016). Factors affecting medication adherence in elderly people. *Patient Preference and Adherence*, *10*, 2117–2125. doi:10.2147/PPA.S118121 PMID:27799748

Jiritano, F., Coco, V. L., Matteucci, M., Fina, D., Willers, A., & Lorusso, R. (2020). Temporary mechanical circulatory support in acute heart failure. *Cardiac Failure Review*, *6*, 6. doi:10.15420/cfr.2019.02 PMID:32257388

Johnson, E. C. B., Ho, K., Yu, G.-Q., Das, M., Sanchez, P. E., Djukic, B., Lopez, I., Yu, X., Gill, M., Zhang, W., Paz, J. T., Palop, J. J., & Mucke, L. (2020). Behavioral and neural network abnormalities in human APP transgenic mice resemble those of App knock-in mice and are modulated by familial Alzheimer's disease mutations but not by inhibition of BACE1. *Molecular Neurodegeneration*, *15*(1), 1–26. doi:10.118613024-020-00393-5 PMID:32921309

Johnson, R., Shaw, J., Berding, J., Gather, M., & Rebstock, M. (2017). European national government approaches to older people's transport system needs. *Transport Policy*, *59*, 17–27. doi:10.1016/j.tranpol.2017.06.005

Johnston, M. C., Crilly, M., Black, C., Prescott, G. J., & Mercer, S. W. (2019). Defining and measuring multimorbidity: A systematic review of systematic reviews. *European Journal of Public Health*, *29*(1), 182–189. doi:10.1093/eurpub/cky098 PMID:29878097

Jolles, J., Verhey, F. R., Riedel, W. J., & Houx, P. J. (1995, December). Cognitive impairment in elderly people: Predisposing factors and implications for experimental drug studies. *Drugs & Aging*, *7*(6), 459–479. doi:10.2165/00002512-199507060-00006 PMID:8601053

Jongsiriyanyong, S., & Limpawattana, P. (2018, December). Mild cognitive impairment in clinical practice: A review article. *American Journal of Alzheimer's Disease and Other Dementias*, *33*(8), 500–507. doi:10.1177/1533317518791401 PMID:30068225

Jungo, K. T., Cheval, B., Sieber, S., Antonia van der Linden, B. W., Ihle, A., Carmeli, C., Chiolero, A., Streit, S., & Cullati, S. (2022). Life-course socioeconomic conditions, multimorbidity and polypharmacy in older adults: A retrospective cohort study. *PLoS One*, *17*(8), e0271298. doi:10.1371/journal.pone.0271298 PMID:35917337

Jurgens, C. Y., Moser, D. K., Armola, R., Carlson, B., Sethares, K., & Riegel, B. (2009). Symptom clusters of heart failure. *Research in Nursing & Health*, *32*(5), 551–560. doi:10.1002/nur.20343 PMID:19650069

Justice, N. J. (2018). The relationship between stress and Alzheimer's disease. *Neurobiology of Stress*, *8*, 127–133. doi:10.1016/j.ynstr.2018.04.002 PMID:29888308

Kalinkovich, A., & Livshits, G. (2017). Sarcopenic obesity or obese sarcopenia: A cross talk between age-associated adipose tissue and skeletal muscle inflammation as a main mechanism of the pathogenesis. *Ageing Research Reviews*, *35*, 200–221. doi:10.1016/j.arr.2016.09.008 PMID:27702700

Kanai, R., Kanemaru, S., Tamura, K. N., Umezawa, N., Yoshida, M., Miwa, T., & Kumazawa, A. (2021). Hearing Outcomes and Complications of Cochlear Implantation in Elderly Patients over 75 Years of Age. *Journal of Clinical Medicine*, *10*, 3123.

Katsuumi, G., Shimizu, I., Yoshida, Y., & Minamino, T. (2018). Vascular senescence in cardiovascular and metabolic diseases. *Frontiers in Cardiovascular Medicine*, *5*, 18. doi:10.3389/fcvm.2018.00018 PMID:29556500

Kaufman, C. E., Grau, L., Begay, R., Reid, M., Goss, C. W., Hicken, B., Shore, J. H., & O'Connell, J. (2022). American indian and alaska native veterans in the indian health service: Health status, utilization, and cost. *PLoS One*, *17*(4), e0266378. doi:10.1371/journal.pone.0266378 PMID:35363822

Kaylie, D. M. (2022). *Effects of Aging on the Ears*. Nose, and Throat.

Keenan, T. D. L., Goldacre, R., & Goldacre, M. J. (2014). Associations between age-related macular degeneration, Alzheimer disease, and dementia: Record linkage study of hospital admissions. *JAMA Ophthalmology*, *132*(1), 63–68. doi:10.1001/jamaophthalmol.2013.5696 PMID:24232933

Kemp, B., Brummel-Smith, K., & Plowman, V. J. (1989). Geriatric rehab program focuses on research, training, and service. *Journal of Rehabilitation*, *55*(4), 9–12.

Kenny, R. A., Romero-Ortuno, R., & Kumar, P. (2017). Falls in older adults. *Medicine*, *45*(1), 28–33. doi:10.1016/j.mpmed.2016.10.007 PMID:28298236

Kim, J. S., Wilson, J. M., & Lee, S. R. (2010). Dietary implications on mechanisms of sarcopenia: Roles of protein, amino acids and antioxidants. *The Journal of Nutritional Biochemistry*, *21*(1), 1–13. doi:10.1016/j.jnutbio.2009.06.014 PMID:19800212

Kim, J., & Parish, A. L. (2017). Polypharmacy and medication management in older adults. *Nursing Clinics*, *52*(3), 457–468. doi:10.1016/j.cnur.2017.04.007 PMID:28779826

Kingston, A., Robinson, L., Booth, H., Knapp, M., & Jagger, C. (2018). Projections of multimorbidity in the older population in England to 2035: Estimates from the Population Ageing and Care Simulation (PACSim) model. *Age and Ageing*, *47*(3), 374–380. doi:10.1093/ageing/afx201 PMID:29370339

Kivimäki, M., Strandberg, T., Pentti, J., Nyberg, S. T., Frank, P., Jokela, M., & Sipilä, P. N. (2022). Body-mass index and risk of obesity-related complex multimorbidity: An observational multicohort study. *The Lancet. Diabetes & Endocrinology*, *10*(4), 253–263. doi:10.1016/S2213-8587(22)00033-X PMID:35248171

Kjellberg, J., Larsen, A. T., Ibsen, R., & Højgaard, B. (2017). The socioeconomic burden of obesity. *Obesity Facts*, *10*(5), 493–502. doi:10.1159/000480404 PMID:29020681

Knapp, M., Iemmi, V., & Romeo, R. (2013). Dementia care costs and outcomes: A systematic review. *International Journal of Geriatric Psychiatry*, *28*(6), 551–561. doi:10.1002/gps.3864 PMID:22887331

Knutson, J. W., & Slavin, R. G. (1995). Sinusitis in the Aged. *Drugs & Aging*, *7*, 310–316.

Koller, D., Schön, G., Schäfer, I., Glaeske, G., van den Bussche, H., & Hansen, H. (2014). Multimorbidity and long-term care dependency—A five-year follow-up. *BMC Geriatrics*, *14*(1), 1–9. doi:10.1186/1471-2318-14-70 PMID:24884813

Kretchy, I. A., Owusu-Daaku, F. T., & Danquah, S. A. (2014). Mental health in hypertension: Assessing symptoms of anxiety, depression, and stress on anti-hypertensive medication adherence. *International Journal of Mental Health Systems*, *8*(1), 1–6. doi:10.1186/1752-4458-8-25 PMID:24987456

Kshatri, J. S., Palo, S. K., Bhoi, T., Barik, S. R., & Pati, S. (2020). Prevalence and Patterns of Multimorbidity Among Rural Elderly: Findings of the AHSETS Study. *Frontiers in Public Health*, *8*, 582663. doi:10.3389/fpubh.2020.582663 PMID:33251177

Kuipers, S. J., Cramm, J. M., & Nieboer, A. P. (2019). The importance of patient-centered care and co-creation of care for satisfaction with care and physical and social well-being of patients with multi-morbidity in the primary care setting. *BMC Health Services Research*, *19*(1), 1–9. doi:10.118612913-018-3818-y PMID:30621688

Kuipers, S. J., Nieboer, A. P., & Cramm, J. M. (2020). Views of patients with multi-morbidity on what is important for patient-centered care in the primary care setting. *BMC Family Practice*, *21*(1), 1–12. doi:10.118612875-020-01144-7 PMID:32336277

Kurdoğlu, Z. (2021). Do the COVID-19 vaccines cause menstrual irregularities. *International Journal of Women's Health and Reproduction Sciences*, *9*(3), 158–159. doi:10.15296/ijwhr.2021.29

Kuring, J. K., Mathias, J. L., & Ward, L. (2018, December 15). Prevalence of depression, anxiety, and PTSD in people with dementia: A systematic review and meta-analysis. *Neuropsychology Review*, 28(4), 393–416. doi:10.100711065-018-9396-2 PMID:30536144

Laali, K. K., Greves, W. J., Correa-Smits, S. J., Zwarycz, A. T., Bunge, S. D., Borosky, G. L., Manna, A., Paulus, A., & Chanan-Khan, A. (2018). Novel fluorinated curcuminoids and their pyrazole and isoxazole derivatives: Synthesis, structural studies, Computational/Docking and in-vitro bioassay. *Journal of Fluorine Chemistry*, 206, 82–98. doi:10.1016/j.jfluchem.2017.11.013

Lainchbury, J. G., Troughton, R. W., Strangman, K. M., Frampton, C. M., Pilbrow, A., Yandle, T. G., Hamid, A. K., Nicholls, M. G., & Richards, A. M. (2009). N-terminal pro–B-type natriuretic peptide-guided treatment for chronic heart failure: Results from the BATTLESCARRED (NT-proBNP–Assisted Treatment To Lessen Serial Cardiac Readmissions and Death) trial. *Journal of the American College of Cardiology*, 55(1), 53–60. doi:10.1016/j.jacc.2009.02.095 PMID:20117364

Landi, F., Liperoti, R., Russo, A., Giovannini, S., Tosato, M., Barillaro, C., Capoluongo, E., Bernabei, R., & Onder, G. (2013). Association of anorexia with sarcopenia in a community-dwelling elderly population: Results from the il SIRENTE study. *European Journal of Nutrition*, 52(3), 1261–1268. doi:10.100700394-012-0437-y PMID:22923016

Langa, K. M., Larson, E. B., Karlawish, J. H., Cutler, D. M., Kabeto, M. U., Kim, S. Y., & Rosen, A. B. (2008, March 1). Trends in the prevalence and mortality of cognitive impairment in the United States: Is there evidence of a compression of cognitive morbidity? *Alzheimer's & Dementia*, 4(2), 134–144. doi:10.1016/j.jalz.2008.01.001 PMID:18631957

Lanté, F., Chafai, M., Raymond, E. F., Salgueiro Pereira, A. R., Mouska, X., Kootar, S., Barik, J., Bethus, I., & Marie, H. (2015). Subchronic glucocorticoid receptor inhibition rescues early episodic memory and synaptic plasticity deficits in a mouse model of Alzheimer's disease. *Neuropsychopharmacology*, 40(7), 1772–1781. doi:10.1038/npp.2015.25 PMID:25622751

Larkin, J., Foley, L., Smith, S. M., Harrington, P., & Clyne, B. (2021). The experience of financial burden for people with multimorbidity: A systematic review of qualitative research. *Health Expectations*, 24(2), 282–295. doi:10.1111/hex.13166 PMID:33264478

Laureys, S., Gosseries, O., & Tononi, G. (Eds.). (2015 Aug 12). *The neurology of consciousness: cognitive neuroscience and neuropathology*. Academic Press.

Le Reste, J. Y., Nabbe, P., Rivet, C., Lygidakis, C., Doerr, C., Czachowski, S., & Assenova, R. (2015). The European general practice research network presents the translations of its comprehensive definition of multimorbidity in family medicine in ten European languages. *PLoS One*, 10(1), e0115796. doi:10.1371/journal.pone.0115796 PMID:25607642

Le, G. N., & Marrone, N. (2017). Age-Related Vestibular Disorders: Implications for Older Adult Patients. Arizona.

Lee, H., & Ailshire, J. (2020). Neighborhood and Housing Conditions and Risk of Falls. *Innovation in Aging*, 4(Suppl 1), 651–652. doi:10.1093/geroni/igaa057.2245

Lee, J. K., Grace, K. A., & Taylor, A. J. (2006). Effect of a pharmacy care program on medication adherence and persistence, blood pressure, and low-density lipoprotein cholesterol: A randomized controlled trial. *Journal of the American Medical Association*, *296*(21), 2563–2571. doi:10.1001/jama.296.21.joc60162 PMID:17101639

Lee, J. K., & Jeong, H. W. (2021, January). Wearing face masks regardless of symptoms is crucial for preventing the spread of COVID-19 in hospitals. *Infection Control and Hospital Epidemiology*, *42*(1), 115–116. doi:10.1017/ice.2020.202 PMID:32372736

Lee, J.-H., Yang, D.-S., Goulbourne, C. N., Im, E., Stavrides, P., Pensalfini, A., ... Berg, M. J. (2022). Faulty autolysosome acidification in Alzheimer's disease mouse models induces autophagic build-up of Aβ in neurons, yielding senile plaques. *Nature Neuroscience*, *25*(6), 688–701. doi:10.1038/1593-022-01084-8 PMID:35654956

Lee, J.-Y., Lee, D. W., Cho, S.-J., Na, D. L., Jeon, H. J., Kim, S.-K., Lee, Y. R., Youn, J.-H., Kwon, M., & Lee, J.-H. (2008). Brief screening for mild cognitive impairment in elderly outpatient clinic: Validation of the Korean version of the Montreal Cognitive Assessment. *Journal of Geriatric Psychiatry and Neurology*, *21*(2), 104–110. doi:10.1177/0891988708316855 PMID:18474719

Lee, S. K. (2019). Epilepsy in the elderly: Treatment and consideration of comorbid diseases. *Journal of Epilepsy Research*, *9*(1), 27–35. doi:10.14581/jer.19003 PMID:31482054

Lehnert, T., Heider, D., Leicht, H., Heinrich, S., Corrieri, S., Luppa, M., Riedel-Heller, S., & König, H.-H. (2011). Health care utilization and costs of elderly persons with multiple chronic conditions. *Medical Care Research and Review: MCRR*, *68*(4), 387–420. doi:10.1177/1077558711399580 PMID:21813576

Lehrer, H., Lin, J.-Y., Kwon, C.-S., Agarwal, P., Mazumdar, M., & Jette, N. (2021). The co-occurrence of dementia in those with epilepsy is associated with 30-day readmission–A population-based study. *Epilepsy & Behavior*, *122*, 108126. doi:10.1016/j.yebeh.2021.108126 PMID:34153638

Leppin, A. L., Montori, V. M., & Gionfriddo, M. R. (2015). Minimally disruptive medicine: A pragmatically comprehensive model for delivering care to patients with multiple chronic conditions. Healthcare.

Leritz, E. C., McGlinchey, R. E., Kellison, I., Rudolph, J. L., & Milberg, W. P. (2011). Cardiovascular disease risk factors and cognition in the elderly. *Current Cardiovascular Risk Reports*, *5*(5), 407–412. doi:10.1007/12170-011-0189-x PMID:22199992

Leung, A., Chi, I., & Lui, Y. H. (2006). A Cross-Cultural Study in Older Adults' Learning Experience. *Asian Journal of Gerontology & Geriatrics*, *1*, 78–83.

Li, K., Huang, T., Zheng, J., Wu, K., & Li, D. (2014). Effect of marine-derived n-3 polyunsaturated fatty acids on C-reactive protein, interleukin 6 and tumor necrosis factor α: A meta-analysis. *PLoS One*, *9*(2), e88103. doi:10.1371/journal.pone.0088103 PMID:24505395

Lin, C.-C., Chiu, M.-J., Hsiao, C.-C., Lee, R.-G., & Tsai, Y.-S. (2006). Wireless health care service system for elderly with dementia. *IEEE Transactions on Information Technology in Biomedicine*, *10*(4), 696–704. doi:10.1109/TITB.2006.874196 PMID:17044403

Liu, H., Yang, Y., Xia, Y., Zhu, W., Leak, R. K., Wei, Z., Wang, J., & Hu, X. (2017). Aging of cerebral white matter. *Ageing Research Reviews*, *34*, 64–76. doi:10.1016/j.arr.2016.11.006 PMID:27865980

Liu, S., Yu, W., & Lü, Y. (2016). The causes of new-onset epilepsy and seizures in the elderly. *Neuropsychiatric Disease and Treatment*, *12*, 1425. doi:10.2147/NDT.S107905 PMID:27382285

Livingston, G., Sommerlad, A., Orgeta, V., Costafreda, S. G., Huntley, J., Ames, D., Ballard, C., Banerjee, S., Burns, A., Cohen-Mansfield, J., Cooper, C., Fox, N., Gitlin, L. N., Howard, R., Kales, H. C., Larson, E. B., Ritchie, K., Rockwood, K., Sampson, E. L., ... Mukadam, N. (2017). Dementia prevention, intervention, and care. *Lancet*, *390*(10113), 2673–2734. doi:10.1016/S0140-6736(17)31363-6 PMID:28735855

Li, W., Yue, T., & Liu, Y. (2020). New understanding of the pathogenesis and treatment of stroke-related sarcopenia. *Biomedicine and Pharmacotherapy*, *131*, 110721. doi:10.1016/j.biopha.2020.110721 PMID:32920517

Li, Z., Zhao, Y. P., & Hu, X. Y. (2016). The association between multimorbidity and medication non-adherence in elderly with hypertension in western China. *Hu Li Za Zhi*, *63*(5), 65. PMID:27699741

Llewelyn, J., & Mitchell, R. (1997). Survival of patients who needed salvage surgery for recurrence after radiotherapy for oral carcinoma. *British Journal of Oral & Maxillofacial Surgery*, *35*, 424–428.

Llop-Medina, L., Fu, Y., Garcés-Ferrer, J., & Doñate-Martínez, A. (2022). Palliative care in older people with multimorbidities: A scoping review on the palliative care needs of patients, carers, and health professionals. *International Journal of Environmental Research and Public Health*, *19*(6), 3195. doi:10.3390/ijerph19063195 PMID:35328881

Locher, J. L., Ritchie, C. S., Roth, D. L., Sen, B., Vickers, K. S., & Vailas, L. I. (2009). Food choice among homebound older adults: Motivations and perceived barriers. *JNHA-The Journal of Nutrition. Health and Aging*, *13*(8), 659–664. PMID:19657547

Lo, J. H. T., Yiu, T., Ong, M. T. Y., & Lee, W. Y. W. (2020). Sarcopenia: Current treatments and new regenerative therapeutic approaches. *Journal of Orthopaedic Translation*, *23*, 38–52. doi:10.1016/j.jot.2020.04.002 PMID:32489859

Lozano-Hernández, C. M., López-Rodríguez, J. A., Leiva-Fernández, F., Calderón-Larrañaga, A., Barrio-Cortes, J., Gimeno-Feliu, L. A., Poblador-Plou, B., & Cura-González, I. (2020). Social support, social context, and nonadherence to treatment in young senior patients with multimorbidity and polypharmacy followed-up in primary care. MULTIPAP Study. *PLoS One*, *15*(6), e0235148. doi:10.1371/journal.pone.0235148 PMID:32579616

Lunedo, S. M. C., Sass, S. M. G., Gomes, A. B., Kanashiro, K., & Bortolon, L. (2008). The Prevalence of the Major ENT Symptoms in an Ambulatorial Geriatric Population. *International Archives of Otorhinolaryngology*, *12*(1), 95–98.

Lupien, S. J., McEwen, B. S., Gunnar, M. R., & Heim, C. (2009). Effects of stress throughout the lifespan on the brain, behaviour and cognition. *Nature Reviews. Neuroscience*, *10*(6), 434–445. doi:10.1038/nrn2639 PMID:19401723

Lv, J., Li, R., Yuan, L., Yang, X.-l., Wang, Y., Ye, Z.-W., & Huang, F.-M. (2022). Research on the frailty status and adverse outcomes of elderly patients with multimorbidity. *BMC Geriatrics*, *22*(1), 560.

MacLaughlin, E. J., Raehl, C. L., Treadway, A. K., Sterling, T. L., Zoller, D. P., & Bond, C. A. (2005). Assessing medication adherence in the elderly: Which tools to use in clinical practice? *Drugs & Aging*, *22*(3), 231–255. doi:10.2165/00002512-200522030-00005 PMID:15813656

Mahbub, M. H., Hase, R., Yamaguchi, N., Hiroshige, K., Harada, N., Bhuiyan, A. N. M., & Tanabe, T. (2020). Acute Effects of Whole-Body Vibration on Peripheral Blood Flow, Vibrotactile Perception and Balance in Older Adults. *International Journal of Environmental Research and Public Health*, *17*(3), 1069. doi:10.3390/ijerph17031069 PMID:32046205

Mahendran, M., Speechley, K. N., & Widjaja, E. (2017). Systematic review of unmet healthcare needs in patients with epilepsy. *Epilepsy & Behavior*, *75*, 102–109. doi:10.1016/j.yebeh.2017.02.034 PMID:28843210

Mahwati, Y. (2014). Determinants of multimorbidity among the elderly population in Indonesia. *Kesmas: Jurnal Kesehatan Masyarakat Nasional*, *9*(2), 187–193. doi:10.21109/kesmas.v9i2.516

Maitre, J., Jully, J. L., Gasnier, Y., & Paillard, T. (2013). Chronic physical activity preserves efficiency of proprioception in postural control in older women. *Journal of Rehabilitation Research and Development*, *50*(6).

Malafarina, V., Uriz-Otano, F., Gil-Guerrero, L., & Iniesta, R. (2013). The anorexia of ageing: Physiopathology, prevalence, associated comorbidity and mortality. A systematic review. *Maturitas*, *74*(4), 293–302. doi:10.1016/j.maturitas.2013.01.016 PMID:23415063

Mangin, D., Bahat, G., Golomb, B. A., Mallery, L. H., Moorhouse, P., Onder, G., Petrovic, M., & Garfinkel, D. (2018). International Group for Reducing Inappropriate Medication Use & Polypharmacy (IGRIMUP): Position statement and 10 recommendations for action. *Drugs & Aging*, *35*(7), 575–587. doi:10.100740266-018-0554-2 PMID:30006810

Mankhong, S., Kim, S., Moon, S., Kwak, H. B., Park, D. H., & Kang, J. H. (2020). Experimental models of sarcopenia: Bridging molecular mechanism and therapeutic strategy. *Cells*, *9*(6), 1385. doi:10.3390/cells9061385 PMID:32498474

Mankia, K., & Emery, P. (2019). Palindromic rheumatism as part of the rheumatoid arthritis continuum. *Nature Reviews. Rheumatology*, *15*(11), 687–695. doi:10.103841584-019-0308-5 PMID:31595059

Marengoni, A., Angleman, S., Melis, R., Mangialasche, F., Karp, A., Garmen, A., Meinow, B., & Fratiglioni, L. (2011). Aging with multimorbidity: A systematic review of the literature. *Ageing Research Reviews*, *10*(4), 430–439. doi:10.1016/j.arr.2011.03.003 PMID:21402176

Mark, R. E., & Sitskoorn, M. M. (2013). Are subjective cognitive complaints relevant in preclinical Alzheimer's disease? A review and guidelines for healthcare professionals. *Reviews in Clinical Gerontology*, *23*(1), 61–74. doi:10.1017/S0959259812000172

Marquetand, J., Bode, L., Fuchs, S., Ernst, J., von Känel, R., & Boettger, S. (2021). Predisposing, and precipitating factors for delirium in the very old (≥ 80 years): A prospective cohort study of 3,076 patients. *Gerontology*, *67*(5), 599–607. doi:10.1159/000514298 PMID:33789299

Martone, A. M., Marzetti, E., Calvani, R., Picca, A., Tosato, M., Bernabei, R., & Landi, F. (2019). Assessment of sarcopenia: From clinical practice to research. *Journal of Gerontology and Geriatrics*, *67*(1), 39–45.

Masnoon, N., Shakib, S., Kalisch-Ellett, L., & Caughey, G. E. (2017). What is polypharmacy? A systematic review of definitions. *BMC Geriatrics*, *17*(1), 230. doi:10.118612877-017-0621-2 PMID:29017448

Mathus-Vliegen, E. M., Basdevant, A., Finer, N., Hainer, V., Hauner, H., Micic, D., Maislos, M., Roman, G., Schutz, Y., Tsigos, C., Toplak, H., Yumuk, V., & Zahorska-Markiewicz, B. (2012). Prevalence, pathophysiology, health consequences and treatment options of obesity in the elderly: A guideline. *Obesity Facts*, *5*(3), 460–483. doi:10.1159/000341193 PMID:22797374

Mavaddat, N., Valderas, J. M., Van Der Linde, R., Khaw, K. T., & Kinmonth, A. L. (2014). Association of self-rated health with multimorbidity, chronic disease and psychosocial factors in a large middle-aged and older cohort from general practice: A cross-sectional study. *BMC Family Practice*, *15*(1), 1–11. doi:10.118612875-014-0185-6 PMID:25421440

Mbuya-Bienge, C., Simard, M., Gaulin, M., Candas, B., & Sirois, C. (2021). Does socio-economic status influence the effect of multimorbidity on the frequent use of ambulatory care services in a universal healthcare system? A population-based cohort study. *BMC Health Services Research*, *21*(1), 1–11. doi:10.118612913-021-06194-w PMID:33676497

McAteer, R., & Wellbery, C. (2013, December 15). Palliative care: Benefits, barriers, and best practices. *American Family Physician*, *88*(12), 807–813. PMID:24364543

McCarthy, C. E. (2021). Sleep disturbance, sleep disorders and co-morbidities in the care of the older person. *Medical Science*, *9*(2), 31. PMID:34063838

McDonagh, T. A., Metra, M., Adamo, M., Gardner, R. S., Baumbach, A., Böhm, M., ... Kathrine Skibelund, A. (2021). 2021 ESC Guidelines for the diagnosis and treatment of acute and chronic heart failure: Developed by the Task Force for the diagnosis and treatment of acute and chronic heart failure of the European Society of Cardiology (ESC) With the special contribution of the Heart Failure Association (HFA) of the ESC. *European Heart Journal*, *42*(36), 3599–3726. doi:10.1093/eurheartj/ehab368 PMID:34447992

McGuirt, W. F., & Davis, S. P. (1995). Demographic portrayal and outcome analysis of head and neck cancer surgery in the elderly. *Archives of Otolaryngology—Head & Neck Surgery*, *121*, 150–154.

McLean, A. J., & Le Couteur, D. G. (2004). Aging biology and geriatric clinical pharmacology. *Pharmacological Reviews*, *56*(2), 163–184. doi:10.1124/pr.56.2.4 PMID:15169926

Mcloughlin, B. C., Miles, A., Webb, T. E., Knopp, P., Eyres, C., Fabbri, A., Humphries, F., & Davis, D. (2020, October). Functional and cognitive outcomes after COVID-19 delirium. *European Geriatric Medicine*, *11*(5), 857–862. doi:10.100741999-020-00353-8 PMID:32666303

McMurray, J. J., Packer, M., Desai, A. S., Gong, J., Lefkowitz, M. P., Rizkala, A. R., & Zile, M. R. (2014). Angiotensin–neprilysin inhibition versus enalapril in heart failure. *N Engl J Med*, *371*, 993-1004.

McPhail, S. M. (2016). Multimorbidity in chronic disease: Impact on health care resources and costs. *Risk Management and Healthcare Policy*, *9*, 143–156. doi:10.2147/RMHP.S97248 PMID:27462182

Meador, J. A. (1995). Cerumen impaction in the elderly. *Journal of Gerontological Nursing*, *21*(12), 43–45.

Meads, D. M., Martin, A., Griffiths, A., Kelley, R., Creese, B., Robinson, L., McDermid, J., Walwyn, R., Ballard, C., & Surr, C. A. (2020). Cost-effectiveness of dementia care mapping in care-home settings: Evaluation of a randomised controlled trial. *Applied Health Economics and Health Policy*, *18*(2), 237–247. doi:10.100740258-019-00531-1 PMID:31701483

Mehta, P., McAuley, D. F., Brown, M., Sanchez, E., Tattersall, R. S., & Manson, J. J. (2020). COVID-19: Consider cytokine storm syndromes and immunosuppression. *Lancet*, *395*(10229), 1033–1034. doi:10.1016/S0140-6736(20)30628-0 PMID:32192578

Mellitus, D. (2005). Diagnosis and classification of diabetes mellitus. *Diabetes Care*, *28*(S37), S5–S10. PMID:15618111

Meneilly, G. S., & Tessier, D. (2001). Diabetes in elderly adults. *The Journals of Gerontology. Series A, Biological Sciences and Medical Sciences*, *56*(1), M5–M13. doi:10.1093/gerona/56.1.M5 PMID:11193234

Meng, L., Chen, D., Yang, Y., Zheng, Y., & Hui, R. (2012). Depression increases the risk of hypertension incidence: A meta-analysis of prospective cohort studies. *Journal of Hypertension*, *30*(5), 842–851. doi:10.1097/HJH.0b013e32835080b7 PMID:22343537

Mercer, S., Furler, J., Moffat, K., Fischbacher-Smith, D., & Sanci, L. (2016). *Multimorbidity: technical series on safer primary care*. World Health Organization.

Meyer, M., Constancias, F., Vogel, T., Kaltenbach, G., & Schmitt, E. (2020). Gait Disorder among Elderly People, Psychomotor Disadaptation Syndrome: Post-Fall Syndrome, Risk Factors and Follow-Up–A Cohort Study of 70 Patients. *Gerontology*, 1–8. PMID:33254165

Michalowsky, B., Xie, F., Eichler, T., Hertel, J., Kaczynski, A., Kilimann, I., Teipel, S., Wucherer, D., Zwingmann, I., Thyrian, J. R., & Hoffmann, W. (2019). Cost-effectiveness of a collaborative dementia care management—Results of a cluster-randomized controlled trial. *Alzheimer's & Dementia, 15*(10), 1296–1308. doi:10.1016/j.jalz.2019.05.008 PMID:31409541

Mielenz, T. J., Kannoth, S., Jia, H., Pullyblank, K., Sorensen, J., Estabrooks, P., Stevens, J. A., & Strogatz, D. (2020). Evaluating a two-level vs. three-level fall risk screening algorithm for predicting falls among older adults. *Frontiers in Public Health, 8*, 8. doi:10.3389/fpubh.2020.00373 PMID:32903603

Mijnarends, D. M., Meijers, J. M., Halfens, R. J., ter Borg, S., Luiking, Y. C., Verlaan, S., Schoberer, D., Cruz Jentoft, A. J., van Loon, L. J. C., & Schols, J. M. (2013). Validity and reliability of tools to measure muscle mass, strength, and physical performance in community-dwelling older people: A systematic review. *Journal of the American Medical Directors Association, 14*(3), 170–178. doi:10.1016/j.jamda.2012.10.009 PMID:23276432

Miller, L. A., Spitznagel, M. B., Alosco, M. L., Cohen, R. A., Raz, N., Sweet, L. H., Colbert, L., Josephson, R., Hughes, J., Rosneck, J., & Gunstad, J. (2012). Cognitive profiles in heart failure: A cluster analytic approach. *Journal of Clinical and Experimental Neuropsychology, 34*(5), 509–520. doi:10.1080/13803395.2012.663344 PMID:22375800

Miller, Y. (2022). Advancements and future directions in research of the roles of insulin in amyloid diseases. *Biophysical Chemistry, 281*, 106720. doi:10.1016/j.bpc.2021.106720 PMID:34823073

Minaglia, C., Giannotti, C., Boccardi, V., Mecocci, P., Serafini, G., Odetti, P., & Monacelli, F. (2019). Cachexia and advanced dementia. *Journal of Cachexia, Sarcopenia and Muscle, 10*(2), 263–277. doi:10.1002/jcsm.12380 PMID:30794350

Misra, A., & Khurana, L. (2008). Obesity and the metabolic syndrome in developing countries. *The Journal of Clinical Endocrinology and Metabolism, 93*(11, supplement_1), s9–s30. doi:10.1210/jc.2008-1595 PMID:18987276

Miyawaki, C. E., Bouldin, E. D., Taylor, C. A., & McGuire, L. C. (2020, August 13). Baby boomers as caregivers: Results from the Behavioral Risk Factor Surveillance System in 44 states, the District of Columbia, and Puerto Rico, 2015–2017. *Preventing Chronic Disease, 17*, E80. doi:10.5888/pcd17.200010 PMID:32790608

Mohammad, A., & Muhammad, S. A. (2017). Audiologic Pattern in Elderly Patients: A Tertiary Care Experience. *International Journal of Open Access Otolaryngology, 1*(1), 1–5.

Mohammed, M., & Li, J. (2022, November). Stroke-Related Sarcopenia among Two Different Developing Countries with Diverse Ethnic Backgrounds (Cross-National Study in Egypt and China). []. Multidisciplinary Digital Publishing Institute.]. *Health Care, 10*(11), 2336. PMID:36421660

Monacelli, F., Signori, A., Marengoni, A., Di Santo, S., Rossi, E., Valsecchi, M. G., Morandi, A., & Bellelli, G. (2022, May 1). of Delirium IS. Delirium and clusters of older patients affected by multimorbidity in acute hospitals. *Journal of the American Medical Directors Association, 23*(5), 885–888. doi:10.1016/j.jamda.2021.10.004 PMID:34798007

Mordi, J. A., & Ciuffreda, K. J. (1998). Static aspects of accommodation: Age and presbyopia. *Vision Research*, *38*(11), 1643–1653. doi:10.1016/S0042-6989(97)00336-2 PMID:9747501

Moreland, B., Kakara, R., & Henry, A. (2020). Trends in nonfatal falls and fall-related injuries among adults aged[3] 65 years—United States, 2012–2018. *Morbidity and Mortality Weekly Report*, *69*(27), 875–881. doi:10.15585/mmwr.mm6927a5 PMID:32644982

Mori, H., Kuroda, A., Ishizu, M., Ohishi, M., Takashi, Y., Otsuka, Y., Taniguchi, S., Tamaki, M., Kurahashi, K., Yoshida, S., Endo, I., Aihara, K., Funaki, M., Akehi, Y., & Matsuhisa, M. (2019). Association of accumulated advanced glycation end-products with a high prevalence of sarcopenia and dynapenia in patients with type 2 diabetes. *Journal of Diabetes Investigation*, *10*(5), 1332–1340. doi:10.1111/jdi.13014 PMID:30677242

Moser, D. K., Lee, K. S., Wu, J. R., Mudd-Martin, G., Jaarsma, T., Huang, T. Y., Fan, X.-Z., Strömberg, A., Lennie, T. A., & Riegel, B. (2014). Identification of symptom clusters among patients with heart failure: An international observational study. *International Journal of Nursing Studies*, *51*(10), 1366–1372. doi:10.1016/j.ijnurstu.2014.02.004 PMID:24636665

Moshé, S. L., Perucca, E., Ryvlin, P., & Tomson, T. (2015). Epilepsy: New advances. *Lancet*, *385*(9971), 884–898. doi:10.1016/S0140-6736(14)60456-6 PMID:25260236

Mozaffarian, D., Kumanyika, S. K., Lemaitre, R. N., Olson, J. L., Burke, G. L., & Siscovick, D. S. (2003). Cereal, fruit, and vegetable fiber intake and the risk of cardiovascular disease in elderly individuals. *Journal of the American Medical Association*, *289*(13), 1659–1666. doi:10.1001/jama.289.13.1659 PMID:12672734

Muchna, A., Najafi, B., Wendel, C. S., Schwenk, M., Armstrong, D. G., & Mohler, J. (2018). Foot problems in older adults: Associations with incident falls, frailty syndrome, and sensor-derived gait, balance, and physical activity measures. *Journal of the American Podiatric Medical Association*, *108*(2), 126–139. doi:10.7547/15-186 PMID:28853612

Murlow, C. D., Aguilar, C., Endicott, J. E., Tuley, M. R., Velez, R., & Charlip, W. S. (1990). Quality of life changes and hearing impairment. *Annals of Internal Medicine*, *113*(3), 188–194. doi:10.7326/0003-4819-113-3-188 PMID:2197909

Murman, D. L. The impact of age on cognition. In Seminars in hearing 2015 Aug (Vol. 36, No. 03, pp. 111-121). Thieme Medical Publishers. doi:10.1055-0035-1555115

Muth, C., van den Akker, M., Blom, J. W., Mallen, C. D., Rochon, J., Schellevis, F. G., & Kirchner, H. (2014). The Ariadne principles: How to handle multimorbidity in primary care consultations. *BMC Medicine*, *12*(1), 1–11. doi:10.118612916-014-0223-1 PMID:25484244

Nagle, B. J., Usita, P. M., & Edland, S. D. (2013). United States medical students' knowledge of Alzheimer disease. *J Educ Eval Health Prof, 10*(4), 10.3352.

National Health Service. (2021). *Symptoms-Alzheimer's disease*. NHS. https://www.nhs.uk/conditions/alzheimers-disease/symptoms/

National Institute for Health and Care Excelllence. (2018). Dementia: assessment, management and support for people living with dementia and their carers. In *NICE guideline [NG97]*. https://www.nice.org.uk/guidance/ng97/chapter/recommendations

Navaratnarajah, A., & Jackson, S. H. (2017). The physiology of ageing. *Medicine, 45*(1), 6–10. doi:10.1016/j.mpmed.2016.10.008 PMID:28065164

Na, W., Kim, J., Chung, B. H., Jang, D. J., & Sohn, C. (2020). Relationship between diet quality and sarcopenia in elderly Koreans: 2008–2011 Korea National Health and Nutrition Examination Survey. *Nutrition Research and Practice, 14*(4), 352–364. doi:10.4162/nrp.2020.14.4.352 PMID:32765815

Nejad, A. G., & Pouya, F. (2004). False beliefs and medication non-compliance in psychiatric patients. *Neuroscience Journal, 9*(2), 124–128. PMID:23377366

NICE. (2016). *Multimorbidity: Clinical assessment and management.* NICE guideline [NG56].

Nichols, E., Szoeke, C. E., Vollset, S. E., Abbasi, N., Abd-Allah, F., Abdela, J., ... Asgedom, S. W. (2019). Global, regional, and national burden of Alzheimer's disease and other dementias, 1990–2016: A systematic analysis for the Global Burden of Disease Study 2016. *Lancet Neurology, 18*(1), 88–106. doi:10.1016/S1474-4422(18)30403-4 PMID:30497964

Nieuwenhuizen, W. F., Weenen, H., Rigby, P., & Hetherington, M. M. (2010). Older adults and patients in need of nutritional support: Review of current treatment options and factors influencing nutritional intake. *Clinical Nutrition (Edinburgh, Lothian), 29*(2), 160–169. doi:10.1016/j.clnu.2009.09.003 PMID:19828215

Nilsson, H., Ekberg, O., Olsson, R., & Hindfelt, B. (1996). Quantitative assessment of oral and pharyngeal function in Parkinson's disease. *Dysphagia, 11*, 144–150.

Ninomiya, T. (2014). Diabetes mellitus and dementia. *Current Diabetes Reports, 14*(5), 1–9. doi:10.100711892-014-0487-z PMID:24623199

Nishijima, D. K., Lin, A. L., Weiss, R. E., Yagapen, A. N., Malveau, S. E., Adler, D. H., Bastani, A., Baugh, C. W., Caterino, J. M., Clark, C. L., Diercks, D. B., Hollander, J. E., Nicks, B. A., Shah, M. N., Stiffler, K. A., Storrow, A. B., Wilber, S. T., & Sun, B. C. (2018). ECG predictors of cardiac arrhythmias in older adults with syncope. *Annals of Emergency Medicine, 71*(4), 452–461. doi:10.1016/j.annemergmed.2017.11.014 PMID:29275946

Nivet, C., Duhalde, V., Beaurain, M., Delobel, P., Quelven, I., & Laurent, A. (2022). Fecal microbiota transplantation for refractory clostridioides difficile infection is effective and well tolerated even in very old subjects: A real-life study. *The Journal of Nutrition, Health & Aging, 26*(3), 290–296. doi:10.100712603-022-1756-1 PMID:35297473

Nozaki, I., Kuriyama, M., Manyepa, P., Zyambo, M. K., Kakimoto, K., & Bärnighausen, T. (2013). False beliefs about ART effectiveness, side effects and the consequences of non-retention and non-adherence among ART patients in Livingstone, Zambia. *AIDS and Behavior, 17*, 122–126. doi:10.100710461-012-0221-2 PMID:22714115

O'Shea, E., & O'Reilly, S. (2000). The economic and social cost of dementia in Ireland. *International Journal of Geriatric Psychiatry*, *15*(3), 208–218. doi:10.1002/(SICI)1099-1166(200003)15:3<208::AID-GPS95>3.0.CO;2-X PMID:10713578

Ogawa, Y., Kaneko, Y., Sato, T., Shimizu, S., Kanetaka, H., & Hanyu, H. (2018). Sarcopenia and muscle functions at various stages of Alzheimer disease. *Frontiers in Neurology*, *9*, 710. doi:10.3389/fneur.2018.00710 PMID:30210435

Oladimeji, M., Asiyanbi, G., Fadeyi, A., Belle, O., Olanipekun, S., & Adekola, O. (2019). ESICM LIVES 2019.

Ologe, F. E., Segun-Busari, S., Abdulraheem, I. S., & Afolabi, A. O. (2005). Ear Diseases in Elderly Hospital Patients in Nigeria. *The Journals of Gerontology. Series A, Biological Sciences and Medical Sciences*, *60A*(3), 404–406.

Onder, G., Vetrano, D. L., Palmer, K., Trevisan, C., Amato, L., Berti, F., & Kruger, P. (2022). Italian guidelines on management of persons with multimorbidity and polypharmacy. *Aging Clinical and Experimental Research*, *34*(5), 989–996. doi:10.100740520-022-02094-z PMID:35249211

Orfila, F., Carrasco-Ribelles, L. A., Abellana, R., Roso-Llorach, A., Cegri, F., Reyes, C., & Reyes, F. (2022). Validation of an electronic frailty index with electronic health records: eFRAGICAP index. *BMC Geriatrics*, *22*(1), 404.

Organization, W. H. (2018). *WHO methods and data sources for life tables 1990-2016.* Global Health Estimates Technical Paper WHO/HIS/IER/GHE.

Oskvig, R. M. (1999). Special Problems in the Elderly. *Chest Journal*, *115*(5), 158S–164S.

Osman, H., & Yamout, R. (2022). Palliative Care in the Arab World. In H. O. Al-Shamsi, I. H. Abu-Gheida, F. Iqbal, & A. Al-Wadhi (Eds.), *Cancer in the Arab World*. Springer. doi:10.1007/978-981-16-7945-2_24

Osterberg, L., & Blaschke, T. (2005). Adherence to medication. *The New England Journal of Medicine*, *353*(5), 487–497. doi:10.1056/NEJMra050100 PMID:16079372

Ownby, R. L., Hertzog, C., Crocco, E., & Duara, R. (2006). Factors related to medication adherence in memory disorder clinic patients. *Aging & Mental Health*, *10*(4), 378 385. doi:10.1080/13607860500410011 PMID:16798630

Pachen, M., Abukar, Y., Shanks, J., Lever, N., & Ramchandra, R. (2021). Regulation of Coronary Blood Flow by the Carotid Body Chemoreceptors in Ovine Heart Failure. *Frontiers in Physiology*, *12*, 709. doi:10.3389/fphys.2021.681135 PMID:34122147

Paciaroni, M., & Bogousslavsky, J. (2013). Connecting cardiovascular disease and dementia: Further evidence. [). Am Heart Assoc.]. *Journal of the American Heart Association*, *2*(6), e000656. doi:10.1161/JAHA.113.000656 PMID:24351703

Packer, M., & Metra, M. (2020). Guideline-directed medical therapy for heart failure does not exist: A non-judgmental framework for describing the level of adherence to evidence-based drug treatments for patients with a reduced ejection fraction. *European Journal of Heart Failure*, *22*(10), 1759–1767. doi:10.1002/ejhf.1857 PMID:32432391

Padrón-Monedero, A., Pastor-Barriuso, R., García López, F. J., Martínez Martín, P., & Damián, J. (2020). Falls and long-term survival among older adults residing in care homes. *PLoS One*, *15*(5), e0231618.

Pagotto, V., & Silveira, E. A. (2014). Methods, diagnostic criteria, cutoff points, and prevalence of sarcopenia among older people. *The Scientific World Journal*, *2014*, 2014. doi:10.1155/2014/231312 PMID:25580454

Pan, Q., Zhang, Y., Long, T., He, W., Zhang, S., Fan, Y., & Zhou, J. (2018). Diagnosis of Vertigo and dizziness syndromes in a neurological outpatient clinic. *European Neurology*, *79*(5-6), 287–294.

Park, H. L., O'Connell, J. E., & Thomson, R. G. (2003, December). A systematic review of cognitive decline in the general elderly population. *International Journal of Geriatric Psychiatry*, *18*(12), 1121–1134. doi:10.1002/gps.1023 PMID:14677145

Patel, S., & Krishnaswami, A. (2015). *The role of pharmacists in the care of older adults with multiple chronic conditions in a multidisciplinary, team-based setting*. Academic Press.

Pathirana, T. I., & Jackson, C. A. (2018). Socioeconomic status and multimorbidity: A systematic review and meta-analysis. *Australian and New Zealand Journal of Public Health*, *42*(2), 186–194. doi:10.1111/1753-6405.12762 PMID:29442409

Payne, J. L., Lyketsos, C. G., Steele, C., Baker, L., Galik, E., Kopunek, S., Steinberg, M., & Warren, A. (1998, November). Relationship of cognitive and functional impairment to depressive features in Alzheimer's disease and other dementias. *The Journal of Neuropsychiatry and Clinical Neurosciences*, *10*(4), 440–447. doi:10.1176/jnp.10.4.440 PMID:9813790

Pel-Littel, R. E., Snaterse, M., Teppich, N. M., Buurman, B. M., van Etten-Jamaludin, F. S., van Weert, J., Minkman, M. M., & Scholte op Reimer, W. J. M. (2021). Barriers and facilitators for shared decision making in older patients with multiple chronic conditions: A systematic review. *BMC Geriatrics*, *21*(1), 1–14. doi:10.118612877-021-02050-y PMID:33549059

Persson, J., Nyberg, L., Lind, J., Larsson, A., Nilsson, L. G., Ingvar, M., & Buckner, R. L. (2006, July 1). Structure–function correlates of cognitive decline in aging. *Cerebral Cortex (New York, N.Y.)*, *16*(7), 907–915. doi:10.1093/cercor/bhj036 PMID:16162855

Peterson, S. J., & Mozer, M. (2017). Differentiating sarcopenia and cachexia among patients with cancer. *Nutrition in Clinical Practice*, *32*(1), 30–39. doi:10.1177/0884533616680354 PMID:28124947

Petrovic, D., de Mestral, C., Bochud, M., Bartley, M., Kivimäki, M., Vineis, P., & Stringhini, S. (2018). The contribution of health behaviors to socioeconomic inequalities in health: A systematic review. *Preventive Medicine*, *113*, 15–31.

Picton, J. D., Marino, A. B., & Nealy, K. L. (2018). Benzodiazepine use and cognitive decline in the elderly. *Bulletin - American Society of Hospital Pharmacists*, *75*(1), e6–e12. doi:10.2146/ajhp160381 PMID:29273607

Pilitsi, E., Farr, O. M., Polyzos, S. A., Perakakis, N., Nolen-Doerr, E., Papathanasiou, A. E., & Mantzoros, C. S. (2019). Pharmacotherapy of obesity: Available medications and drugs under investigation. *Metabolism: Clinical and Experimental*, *92*, 170–192. doi:10.1016/j.metabol.2018.10.010 PMID:30391259

Pilotto, A., Cristillo, V., Cotti Piccinelli, S., Zoppi, N., Bonzi, G., Sattin, D., Schiavolin, S., Raggi, A., Canale, A., Gipponi, S., Libri, I., Frigerio, M., Bezzi, M., Leonardi, M., & Padovani, A. (2021, December). Long-term neurological manifestations of COVID-19: Prevalence and predictive factors. *Neurological Sciences*, *42*(12), 4903–4907. doi:10.100710072-021-05586-4 PMID:34523082

Poewe, W., Gauthier, S., Aarsland, D., Leverenz, J. B., Barone, P., Weintraub, D., Tolosa, E., & Dubois, B. (2008). Diagnosis and management of Parkinson's disease dementia. *International Journal of Clinical Practice*, *62*(10), 1581–1587. doi:10.1111/j.1742-1241.2008.01869.x PMID:18822028

Ponikowski, P., Chua, T. P., Anker, S. D., Francis, D. P., Doehner, W., Banasiak, W., Poole-Wilson, P. A., Piepoli, M. F., & Coats, A. J. (2001). Peripheral chemoreceptor hypersensitivity: An ominous sign in patients with chronic heart failure. *Circulation*, *104*(5), 544–549. doi:10.1161/hc3101.093699 PMID:11479251

Powis, J., Jackson Leach, R., Barata Cavalcanti, O., & Lobstein, T. (2021). *Clinical care for obesity*. Available at: data.worldobesity.org/publications/wof-health-systems-final.pdf

Prados-Torres, A., del Cura-González, I., Prados-Torres, D., López-Rodríguez, J. A., Leiva-Fernández, F., Calderón-Larrañaga, A., & Pico-Soler, V. (2017). Effectiveness of an intervention for improving drug prescription in primary care patients with multimorbidity and polypharmacy: Study protocol of a cluster randomized clinical trial (Multi-PAP project). *Implementation Science; IS*, *12*(1), 1–10. doi:10.118613012-017-0584-x PMID:28449721

Prince, M. J., Wimo, A., Guerchet, M. M., Ali, G. C., Wu, Y. T., & Prina, M. (2015). *World Alzheimer Report 2015-The Global Impact of Dementia: An analysis of prevalence, incidence, cost, and trends*. WAA.

Prince, M. J., Wimo, A., Guerchet, M. M., Ali, G. C., Wu, Y.-T., & Prina, M. (2015). World Alzheimer Report 2015-The Global Impact of Dementia: An analysis of prevalence, incidence, cost and trends.

Prince, M. J., Wu, F., Guo, Y., Robledo, L. M. G., O'Donnell, M., Sullivan, R., & Yusuf, S. (2015). The burden of disease in older people and implications for health policy and practice. *Lancet*, *385*(9967), 549–562.

Prince, M., Ali, G. C., Guerchet, M., Prina, A. M., Albanese, E., & Wu, Y. T. (2016, December). Recent global trends in the prevalence and incidence of dementia, and survival with dementia. *Alzheimer's Research & Therapy*, *8*(1), 1–3. doi:10.118613195-016-0188-8 PMID:27473681

Qassem, T., Aly-ElGabry, D., Alzarouni, A., Abdel-Aziz, K., & Danilo, A. (2021). Psychiatric comorbidities in post-traumatic stress disorder: Detailed findings from the adult psychiatric morbidity survey in the english population. *The Psychiatric Quarterly*, *92*(1), 321–330. doi:10.100711126-020-09797-4 PMID:32705407

Rana, A. K. M. M., Kabir, Z. N., Lundborg, C. S., & Wahlin, A. (2010). Health Education Improves Both Arthritis-related Illness and Self-rated Health: An Intervention Study Among Older People in Rural Bangladesh. *Public Health*, *124*(12), 705–712. doi:10.1016/j.puhe.2010.07.005 PMID:21056439

Rathert, C., Wyrwich, M. D., & Boren, S. A. (2013). Patient-centered care and outcomes: A systematic review of the literature. *Medical Care Research and Review: MCRR*, *70*(4), 351–379. doi:10.1177/1077558712465774 PMID:23169897

Rayman, G., Akpan, A., Cowie, M., Evans, R., Patel, M., Posporelis, S., & Walsh, K. (2022). Managing patients with comorbidities: Future models of care. *Future Healthcare Journal*, *9*(2), 101–105. doi:10.7861/fhj.2022-0029 PMID:35928198

Rea, I. M. (2017). Towards ageing well: Use it or lose it: Exercise, epigenetics and cognition. *Biogerontology*, *18*(4), 679–691.

Rejeski, W. J., Marsh, A. P., Chmelo, E., & Rejeski, J. J. (2010). Obesity, intentional weight loss and physical disability in older adults. *Obesity Reviews*, *11*(9), 671–685. doi:10.1111/j.1467-789X.2009.00679.x PMID:19922431

Renzi, A., Verrusio, W., Messina, M., & Gaj, F. (2020, November). Psychological intervention with elderly people during the COVID-19 pandemic: The experience of a nursing home in Italy. *Psychogeriatrics*, *20*(6), 918–919. doi:10.1111/psyg.12594 PMID:32770596

Resolution WHA67. (2014). *19. Strengthening of palliative care as a component of comprehensive care throughout the life course*. Sixty-seventh World Health Assembly.

Ribarič, S. (2022). Physical exercise, a potential non-pharmacological intervention for attenuating neuroinflammation and cognitive decline in Alzheimer's disease patients. *International Journal of Molecular Sciences*, *23*(6), 3245. doi:10.3390/ijms23063245 PMID:35328666

Rice, J. B., White, A. G., Scarpati, L. M., Wan, G., & Nelson, W. W. (2017). Long-term systemic corticosteroid exposure: A systematic literature review. *Clinical Therapeutics*, *39*(11), 2216–2229.

Richardson, W. C., Berwick, D., Bisgard, J., Bristow, L., Buck, C., & Cassel, C. (2001). *Institute of medicine. Crossing the quality chasm: a new health system for the 21st century*. National Academy Press.

Rimm, A. (2014). Prevalence of obesity in the United States. *Journal of the American Medical Association*, *312*(2), 189–189. doi:10.1001/jama.2014.6219 PMID:25005660

Robinson, S., Cooper, C., & Sayer, A. A. (2017). Nutrition and sarcopenia: a review of the evidence and implications for preventive strategies. *Clinical Nutrition and Aging*, 3-15.

Robinson, S. M., Reginster, J. Y., Rizzoli, R., Shaw, S. C., Kanis, J. A., Bautmans, I., Bischoff-Ferrari, H., Bruyère, O., Cesari, M., Dawson-Hughes, B., Fielding, R. A., Kaufman, J. M., Landi, F., Malafarina, V., Rolland, Y., van Loon, L. J., Vellas, B., Visser, M., Cooper, C., ... Rueda, R. (2018). Does nutrition play a role in the prevention and management of sarcopenia? *Clinical Nutrition (Edinburgh, Lothian)*, *37*(4), 1121–1132. doi:10.1016/j.clnu.2017.08.016 PMID:28927897

Rodriguez-Blazquez, C., João Forjaz, M., Gimeno-Miguel, A., Bliek-Bueno, K., Poblador-Plou, B., Pilar Luengo-Broto, S., & Rodríguez-Acuña, R. (2020). Assessing the pilot implementation of the integrated multimorbidity care model in five European settings: Results from the joint action CHRODIS-PLUS. *International Journal of Environmental Research and Public Health*, *17*(15), 5268. doi:10.3390/ijerph17155268 PMID:32707791

Roger, V. L., Go, A. S., Lloyd-Jones, D. M., Adams, R. J., Berry, J. D., Brown, T. M., & Ford, E. S. (2011). Executive summary: Heart disease and stroke statistics—2011 update. *Circulation*, *123*(4), 459–463. doi:10.1161/CIR.0b013e3182009701 PMID:21160056

Rolski, F., & Błyszczuk, P. (2020). Complexity of TNF-α signaling in heart disease. *Journal of Clinical Medicine*, *9*(10), 3267. doi:10.3390/jcm9103267 PMID:33053859

Román, G. C. (2003). Vascular dementia: distinguishing characteristics, treatment, and prevention. *Journal of the American Geriatrics Society, 51*(5s2), S296–S304.

Romano, A., & Romano, R. (2020). Gas Exchange and Control of Breathing in Elderly and End-of-Life Diseases. In *Ventilatory Support and Oxygen Therapy in Elder, Palliative and End-of-Life Care Patients* (pp. 15–20). Springer.

Romano, E., Ma, R., Vancampfort, D., Firth, J., Felez-Nobrega, M., Haro, J. M., Stubbs, B., & Koyanagi, A. (2021). Multimorbidity and obesity in older adults from six low-and middle-income countries. *Preventive Medicine*, *153*, 106816. doi:10.1016/j.ypmed.2021.106816 PMID:34599928

Rossi, S. (2018). *AMH Aged Care companion*. Adelaide: Australian Medicines Handbook Pty Ltd. Available at www.amh.nct.au

Roy, N., Kim, J., Courey, M., & Cohen, S. M. (2016). Voice disorders in the elderly: A national database study. *The Laryngoscope*, *126*, 421–428.

Roy, N., Stemple, J. C., Merrill, R. M., & Thomas, L. (2007). Epidemiology of voice disorders in the elderly: Preliminary findings. *The Laryngoscope*, *117*, 628–633.

Rubino, F., Puhl, R. M., Cummings, D. E., Eckel, R. H., Ryan, D. H., Mechanick, J. I., Nadglowski, J., Ramos Salas, X., Schauer, P. R., Twenefour, D., Apovian, C. M., Aronne, L. J., Batterham, R. L., Berthoud, H.-R., Boza, C., Busetto, L., Dicker, D., De Groot, M., Eisenberg, D, & Dixon, J. B. (2020). Joint international consensus statement for ending stigma of obesity. *Nature Medicine*, *26*(4), 485–497. doi:10.103841591-020-0803-x PMID:32127716

Rubiño, J. A., Gamundí, A., Akaarir, M., Canellas, F., Rial, R., & Nicolau, M. C. (2020). Bright Light Therapy and Circadian Cycles in Institutionalized Elders. *Frontiers in Neuroscience*, 14.

Ryan, A., Wallace, E., O'Hara, P., & Smith, S. M. (2015). Multimorbidity and functional decline in community-dwelling adults: A systematic review. *Health and Quality of Life Outcomes*, *13*(1), 1–13. doi:10.118612955-015-0355-9 PMID:26467295

Sabaté, E., & Sabaté, E. (Eds.). (2003). *Adherence to long-term therapies: evidence for action.* World Health Organization.

Sabin, S. L., Rosenfeld, R. M., Sundaram, K., Har-EI, G., & Lucente, F. E. (1999). The impact of comorbidity and age on survival with laryngeal cancer. *Ear, Nose, and Throat Journal*, *78*(8), 578–584.

Saftari, L. N., & Kwon, O. S. (2018). Ageing vision and falls: A review. *Journal of Physiological Anthropology*, *37*(1), 1–14.

Salari, P., O'Mahony, C., Henrard, S., Welsing, P., Bhadhuri, A., Schur, N., Roumet, M., Beglinger, S., Beck, T., Jungo, K. T., Byrne, S., Hossmann, S., Knol, W., O'Mahony, D., Spinewine, A., Rodondi, N., & Schwenkglenks, M. (2022). Cost-effectiveness of a structured medication review approach for multimorbid older adults: Within-trial analysis of the OPERAM study. *PLoS One*, *17*(4), e0265507. doi:10.1371/journal.pone.0265507 PMID:35404990

Salisbury, C. (2012). Multimorbidity: Redesigning health care for people who use it. *Lancet*, *380*(9836), 7–9. doi:10.1016/S0140-6736(12)60482-6 PMID:22579042

Salisbury, C., Johnson, L., Purdy, S., Valderas, J. M., & Montgomery, A. A. (2011). Epidemiology and impact of multimorbidity in primary care: A retrospective cohort study. *The British Journal of General Practice*, *61*(582), e12–e21. doi:10.3399/bjgp11X548929 PMID:21401985

Salisbury, C., Man, M.-S., Bower, P., Guthrie, B., Chaplin, K., Gaunt, D. M., & Hollinghurst, S. (2018). Management of multimorbidity using a patient-centred care model: A pragmatic cluster-randomised trial of the 3D approach. *Lancet*, *392*(10141), 41–50. doi:10.1016/S0140-6736(18)31308-4 PMID:29961638

Salive, M. E. (2013). Multimorbidity in older adults. *Epidemiologic Reviews*, *35*(1), 75–83. doi:10.1093/epirev/mxs009 PMID:23372025

Salthouse, T. A. (2009, April 1). When does age-related cognitive decline begin? *Neurobiology of Aging*, *30*(4), 507–514. doi:10.1016/j.neurobiolaging.2008.09.023 PMID:19231028

Salyer, J., Flattery, M., & Lyon, D. E. (2019). Heart failure symptom clusters and quality of life. *Heart & Lung*, *48*(5), 366–372. doi:10.1016/j.hrtlng.2019.05.016 PMID:31204015

Sampson, E. L., Blanchard, M. R., Jones, L., Tookman, A., & King, M. (2009). Dementia in the acute hospital: Prospective cohort study of prevalence and mortality. *The British Journal of Psychiatry*, *195*(1), 61–66. doi:10.1192/bjp.bp.108.055335 PMID:19567898

Sara, H. H., Chowdhury, M. A. B., & Haque, M. A. (2018). Multimorbidity among elderly in Bangladesh. *Aging Medicine*, *1*(3), 267–275.

Sari, R. K., Sutiadiningsih, A., Zaini, H., Meisarah, F., & Hubur, A. A. (2020). Factors affecting cognitive intelligence theory. *Journal of Critical Reviews*, *7*(17), 402–410.

Saudi Palliative Care National Clinical Guideline for Oncology. (n.d.). SHC. shc.gov.sa/ar/NCC/Documents/Saudi%20Palliative%20Care%20National%20Clinical%20 Guideline%20for%20Oncology.pdf

Saunders, C. (2000). The evolution of palliative care. *Patient Education and Counseling*, *41*(1), 7–13. doi:10.1016/S0738-3991(00)00110-5 PMID:10900362

Savaskan, E. (2012, December 1). Delirium and multimorbidity in the elderly. *Praxis (Bern)*, *101*(25), 1633–1636. doi:10.1024/1661-8157/a001147 PMID:23233102

Savva, G. M., & Stephan, B. C. M. (2010). Epidemiological studies of the effect of stroke on incident dementia: A systematic review. *Stroke*, *41*(1), e41–e46. doi:10.1161/STROKEAHA.109.559880 PMID:19910553

Schapmire, T. J., Head, B. A., Nash, W. A., Yankeelov, P. A., Furman, C. D., Wright, R. B., & Faul, A. C. (2018). Overcoming barriers to interprofessional education in gerontology: The interprofessional curriculum for the care of older adults. *Advances in Medical Education and Practice*, *9*, 109.

Schjødt, K., Erlang, A. S., Starup-Linde, J., & Jensen, A. L. (2022). Older hospitalised patients' experience of involvement in discharge planning. *Scandinavian Journal of Caring Sciences*, *36*(1), 192–202. doi:10.1111cs.12977 PMID:33694211

Scholl, I., Zill, J. M., Härter, M., & Dirmaier, J. (2014). An integrative model of patient-centeredness–a systematic review and concept analysis. *PLoS One*, *9*(9), e107828. doi:10.1371/journal.pone.0107828 PMID:25229640

Sciomer, S., Moscucci, F., Maffei, S., Gallina, S., & Mattioli, A. V. (2019). Prevention of cardiovascular risk factors in women: The lifestyle paradox and stereotypes we need to defeat. *European Journal of Preventive Cardiology*, *26*(6), 609–610.

Seferović, P. M., Polovina, M., Adlbrecht, C., Bělohlávek, J., Chioncel, O., Goncalvesova, E., Milinković, I., Grupper, A., Halmosi, R., Kamzola, G., Koskinas, K. C., Lopatin, Y., Parkhomenko, A., Põder, P., Ristić, A. D., Šakalytė, G., Trbušić, M., Tundybayeva, M., Vrtovec, B, & Coats, A. J. (2021). Navigating between Scylla and Charybdis: Challenges and strategies for implementing guideline-directed medical therapy in heart failure with reduced ejection fraction. *European Journal of Heart Failure*, *23*(12), 1999–2007. doi:10.1002/ejhf.2378 PMID:34755422

Seixas, M. B., Almeida, L. B., Trevizan, P. F., Martinez, D. G., Laterza, M. C., Vanderlei, L. C. M., & Silva, L. P. (2020). Effects of inspiratory muscle training in older adults. *Respiratory Care*, *65*(4), 535–544.

Selkoe, D. J. (1994). Cell biology of the amyloid beta-protein precursor and the mechanism of Alzheimer's disease. *Annual Review of Cell Biology*, *10*(1), 373–403. doi:10.1146/annurev. cb.10.110194.002105 PMID:7888181

Semba, R. D., Ferrucci, L., Sun, K., Walston, J., Varadhan, R., Guralnik, J. M., & Fried, L. P. (2007). Oxidative stress and severe walking disability among older women. *The American Journal of Medicine*, *120*(12), 1084–1089. doi:10.1016/j.amjmed.2007.07.028 PMID:18060930

Sembiah, S., Dasgupta, A., Taklikar, C. S., Paul, B., Bandyopadhyay, L., Burman, J., & Subbakrishna, N. (2022). Gender inequalities in prevalence, pattern and predictors of multimorbidity among geriatric population in rural West Bengal. *Journal of Family Medicine and Primary Care*, *11*(8), 4555–4561. doi:10.4103/jfmpc.jfmpc_565_21 PMID:36352948

Sengoku, R. (2020). Aging and Alzheimer's disease pathology. *Neuropathology*, *40*(1), 22–29.

Serrano, V., Spencer-Bonilla, G., Boehmer, K. R., & Montori, V. M. (2017). Minimally disruptive medicine for patients with diabetes. *Current Diabetes Reports*, *17*(11), 1–7. doi:10.100711892-017-0935-7 PMID:28942581

Shah, K., Wingkun, N. J. G., Lambert, C. P., & Villareal, D. T. (2008). Weight loss Therapy Improves Endurance Capacity in Obese Older Adults. *Journal of the American Geriatrics Society*, *56*(6), 1157–1159. doi:10.1111/j.1532-5415.2008.01699.x PMID:18554372

Shaker, R., Ren, J., Zamir, Z., Sarna, A., Liu, J., & Sui, Z. (1994). Effect of aging, position, and temperature on the threshold volume triggering pharyngeal swallows. *Gastroenterology*, *107*(2), 396–402.

Sharma, P., & Maurya, P. (2022). Gender differences in the prevalence and pattern of disease combination of chronic multimorbidity among Indian elderly. *Ageing International*, *47*(2), 265–283. doi:10.100712126-021-09419-9

Sharma, P., Sharma, A., Fayaz, F., Wakode, S., & Pottoo, F. H. (2020). Biological Signatures of Alzheimer's Disease. *Current Topics in Medicinal Chemistry*, *20*(9), 770–781.

Shead, V. L., Rodriguez, R. L., Dreeben, S. J., McBride, S. A., Byrne, G., & Pachana, N. (2021). Anxiety in older adults across care settings. *Anxiety in older people: Clinical and research perspectives*, 157-172.

Shea, M. K., Houston, D. K., Nicklas, B. J., Messier, S. P., Davis, C. C., Miller, M. E., Harris, T. B., Kitzman, D. W., Kennedy, K., & Kritchevsky, S. B. (2010). The effect of randomization to weight loss on total mortality in older overweight and obese adults: The ADAPT Study. *Journals of Gerontology Series A: Biomedical Sciences and Medical Sciences*, *65*(5), 519–525. doi:10.1093/gerona/glp217 PMID:20080875

Sherzai, D., Losey, T., Vega, S., & Sherzai, A. (2014). Seizures and dementia in the elderly: Nationwide Inpatient Sample 1999–2008. *Epilepsy & Behavior*, *36*, 53–56. doi:10.1016/j. yebeh.2014.04.015 PMID:24857809

Shih, J. J., Fountain, N. B., Herman, S. T., Bagic, A., Lado, F., Arnold, S., Zupanc, M. L., Riker, E., & Labiner, D. M. (2018). Indications and methodology for video-electroencephalographic studies in the epilepsy monitoring unit. *Epilepsia*, *59*(1), 27–36. doi:10.1111/epi.13938 PMID:29124760

Shruthi, R., Jyothi, R., Pundarikaksha, H. P., Nagesh, G. N., & Tushar, T. J. (2016). A study of medication compliance in geriatric patients with chronic illnesses at a tertiary care hospital. *Journal of Clinical and Diagnostic Research: JCDR*, *10*(12), FC40. doi:10.7860/JCDR/2016/21908.9088 PMID:28208878

Siervo, M., Oggioni, C., Jakovljevic, D. G., Trenell, M., Mathers, J. C., Houghton, D., Celis-Morales, C., Ashor, A. W., Ruddock, A., Ranchordas, M., Klonizakis, M., & Williams, E. A. (2016). Dietary nitrate does not affect physical activity or outcomes in healthy older adults in a randomized, cross-over trial. *Nutrition Research (New York, N.Y.)*, *36*(12), 1361–1369. doi:10.1016/j.nutres.2016.11.004 PMID:27890482

Silbersweig, D., Safar, L. T., & Daffner, K. R. (2020). *Neuropsychiatry and Behavioral Neurology*. Principles and Practice. McGraw Hill Professional.

Silverberg, D. S., Wexler, D., & Iaina, A. (2002). The importance of anemia and its correction in the management of severe congestive heart failure. *European Journal of Heart Failure*, *4*(6), 681–686. doi:10.1016/S1388-9842(02)00115-0 PMID:12453537

Simmonds, M., Llewellyn, A., Owen, C. G., & Woolacott, N. (2016). Predicting adult obesity from childhood obesity: A systematic review and meta-analysis. *Obesity Reviews*, *17*(2), 95–107. doi:10.1111/obr.12334 PMID:26696565

Sinclair, A. J., & Abdelhafiz, A. H. (2022). Multimorbidity, Frailty and Diabetes in Older People–Identifying Interrelationships and Outcomes. *Journal of Personalized Medicine*, *12*(11), 1911. doi:10.3390/jpm12111911 PMID:36422087

Singam, N. S. V., Fine, C., & Fleg, J. L. (2020). Cardiac changes associated with vascular aging. *Clinical Cardiology*, *43*(2), 92–98.

Skinner, M. W., Andrews, G. J., & Cutchin, M. P. (Eds.). (2017). *Geographical gerontology: Perspectives, concepts, approaches*. Routledge.

Smith, S. M., Wallace, E., Salisbury, C., Sasseville, M., Bayliss, E., & Fortin, M. (2018). A core outcome set for multimorbidity research (COSmm). *Annals of Family Medicine*, *16*(2), 132–138. doi:10.1370/afm.2178 PMID:29531104

Sogebi, O. A. (2013). Profile of ear diseases among elderly patients in Sagamu, South-Western Nigeria. *Nigerian Journal of Medicine*, *22*(3), 257.

Sogebi, O. A., Ariba, A. J., Otulana, T. O., & Osalusi, B. S. (2014). Vestibular disorders in elderly patients: Characteristics, causes and consequences. *The Pan African Medical Journal*, *19*, 146.

Solari, E., Marcozzi, C., Ottaviani, C., Negrini, D., & Moriondo, A. (2022). Draining the Pleural Space: Lymphatic Vessels Facing the Most Challenging Task. *Biology (Basel)*, *11*(3), 419. doi:10.3390/biology11030419 PMID:35336793

Soley-Bori, M., Ashworth, M., Bisquera, A., Dodhia, H., Lynch, R., Wang, Y., & Fox-Rushby, J. (2021). Impact of multimorbidity on healthcare costs and utilisation: A systematic review of the UK literature. *The British Journal of General Practice*, *71*(702), e39–e46. doi:10.3399/bjgp20X713897 PMID:33257463

Song, E. K., Moser, D. K., Rayens, M. K., & Lennie, T. A. (2010). Symptom clusters predict event-free survival in patients with heart failure. *The Journal of Cardiovascular Nursing*, *25*(4), 284–291. doi:10.1097/JCN.0b013e3181cfbcbb PMID:20539163

Son, Y. J., & Won, M. H. (2017). Depression and medication adherence among older Korean patients with hypertension: Mediating role of self-efficacy. *International Journal of Nursing Practice*, *23*(3), e12525. doi:10.1111/ijn.12525 PMID:28194846

Southworth, E., & Parsi, K. (2018). How Should a Physician Counsel a Vegan Patient With IBD Who Might Benefit From Supplements? *AMA Journal of Ethics*, *20*(11), 1025–1032. doi:10.1001/amajethics.2018.1025 PMID:30499430

Sreenivas, V., Natashya, H. S., & Sumy, P. (2021). The Role of Comorbidities in Benign Paroxysmal Positional Vertigo. *Ear, Nose, and Throat Journal*, *100*(5), NP225–NP230.

St John Sutton, M. G., Plappert, T., Abraham, W. T., Smith, A. L., DeLurgio, D. B., Leon, A. R., Loh, E., Kocovic, D. Z., Fisher, W. G., Ellestad, M., Messenger, J., Kruger, K., Hilpisch, K. E., & Hill, M. R. (2003). Effect of cardiac resynchronization therapy on left ventricular size and function in chronic heart failure. *Circulation*, *107*(15), 1985–1990. doi:10.1161/01.CIR.0000065226.24159.E9 PMID:12668512

Stachler, R. J., Francis, D. O., Schwartz, S. R., Damask, C. C., Digoy, G. P., Krouse, H. J., & McCoy, S. J. (2018). Clinical Practice Guideline: Hoarseness (Dysphonia) (Update). *Otolaryngology - Head and Neck Surgery*, *00*(0), 1–42.

Stambler, I. (2017). Recognizing degenerative aging as a treatable medical condition: Methodology and policy. *Aging and Disease*, *8*(5), 583.

Starfield, B., Lemke, K. W., Herbert, R., Pavlovich, W. D., & Anderson, G. (2005). Comorbidity and the use of primary care and specialist care in the elderly. *Annals of Family Medicine*, *3*(3), 215–222. doi:10.1370/afm.307 PMID:15928224

Starr, K. N. P., & Bales, C. W. (2015). Excessive body weight in older adults. *Clinics in Geriatric Medicine*, *31*(3), 311–326. doi:10.1016/j.cger.2015.04.001 PMID:26195092

Stephens, S. D., Callaghan, D. E., Hogan, S., Meredith, R., Rayment, A., & Davis, A. C. (1990). Hearing disability in people aged 50-65: Effectiveness and acceptability of rehabilitative intervention. *British Medical Journal*, *300*(6723), 508–511. doi:10.1136/bmj.300.6723.508 PMID:2107929

Steptoe, A., Jackson, S. E., & Wardle, J. (2016). Sexual activity and concerns in people with coronary heart disease from a population-based study. *Heart (British Cardiac Society)*, *102*(14), 1095–1099. doi:10.1136/heartjnl-2015-308993 PMID:27126394

Stewart, R., Xue, Q. L., Masaki, K., Petrovitch, H., Ross, G. W., White, L. R., & Launer, L. J. (2009, August 1). Change in blood pressure and incident dementia: A 32-year prospective study. *Hypertension, 54*(2), 233–240. doi:10.1161/HYPERTENSIONAHA.109.128744 PMID:19564551

Stoever, K., Heber, A., Eichberg, S., Zijlstra, W., & Brixius, K. (2015). Changes of Body Composition, Muscular Strength and Physical Performance Due to Resistance Training in Older Persons with Sarcopenic Obesity. *The Journal of Frailty & Aging, 4*(4), 216–222. PMID:27031021

Stott, D. J., & Young, J. (2012). Across the pond'–a response to the NICE guidelines for management. *Lancet, 380*, 37–43.

Stott, D. J., & Young, J. (2017). 'Across the pond'—A response to the NICE guidelines for management of multi-morbidity in older people. *Age and Ageing, 46*(3), 343–345. doi:10.1093/ageing/afx031 PMID:28369219

Street, R. L. Jr, Gordon, H. S., Ward, M. M., Krupat, E., & Kravitz, R. L. (2005). Patient participation in medical consultations: Why some patients are more involved than others. *Medical Care, 43*(10), 960–969. doi:10.1097/01.mlr.0000178172.40344.70 PMID:16166865

Suzuki, K. (2013). „Garfinkel, S. N „Critchley, HD, & Se exteroceptive and interoceptive domains modulates ropsychologic1, 5*(13), 2909-2917.

Tadeu, A. C. R., de Figueiredo, I. J., & Santiago, L. M. (2020). Multimorbidity and consultation time: A systematic review. *BMC Family Practice, 21*(1), 1–8. doi:10.118612875-020-01219-5 PMID:32723303

Tafiadis, D., Chronopoulos, S. K., Helidoni, M. E., Kosma, E. I., Voniati, L., & Papadopoulos, P. … Velegrakis, G. A. (2019). Checking for voice disorders without clinical intervention : The Greek and global VHI thresholds for voice disordered patients. *Scientific Reports, 9*, 1–9. doi:10.1038/s41598-019-45758-z

Takeuchi, S., Kohno, T., Goda, A., Shiraishi, Y., Kawana, M., Saji, M., Nagatomo, Y., Nishihata, Y., Takei, M., Nakano, S., Soejima, K., Kohsaka, S., & Yoshikawa, T. West Tokyo Heart Failure Registry Investigators. (2022). Multimorbidity, guideline-directed medical therapies, and associated outcomes among hospitalized heart failure patients. *ESC Heart Failure, 9*(4), 2500–2510. doi:10.1002/ehf2.13954 PMID:35561100

Tan, C. S. (2020). The need of patient education to improve medication adherence among hypertensive patients. *Malaysian Journal of Pharmacy, 6*(1), 1–5. doi:10.52494/MOEL1486

Tate, R. B., Swift, A. U., & Bayomi, D. J. (2013). Older men's lay definitions of successful aging over time: The Manitoba follow-up study. *International Journal of Aging & Human Development, 76*(4), 297–322. doi:10.2190/AG.76.4.b PMID:23855184

Tavares-Júnior, J. W., de Souza, A. C., Borges, J. W., Oliveira, D. N., Siqueira-Neto, J. I., Sobreira-Neto, M. A., & Braga-Neto, P. (2022, April 18). COVID-19 associated cognitive impairment: A systematic review. *Cortex, 152*, 77–97. doi:10.1016/j.cortex.2022.04.006 PMID:35537236

Taylor, C. J., Harrison, C., Britt, H., Miller, G., & Hobbs, F. R. (2017). Heart failure and multimorbidity in Australian general practice. *Journal of Comorbidity*, 7(1), 44–49. doi:10.15256/joc.2017.7.106 PMID:29090188

Teipel, S., Babiloni, C., Hoey, J., Kaye, J., Kirste, T., & Burmeister, O. K. (2016). Information and communication technology solutions for outdoor navigation in dementia. *Alzheimer's & Dementia*, 12(6), 695–707. doi:10.1016/j.jalz.2015.11.003 PMID:26776761

Thoits, P. A. (2013). Self, identity, stress, and mental health. Handbook of the sociology of mental health, 357-377.

Thomas, M., Khariton, Y., Fonarow, G. C., Arnold, S. V., Hill, L., Nassif, M. E., Sharma, P. P., Butler, J., Thomas, L., Duffy, C. I., DeVore, A. D., Hernandez, A., Albert, N. M., Patterson, J. H., Williams, F. B., McCague, K., & Spertus, J. A. (2019). Association of changes in heart failure treatment with patients' health status: Real-world evidence from CHAMP-HF. *JACC. Heart Failure*, 7(7), 615–625. doi:10.1016/j.jchf.2019.03.020 PMID:31176672

Tieland, M., Trouwborst, I., & Clark, B. C. (2018). Skeletal muscle performance and ageing. *Journal of Cachexia, Sarcopenia and Muscle*, 9(1), 3–19.

Tonelli, M., Wiebe, N., Straus, S., Fortin, M., Guthrie, B., James, M. T., Klarenbach, S. W., Tam-Tham, H., Lewanczuk, R., Manns, B. J., & Quan, H. (2017, August 14). Multimorbidity, dementia and health care in older people: A population-based cohort study. *Canadian Medical Association Open Access Journal.*, 5(3), E623–E631. PMID:28811281

Toots, A., Wiklund, R., Littbrand, H., Nordin, E., Nordström, P., Lundin-Olsson, L., & Rosendahl, E. (2019). The effects of exercise on falls in older people with dementia living in nursing homes: A randomized controlled trial. *Journal of the American Medical Directors Association, 20*(7), 835-842.

Tornero-Quiñones, I., Sáez-Padilla, J., Espina Díaz, A., Abad Robles, M. T., & Sierra Robles, Á. (2020). Functional ability, frailty and risk of falls in the elderly: Relations with autonomy in daily living. *International Journal of Environmental Research and Public Health*, 17(3), 1006.

Tosato, M., Marzetti, E., Cesari, M., Savera, G., Miller, R. R., Bernabei, R., Landi, F., & Calvani, R. (2017). Measurement of muscle mass in sarcopenia: From imaging to biochemical markers. *Aging Clinical and Experimental Research*, 29(1), 19–27. doi:10.100740520-016-0717-0 PMID:28176249

Trevena, L. (2018). Minimally disruptive medicine for patients with complex multimorbidity. *Australian Journal of General Practice*, 47(4), 175–179. doi:10.31128/AFP-10-17-4374 PMID:29621856

Truby, L. K., & Rogers, J. G. (2020). Advanced heart failure: Epidemiology, diagnosis, and therapeutic approaches. *Heart Failure*, 8(7), 523–536. PMID:32535126

Tsay, A. J. (2018). The internet, ethics, and false beliefs in health care. *AMA Journal of Ethics*, 20(11), 1003–1006. doi:10.1001/amajethics.2018.1003

Tsuji, K., Velázquez-Villaseñor, L., Rauch, S. D., Glynn, R. J., Wall, C., & Merchant, S. N. (2000). Temporal bone studies of the human peripheral vestibular system. Aminoglycoside ototoxicity. *The Annals of Otology, Rhinology & Laryngology. Supplement, 181,* 20–25.

Turana, Y., Tengkawan, J., Chia, Y. C., Shin, J., Chen, C. H., Park, S., Tsoi, K., Buranakitjaroen, P., Soenarta, A. A., Siddique, S., Cheng, H.-M., Tay, J. C., Teo, B. W., Wang, T.-D., & Kario, K. (2021). Mental health problems and hypertension in the elderly: Review from the HOPE Asia Network. *Journal of Clinical Hypertension, 23*(3), 504–512. doi:10.1111/jch.14121 PMID:33283971

UK, N. G. C. (2016). *Multimorbidity: assessment, prioritisation and management of care for people with commonly occurring multimorbidity.* UK.

Ungvari, Z., Tarantini, S., Donato, A. J., Galvan, V., & Csiszar, A. (2018). Mechanisms of vascular aging. *Circulation Research, 123*(7), 849–867.

Upadhyay, J., Farr, O., Perakakis, N., Ghaly, W., & Mantzoros, C. (2018). Obesity as a disease. *Medicina Clínica, 102*(1), 13–33. PMID:29156181

Üstün, B., & Kennedy, C. (2009, June 1). What is "functional impairment"? Disentangling disability from clinical significance. *World Psychiatry; Official Journal of the World Psychiatric Association (WPA), 8*(2), 82–85. doi:10.1002/j.2051-5545.2009.tb00219.x PMID:19516924

van den Akker, M., Buntinx, F., & Knottnerus, J. A. (1996). Comorbidity or multimorbidity: What's in a name? A review of literature. *The European Journal of General Practice, 2*(2), 65–70. doi:10.3109/13814789609162146

van den Anker, J., Reed, M. D., Allegaert, K., & Kearns, G. L. (2018). Developmental changes in pharmacokinetics and pharmacodynamics. *Journal of Clinical Pharmacology, 58,* S10–S25.

Van Gaal, L. F., Mertens, I. L., & De Block, C. E. (2006). Mechanisms linking obesity with cardiovascular disease. *Nature, 444*(7121), 875–880. doi:10.1038/nature05487 PMID:17167476

van Onna, M., & Boonen, A. (2016). The challenging interplay between rheumatoid arthritis, ageing and comorbidities. *BMC Musculoskeletal Disorders, 17*(1), 184.

Van Rijckevorsel, K. (2006). Cognitive problems related to epilepsy syndromes, especially malignant epilepsies. *Seizure, 15*(4), 227–234. doi:10.1016/j.seizure.2006.02.019 PMID:16563807

Van Straaten, E. C. W., Scheltens, P., & Barkhof, F. (2004). MRI and CT in the diagnosis of vascular dementia. *Journal of the Neurological Sciences, 226*(1–2), 9–12. doi:10.1016/j.jns.2004.09.003 PMID:15537511

Vankova, H., Holmerova, I., & Volicer, L. (2021). Geriatric depression and inappropriate medication: Benefits of interprofessional team cooperation in nursing homes. *International Journal of Environmental Research and Public Health, 18*(23), 12438. doi:10.3390/ijerph182312438 PMID:34886164

Vannorsdall, T. D., Brigham, E., Fawzy, A., Raju, S., Gorgone, A., Pletnikova, A., Lyketsos, C. G., Parker, A. M., & Oh, E. S. (2022, March 1). Cognitive dysfunction, psychiatric distress, and functional decline after COVID-19. *Journal of the Academy of Consultation-liaison Psychiatry*, *63*(2), 133–143. doi:10.1016/j.jaclp.2021.10.006 PMID:34793996

Vargo, D. L., Kramer, W. G., Black, P. K., Smith, W. B., Serpas, T., & Brater, D. C. (1995). Bioavailability, pharmacokinetics, and pharmacodynamics of torsemide and furosemide in patients with congestive heart failure. *Clinical Pharmacology and Therapeutics*, *57*(6), 601–609. doi:10.1016/0009-9236(95)90222-8 PMID:7781259

Vassar, M., Jellison, S., Wendelbo, H., Wayant, C., Gray, H., & Bibens, M. (2019). Using the CONSORT statement to evaluate the completeness of reporting of addiction randomised trials: A cross-sectional review. *BMJ Open*, *9*(9), e032024. doi:10.1136/bmjopen-2019-032024 PMID:31494625

Veronese, N., Stubbs, B., Noale, M., Solmi, M., Pilotto, A., Vaona, A., & Maggi, S. (2017). Polypharmacy is associated with higher frailty risk in older people: An 8-year longitudinal cohort study. *Journal of the American Medical Directors Association*, *18*(7), 624–628.

Vetrano, D. L., Foebel, A. D., Marengoni, A., Brandi, V., Collamati, A., Heckman, G. A., Hirdes, J., Bernabei, R., & Onder, G. (2016). Chronic diseases and geriatric syndromes: The different weight of comorbidity. *European Journal of Internal Medicine*, *27*, 62–67. doi:10.1016/j.ejim.2015.10.025 PMID:26643938

Vetrano, D. L., Rizzuto, D., Calderón-Larrañaga, A., Onder, G., Welmer, A.-K., Bernabei, R., Marengoni, A., & Fratiglioni, L. (2018). Trajectories of functional decline in older adults with neuropsychiatric and cardiovascular multimorbidity: A Swedish cohort study. *PLoS Medicine*, *15*(3), e1002503. doi:10.1371/journal.pmed.1002503 PMID:29509768

Vetrano, D. L., Roso-Llorach, A., Fernández, S., Guisado-Clavero, M., Violán, C., Onder, G., Fratiglioni, L., Calderón-Larrañaga, A., & Marengoni, A. (2020). Twelve-year clinical trajectories of multimorbidity in a population of older adults. *Nature Communications*, *11*(1), 3223. doi:10.103841467-020-16780-x PMID:32591506

Villareal, D. T., Chode, S., Parimi, N., Sinacore, D. R., Hilton, T., Armamento-Villareal, R., Napoli, N., Qualls, C., & Shah, K. (2011). Weight loss, exercise, or both and physical function in obese older adults. *The New England Journal of Medicine*, *364*(13), 1218–1229. doi:10.1056/NEJMoa1008234 PMID:21449785

Vincent, G. K. (2010). *The next four decades: The older population in the United States: 2010 to 2050*. US Department of Commerce, Economics and Statistics Administration.

Violán, C., Fernández-Bertolín, S., Guisado-Clavero, M., Foguet-Boreu, Q., Valderas, J. M., Vidal Manzano, J., Roso-Llorach, A., & Cabrera-Bean, M. (2020). Five-year trajectories of multimorbidity patterns in an elderly Mediterranean population using Hidden Markov Models. *Scientific Reports*, *10*(1), 16879. doi:10.103841598-020-73231-9 PMID:33037233

Vosoughi, K., Atieh, J., Khanna, L., Khoshbin, K., Prokop, L. J., Davitkov, P., Murad, M. H., & Camilleri, M. (2021). Association of glucagon-like peptide 1 analogs and agonists administered for obesity with weight loss and adverse events: A systematic review and network meta-analysis. *EClinicalMedicine*, *42*, 101213. doi:10.1016/j.eclinm.2021.101213 PMID:34877513

Wakimoto, P., & Block, G. (2001). Dietary intake, dietary patterns, and changes with age: An epidemiological perspective. *The Journals of Gerontology. Series A, Biological Sciences and Medical Sciences*, *56*(suppl_2), 65–80. doi:10.1093/gerona/56.suppl_2.65 PMID:11730239

Walrand, S., Guillet, C., Salles, J., Cano, N., & Boirie, Y. (2011). Physiopathological mechanism of sarcopenia. *Clinics in Geriatric Medicine*, *27*(3), 365–385. doi:10.1016/j.cger.2011.03.005 PMID:21824553

Wang, T., Yuan, F., Chen, Z., Zhu, S., Chang, Z., Yang, W., Deng, B., Que, R., Cao, P., Chao, Y., Chan, L., Pan, Y., Wang, Y., Xu, L., Lyu, Q., Chan, P., Yenari, M. A., Tan, E.-K., & Wang, Q. (2020). Vascular, inflammatory and metabolic risk factors in relation to dementia in Parkinson's disease patients with type 2 diabetes mellitus. *Aging (Albany NY)*, *12*(15), 15682–15704. doi:10.18632/aging.103776 PMID:32805719

Wang, Y., Huang, H., & Chen, G. (2020). Effects of lighting on ECG, visual performance and psychology of the elderly. *Optik (Stuttgart)*, *203*, 164063.

Ward, Z. J., Bleich, S. N., Cradock, A. L., Barrett, J. L., Giles, C. M., Flax, C., Long, M. W., & Gortmaker, S. L. (2019). Projected US state-level prevalence of adult obesity and severe obesity. *The New England Journal of Medicine*, *381*(25), 2440–2450. doi:10.1056/NEJMsa1909301 PMID:31851800

Welsh, T. J. (2019). Multimorbidity in people living with dementia. *Case Reports in Women's Health*, (Jul), 23. PMID:31193805

Whitty, C. J., MacEwen, C., Goddard, A., Alderson, D., Marshall, M., Calderwood, C., & Stokes-Lampard, H. (2020). *Rising to the challenge of multimorbidity* (Vol. 368). British Medical Journal Publishing Group.

WHO. (1997). *Obesity: preventing and managing the global epidemic. Report of a WHO consultation on obesity*. WHO.

WHO. (2000). Obesity: Preventing and managing the global epidemic. *World Health Organization Technical Report Series*, *894*, 1–253. PMID:11234459

WHO. (2022). *Draft recommendations for the prevention and management of obesity over the life course, including potential targets*. WHO. www.who.int/teams/noncommunicable-diseases/governance/obesityrecommendations

Wilcox, C. S., Testani, J. M., & Pitt, B. (2020). Pathophysiology of diuretic resistance and its implications for the management of chronic heart failure. *Hypertension*, *76*(4), 1045–1054. doi:10.1161/HYPERTENSIONAHA.120.15205 PMID:32829662

Willadsen, T. G., Bebe, A., Køster-Rasmussen, R., Jarbøl, D. E., Guassora, A. D., Waldorff, F. B., Reventlow, S., & Olivarius, N. F. (2016). The role of diseases, risk factors and symptoms in the definition of multimorbidity–a systematic review. *Scandinavian Journal of Primary Health Care*, *34*(2), 112–121. doi:10.3109/02813432.2016.1153242 PMID:26954365

Williams, K. N., & Kemper, S. (2010, May 1). Interventions to reduce cognitive decline in aging. *Journal of Psychosocial Nursing and Mental Health Services*, *48*(5), 42–51. doi:10.3928/02793695-20100331-03 PMID:20415290

Williams, S. C. (2013). Alzheimer's disease: Mapping the brain's decline. *Nature*, *502*(7473), S84–S85. doi:10.1038/502S84a PMID:24187700

Wing, R. R., Phelan, S., & Tate, D. (2002). The role of adherence in mediating the relationship between depression and health outcomes. *Journal of Psychosomatic Research*, *53*(4), 877–881. doi:10.1016/S0022-3999(02)00315-X PMID:12377297

Winkler, S., Garg, A. K., Mekayarajjananonth, T., Bakaeen, L. G., & Khan, E. (1999). Depressed taste and smell in geriatric patients. *The Journal of the American Dental Association*, *130*(12), 1759–1765.

Witham, M. D., & Avenell, A. (2010). Interventions to achieve long-term weight loss in obese older people: A systematic review and meta-analysis. *Age and Ageing*, *39*(2), 176–184. doi:10.1093/ageing/afp251 PMID:20083615

Wleklik, M., Uchmanowicz, I., Jankowska, E. A., Vitale, C., Lisiak, M., Drozd, M., Pobrotyn, P., Tkaczyszyn, M., & Lee, C. (2020). Multidimensional approach to frailty. *Frontiers in Psychology*, *11*, 564. doi:10.3389/fpsyg.2020.00564 PMID:32273868

Wolffsohn, J. S., & Davies, L. N. (2019). Presbyopia: Effectiveness of correction strategies. *Progress in Retinal and Eye Research*, *68*, 124–143.

Wong, C. Y., Chaudhry, S. I., Desai, M. M., & Krumholz, H. M. (2011). Trends in comorbidity, disability, and polypharmacy in heart failure. *The American Journal of Medicine*, *124*(2), 136–143. doi:10.1016/j.amjmed.2010.08.017 PMID:21295193

Woo MS, Malsy J, Pöttgen J, Seddiq Zai S, Ufer F, Hadjilaou A, Schmiedel S, Addo MM, Gerloff C, Heesen C, Schulze Zur Wiesch J. (2020). Frequent neurocognitive deficits after recovery from mild COVID-19. *Brain communications, 2*(2).

Woods, B., Aguirre, E., Spector, A. E., & Orrell, M. (2012). Cognitive stimulation to improve cognitive functioning in people with dementia. *Cochrane Database of Systematic Reviews*, *2*. doi:10.1002/14651858.CD005562.pub2 PMID:22336813

Woo, P., Casper, J., Colton, R., & Brewer, D. (1992). Dysphonia in the aging: Physiology versus disease. *The Laryngoscope*, *102*, 139–144.

Woo, Y. S., Shin, G. I., & Park, H. Y. (2020). Comparative Analysis of Differences in Reaction Time and Divided Attention with Elderly Age: Using the Driving Ability Assessment Tool. *Therapeutic Science for Rehabilitation*, *9*(3), 53–61.

World Health Organization. (2004). International Statistical Classification of Diseases and related health problems: Alphabetical index (Vol. 1, 2, 3). World Health Organization.

World Health Organization. (2011). *Waist circumference and waist-hip ratio: report of a WHO expert consultation.* WHO.

World Health Organization. (2017, December 12). *Mental health of older adults.* WHO.

World Health Organization. (2018). *Integrating palliative care and symptom relief into primary health care: a WHO guide for planners, implementers, and managers.* WHO.

World Obesity Federation. (2021). *Obesity is a disease.* WOF. www.worldobesityday.org/assets/downloads/Obesity_Is_a_Disease.pdf

Wormser, D., Di Angelantonio, E., Sattar, N., Collins, R., Thompson, S., & Danesh, J. (2011). Body-mass index, abdominal adiposity, and cardiovascular risk–Authors' reply. *Lancet, 378*(9787), 228. doi:10.1016/S0140-6736(11)61122-7

Wu, Y., Xu, X., Chen, Z., Duan, J., Hashimoto, K., Yang, L., Liu, C., & Yang, C. (2020, July 1). Nervous system involvement after infection with COVID-19 and other coronaviruses. *Brain, Behavior, and Immunity, 87*, 18–22. doi:10.1016/j.bbi.2020.03.031 PMID:32240762

Xu, J., Wang, J., Wimo, A., Fratiglioni, L., & Qiu, C. (2017). The economic burden of dementia in China, 1990–2030: Implications for health policy. *Bulletin of the World Health Organization, 95*(1), 18–26. doi:10.2471/BLT.15.167726 PMID:28053361

Yanai, H. (2015). Nutrition for sarcopenia. *Journal of Clinical Medicine Research, 7*(12), 926–931. doi:10.14740/jocmr2361w PMID:26566405

Yaribeygi, H., Panahi, Y., Sahraei, H., Johnston, T. P., & Sahebkar, A. (2017). The impact of stress on body function: A review. *EXCLI Journal, 16*, 1057. PMID:28900385

Yarnall, A. J., Sayer, A. A., Clegg, A., Rockwood, K., Parker, S., & Hindle, J. V. (2017). New horizons in multimorbidity in older adults. *Age and Ageing, 46*(6), 882–888. doi:10.1093/ageing/afx150 PMID:28985248

Ye, L., Wen, Y., Chen, Y., Yao, J., Li, X., Liu, Y., Song, J., & Sun, Z. (2020). Diagnostic reference values for sarcopenia in Tibetans in China. *Scientific Reports, 10*(1), 3067. doi:10.103841598-020-60027-0 PMID:32080301

Yin, M., Zhang, H., Liu, Q., Ding, F., Deng, Y., Hou, L., Wang, H., Yue, J., & He, Y. (2021). Diagnostic performance of clinical laboratory indicators with sarcopenia: Results from the west China health and aging trend study. *Frontiers in Endocrinology, 12*, 785045. doi:10.3389/fendo.2021.785045 PMID:34956096

Yokoyama, Y., Kitamura, A., Seino, S., Kim, H., Obuchi, S., Kawai, H., Hirano, H., Watanabe, Y., Motokawa, K., Narita, M., & Shinkai, S. (2021). Association of nutrient-derived dietary patterns with sarcopenia and its components in community-dwelling older Japanese: A cross-sectional study. *Nutrition Journal, 20*(1), 1–10. doi:10.118612937-021-00665-w PMID:33461556

Yu, D. S. F., Li, P. W. C., & Chong, S. O. K. (2018). Symptom cluster among patients with advanced heart failure: A review of its manifestations and impacts on health outcomes. *Current Opinion in Supportive and Palliative Care*, *12*(1), 16–24. doi:10.1097/SPC.0000000000000316 PMID:29176333

Zamboni, M., & Mazzali, G. (2012). Obesity in the elderly: An emerging health issue. *International Journal of Obesity*, *36*(9), 1151–1152. doi:10.1038/ijo.2012.120 PMID:22964828

Zamboni, M., Mazzali, G., Brunelli, A., Saatchi, T., Urbani, S., Giani, A., Rossi, A. P., Zoico, E., & Fantin, F. (2022). The Role of Crosstalk between Adipose Cells and Myocytes in the Pathogenesis of Sarcopenic Obesity in the Elderly. *Cells*, *11*(21), 3361. doi:10.3390/cells11213361 PMID:36359757

Zamboni, M., Mazzali, G., Zoico, E., Harris, T. B., Meigs, J. B., Di Francesco, V., Fantin, F., Bissoli, L., & Bosello, O. (2005). Health consequences of obesity in the elderly: A review of four unresolved questions. *International Journal of Obesity*, *29*(9), 1011–1029. doi:10.1038j. ijo.0803005 PMID:15925957

Zemedikun, D. T., Gray, L. J., Khunti, K., Davies, M. J., & Dhalwani, N. N. (2018). Patterns of multimorbidity in middle-aged and older adults: An analysis of the UK biobank data. *Mayo Clinic Proceedings*, *93*(7), 857–866. doi:10.1016/j.mayocp.2018.02.012 PMID:29801777

Zhang, C., Kuo, C.-C., Moghadam, S. H., Monte, L., Campbell, S. N., Rice, K. C., Sawchenko, P. E., Masliah, E., & Rissman, R. A. (2016). Corticotropin-releasing factor receptor-1 antagonism mitigates beta amyloid pathology and cognitive and synaptic deficits in a mouse model of Alzheimer's disease. *Alzheimer's & Dementia*, *12*(5), 527–537. doi:10.1016/j.jalz.2015.09.007 PMID:26555315

Zhang, L., Shooshtari, S., St. John, P., & Menec, V. H. (2022, November 10). Multimorbidity and depressive symptoms in older adults and the role of social support: Evidence using Canadian Longitudinal Study on Aging (CLSA) data. *PLoS One*, *17*(11), e0276279. doi:10.1371/journal. pone.0276279 PMID:36355773

Zhang, Y., Chen, Y., & Ma, L. (2018). Depression and cardiovascular disease in elderly: Current understanding. *Journal of Clinical Neuroscience*, *47*, 1–5. doi:10.1016/j.jocn.2017.09.022 PMID:29066229

Zhang, Z., Adappa, N. D., Lautenbach, E., Chiu, A. G., Doghramji, L., Howland, T. J., & ... . (2014). The effect of diabetes mellitus on chronic rhinosinusitis and sinus surgery outcome. *International Forum of Allergy & Rhinology*, *4*(4), 315–320.

Zhou, H., Lu, S., Chen, J., Wei, N., Wang, D., Lyu, H., Shi, C., & Hu, S. (2020, October 1). The landscape of cognitive function in recovered COVID-19 patients. *Journal of Psychiatric Research*, *129*, 98–102. doi:10.1016/j.jpsychires.2020.06.022 PMID:32912598

About the Contributors

Adil Alharthi is a consultant internist Saudi board in Internal Medicine 2009 and currently working in Waddi Addawasir Military Hospital. Interested in several areas of Medicine e.g. Multimorbity, HTN, Geriatrics, SCD, Pregnancy induced Medical complications and others.

***

Hamza is pursuing a Ph.D. in Clinical Psychology, Department of Psychiatry, J.N. Medical College & Hospital, Aligarh Muslim University, Aligarh, U.P., India. She has qualified national level NTA-NET and GATE in Psychology. She has presented several research papers at various national and international conferences and seminars. Her interest areas are psychosocial management of mood disorders, primary headaches (migraine, tension-type headaches), and neurodevelopmental disorders (ASD & ADHD).

Deoshree Akhouri is working as an Associate Professor (Clinical Psychology) in the department of Psychiatry at J.N. Medical College & Hospital. She has completed her M.Phil (Medical & Clinical Psychology) from Ranchi Institute of Neuro-Psychiatry & Allied Sciences (RINPAS), Kanke, Ranchi Jharkhand, and has done her Ph.D. from Ranchi University. She is a registered Clinical Psychologist from the rehabilitation Council of India (CRR A13695). Her interest areas are Psychotherapy, mindfulness meditation, hypnotherapy, psychodiagnostics, and psychometrics in various psychiatric conditions, and forensic psychology. She has published more than 50 articles in various national and international journals.

Mohammad Akram is a Students' Counselor at the Department of Psychology, Aligarh Muslim University, Aligarh (India). He has a deep interest in guidance and counseling, research, and the standardization of psychological tools. He obtained a doctoral degree from the Aligarh Muslim University, based on his research "Impact of Academic Stress and Hardiness on Achievement Motivation and Problem

Solving Behavior of Adolescents. He also has Post Graduate Diploma in Guidance & Counseling. He has contributed a number of theoretical articles and empirical papers in refereed and peer-reviewed journals of psychology. He has co-authored a book on Dimensions of Well-being. His fields of specialization are Educational Psychology, Social Psychology, and Counseling Psychology.

Abdulaziz Alghamdi is an MD, 1998 KAUH Saudi board of Urology, 2009 Urology Consultant, 2012 Division Head of Urology, 2015.

Khalid Almotari is a Consultant in Family Medicine since 2010, Saudi and Arab Board of family medicine, master in medical education, master in health administration, trainer and academic supervisor in the program of family medicine, previous director of family medicine and currently director of health education department at King Fahad Armed Forces hospital, Jeddah,Saudi Arabia

Aisha Alshehri is a Clinical Pharmacy Specialist, American Board Certified Pharmacotherpy Specialist (BCPS), King Fahad Armed Forces Hospital-Jeddah.

Samuel Ayodele's mission statement is to work with the fear of God in order to enhance a career and render a selfless service with touch of excellence and proficiency, having competency in a vast array of otorhinolaryngological skills, techniques, research and academics; as well as promoting ear, nose and throat health care through advocacy. Specialty: Otorhinolaryngologist (Ent /Head & Neck Surgery) Interests: Rhinology, Otology, Laryngology, Head & Neck Surgery, Endoscopic Ent Surgery. Date and Place of Birth: 14th October, 1984. Ilorin, Kwara, Nigeria. Sex: Male Nationality: Nigerian State of Origin Kogi Local Govt. Area: Yagba West Marital Status: Married Institutions Attended (with dates): 1 post-graduate education West African College of Surgeons/National Postgraduate Medical College of Nigeria: Faculty of Otorhinolaryngology/Head and Neck Surgery 2012-2019 2 University Education 1st Degree: University of Ilorin, 2003-2010 Ilorin, Nigeria 3 secondary education Titcombe College, Egbe, Kogi State, Nigeria 1995 - 2001 4 primary education ECWA School 1 Oke Egbe, Egbe Kogi State, Nigeria. 1991-1995 Trinity Nursery and Primary School, GRA, Ilorin, Kwara state, Nigeria: 1988- 1991 Academic/Professional Qualifications (with dates): o Doctor of Medicine in Otorhinolaryngology (in view) o Fundamentals of Global Health Research (Certs. FGHR) ..... June 2021 o Project Management in Global Health (Certs. PMGH) --- September 2020 o Leadership and Management in Health (Certs. LMIH) --- December 2019 o Fellow, National Postgraduate Medical College of Nigeria (FMCORLHNS) --- December 2019 o Fellow, West African College of Surgeons in Otorhinolaryngology (FWACS) ---April 2019 o Bachelor of Medicine

& Bachelor of Surgery (MB; BS) ---May 2010 o West African Examination Council (WAEC) / Senior School Certificate (SSC) ---June 2001 Work Experience (with dates): Hospital ENT Consultant (Otorhinolaryngology, Head and Neck Surgery) Department of ORL, Obafemi Awolowo University Teaching Hospital Complex, Ile-Ife. September 2021-Present Department of ENT, Federal Medical Centre, Lokoja: April – September 2021 Department of ENT, General Hospital, Katsina: January 2020 – March 2021 Post-Fellowship Senior Registrar (Otorhinolaryngology) April 2019 – December 2019 o Teaching Junior Residents and Medical Students Chief Resident (Department of Otorhinolaryngology): April 2017 – March 2018 Senior Registrar (Otorhinolaryngology) University of Ilorin Teaching Hospital: April 2016 – March 2019 Associate Tutor in Ear, Nose & Throat Surgery School of Post-Basic Nursing and Community Health Officer Training Institute, UITH, Ilorin: August 2015 - October 2015 Registrar (Otorhinolaryngology) University of Ilorin Teaching Hospital: July 2012 - March 2016 Youth Corps Medical Officer National Youth Service Corps: July. 2011 - June. 2012 Internship (Federal Medical Centre, Lokoja): June 2010 – June 2011.

Tabassum Bashir is pursuing PhD in clinical psychology at department of Psychiatry, J.N Medical College and Hospital, AMU, Aligarh, India. Her research explores several aspects of loops between old versus contemporary therapeutics modules in the management of patients with Alcohol or orther substances related disorders. She is broadly interested in the assessment and management of patients with diverse mental disorders. She has presented research papers at national and international level, published chapters in renowned book publication and attended several seminars and symposium.

Aikaterini Christogianni has a Ph.D. in Experimental and Thermal Physiology from Loughborough University in the UK. She received her MSc in Clinical Neuropsychology at the University of Groningen in the Netherlands during which she was trained in neuropsychological testing procedures, screening, diagnosing, and motoring people with neurological and mental health diseases/disorders. She is interested in improving the quality of life of patients in healthcare systems.

Karen Cordovil graduated in Nutrition from the State University of Rio de Janeiro (UERJ/2006). She completed the Multiprofessional Residency in Family Health at the National School of Public Health Sergio Arouca of Oswaldo Cruz Foundation (ENSP/FIOCRUZ). She received a Master of Science from UERJ (2016). She has experience in Nutrition in Hematology, having more than 12 years of studies dedicated to Nutrition and Sickle Cell Disease. She made a career as a Public Servant at the Health Foundation (FS/SES/RJ) in the State Institute of Hematology Arthur

Siqueira Cavalcanti (HEMORIO/SES/RJ). She also participated as Preceptor of the Program Supervised Internship in Clinical Nutrition at HEMORIO for undergraduate students in Nutrition. Currently, Karen Cordovil is an Excellence Program Scholar Academic (PROEX/CAPES) and Doctoral Student of the Postgraduate Program in Epidemiology at the ENSP/FIOCRUZ. In 2008, Karen received the award for the best scientific work in the postgraduate course in Clinical Nutrition at UFRJ. In 2019, Karen received the UNEGRO Resistance Award at the Legislative Assembly of Rio de Janeiro.

Francesco Zagami was born on January 5, 1954, in Fiumefreddo di Sicilia (Catania), Sicily, and after he attended High School in Giarre (Catania), in 1972 began his medical studies at Catania University and then on July 14 1978 received his M.D. "summa cum laude". After Board Examination (Catania) and qualifying period in clinical pathology in Garibaldi hospital Catania he was engaged on November 7 1979 as a ClinicalPathologist assistant at public hospital Randazzo (Catania). In 1980 he went periodically to the Virologydepartment of the "D. Cotugno" hospital in Naples, where he worked with Prof. Giulio Tarro as a voluntary association in his group of viro-oncology research until 1990. On July 20, 1984, he obtain in CataniaUniversity postgraduate with in Clinical Biology. He is the author, alone or in the group, of 76 medical scientific articles published in specialized journals or in medical books, and has been a speaker in over 150 national or international medical congresses. A fraction of his articles are online in: and, as an independent researcher, while for help-forum see: . Recently is USMLEmember Toronto, Ontario, Canada, PathLabTalk – USA, The American Society of Hematology WashingtonDC – USA, and Journal of Medical Association Thailand and China.Address email: francesco_zagami@virgilio.it and cell. Mobile 0039.329.1809146.

Zarnish Habib is an author and entrepreneur with a degree from Uni. Of Leeds, UK. Habib has written books and papers on various niche including business, nursing, self-help, and fantasy. Habib also teaches in workshops and groups of writers and authors.

Masato Hada has a Bachelor of Medicine and Pharmacy Medical Doctor at Masato Hada's Lab. Retired Surgeon. Currently, he is fully committed to the spread of severe COVID-19 pneumonia treatment.

Muhammad Haider has an MBBS, MRCP (Irland), FCPS (Pakistan); Consultant Internist, KFAFH, Jeddah.

Catherine Hayes qualified in podiatric Medicine in 1992 and was a Founding Fellow of the Faculty of Podiatric Medicine (Royal College of Physicians and Surgeons, Glasgow) in 2012 following the award of Fellowship of the College of Podiatry and General Practice (London) in 2010. She undertakes pedagogic scholarship and research and is Programme Leader for the University of Sunderland's Professional Doctorate suite of pathways at City Campus, Sunderland. Catherine is a UK National Teaching Fellow and is Principal Fellow of Higher Education Advance.

Tabish Igbal completed six years integrated cardiology postgraduate programme from National Institute of Cardiovascular Diseases under Medical University, Dhaka, Bangladesh. Formerly attached with AMRI Hospital, Kolkata, India. Presently working in Armed forces hospital Wadi ad-Dawasir as consultant cardiologist in the department of medicine.

Ayesha Jamal did her M.B.B.S from Rehman medical college in the year 2020 with a distinction in OBGYN .During her final year electives she worked with an eminent oncologist in the US in Hospice Care. She later moved to Canada and joined Red Cross. She is currently working as a clinical assistant in Canada . She aspires to bring a change by contributing in geriatric medicine and hospice care

Sheraz Jamal Khan Secretary, Faculty of General Medicine, College of Physicians and Surgeons, Pakistan. Professor of Medicine, Hayatabad Medical Complex, Peshawar, Pakistan.

Danyah Katlan, PharmD, BCPS Senior Clinical Pharmacist at King Fahad Armed Forces Hospital (KFAFH) Jeddah, Saudi Arabia Danyah Katlan is the Head of Clinical Pharmacy Department at KFAFH. Hematology/Oncology specialized clinical pharmacist. Accomplished ASHP accredited PGY1 program at King Abdulaziz Medical City-Jeddah then worked as Internal Medicine Clinical Pharmacist for 2 years. Afterthat she obtained her PGY2 in hematology/oncology subspecialty

Taha Musa is a leading staff in Biomedical Research Institute, Darfur University College, Nyala, Sudan. He is researcher and promoter of disease awareness and health sciences in developing countries. He has more than 140 publications and exactly 1243 citations.

Gulfisha Qureshi Completed her Doctoral degree in Applied Psychology from Aligarh Muslim University and most of her research work on mental health, resilience and widowhood in Indian context. Additionally, she passed the national level competitive exam (NET) in India. She is actively involved in social psychology, health psychology and women studies. Recently she published a " staking experience scale".

Rimsha Razzaq is currently working on transcriptome analysis, molecular docking and in-silico drug designing in SBB, PU, Lahore. Previously, I have worked on infectious diseases particularly w.r.t Escherichia coli (prevalence of integrons in different phylogenetic groups of E.coli).

Mohammed Reyazuddin has done MBBS and MD in Psychiatry from Jawaharlal Nehru Medical College in 2006 and 2012 respectively. Currently, he is working as an Assistant Professor of Psychiatry at J.N. Medical College. He had also worked as a consultant psychiatrist in the National Mental health Programme at the district hospital, Aligarh. His interest areas include movement disorders, seizure disorders, and neurodegenerative disorders.

Zafar Rizvi completed doctoral degree in social psychology and most of his research work on Procrastination, stress, anxiety and flourishing on medical students and cancer patients. He is also actively Involved in an interdisciplinary field of psychology (Philosophy of neuroscience, Philosophy of psychology, cognitive psychology, Neuroscience and Artificial Intelligence). Currently, he is working on Philosophy of psychology in which he is trying to find out the answers about "we" and "I" through phenomenological approaches, Existential approach, Reductionism, ontology, meta physical approaches. He is also interested in Artificial Intelligence and working on consciousness studies. Other works in progress on consciousness studies. Recently his Interviews Published in Newspaper's e.g., Times of India, The Indian Express and Outlook, Hindustan times on various psychological related topics.

Khawar Shabbir is a highly accomplished pharmacist with more than 30 years of professional experience in both hospital and community setting, had eceived accolades and commendation throughout my career for exceptional patient service and strong work ethics. I have gained excellent communication and interpersonal skills alongside the ability to solve drug related problems and handle challenging situations. I am no stranger to pharmacy practice including but not limited to, clinical pharmacy practice, hospital pharmacy practice, community practice, clinical consultant pharmacy practice, health educator consultant speaker, medication dispensing and medication therapy monitoring. I have democrated sound understanding of the principles underlying pharmaceutical care with an ability to recognize therapeutic incompatibilities. I was appointed as Adjunct Clinical Assistant Professor to supervise training for sixth year PharmD students of King Abdulaziz University for 12 years and was awarded certificates of participation and appreciation. In recognition to my contribution toward the Pharmacy profession for more than 25 hyears, Ontario College of Pharmacists Canada has awarded me certificate of Emeritus.

Mian Mufareh Shah did his MBBS from Khyber Medical University in the year 2012 and his FCPS from College of Physician and Surgeons Pakistan. He worked as registrar, Speciality registrar and now Assistant Professor at Post Graduate Medical Institute, Hayatabad Medical Complex Peshawar, Pakistan in the department of Internal Medicine. He has been trained in various disciples of internal Medicine. He is an avid researcher, teacher and clinician. He teaches and trains both undergraduates and postgraduates and as a faculty member works on administrative, academic and research positions. He has been a mastertrainer for pharmacists and is an integral member of international trials and antibiotic stewardship program

Alaa Shahbar, Pharm.D, BCPS Umm Alqura University, Faculty of Pharmacy, Clinical Pharmacy Department, Makkah, Saudi Arabia Alaa Shahbar is a teaching assistant in Umm alqura university, practicing oncology and hematology clinical pharmacy at umm alqura affiliated hospitals. Alaa has obtained his PGY-2 in oncology and hematology pharmacy at king Abdulaziz Medical City-Jeddah in 2022.

Ahmad Sheraz is currently working on a vaccine development program in SBS, PU, Lahore. Previously, Sheraz has worked on infectious diseases, particularly w.r.t Staphylococcus aureus (association of integrons with drug resistance genes).

Suhaiza Suroya is a doctoral researcher at the School of Design and Creative Arts, Loughborough University, U.K. She holds a Master of Art & Design with a specialisation in Visual Communication and New Media. Since then, she works as a lecturer in Graphic Design & Digital Media in the Faculty of Art & Design, Universiti Teknologi MARA, Malaysia from the year 2009. She also has a background in Business Administration (Hons) in Marketing, 2004. Her current research focuses on the study of typographic customisation in the context of legibility and readability and its application to dyslexic reading and other forms of learning disabilities.

Index

A

C

D

E

F

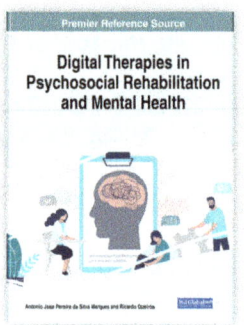
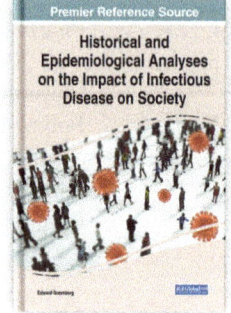
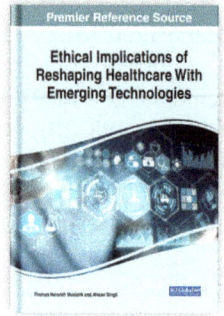
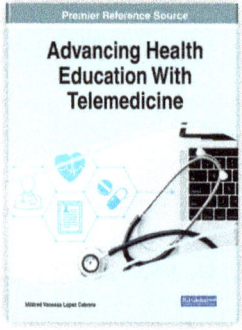
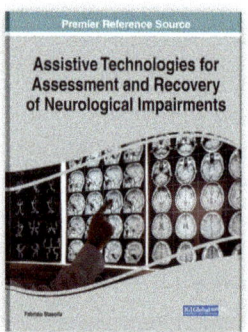
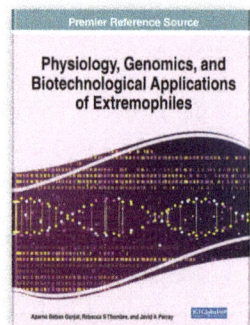
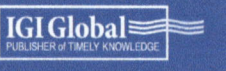

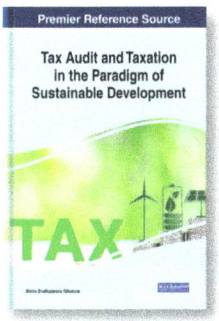
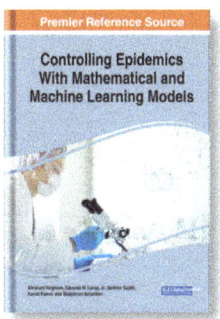
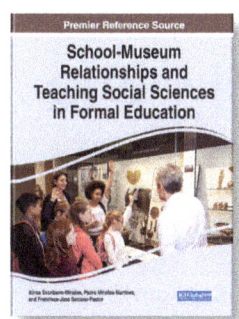
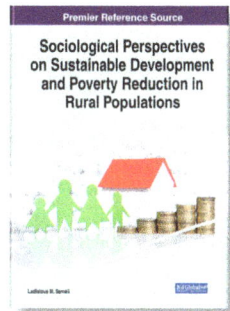

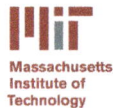 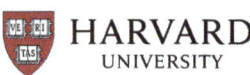 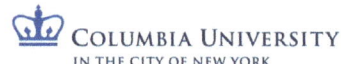 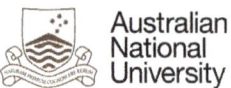
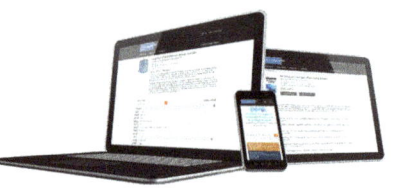
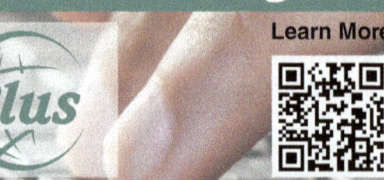

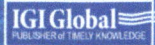
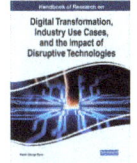
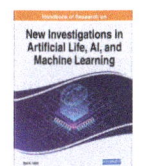
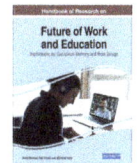
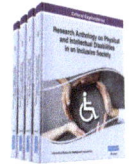
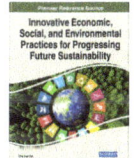
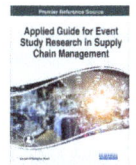
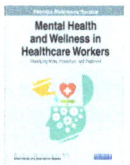
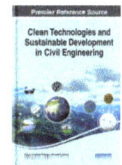

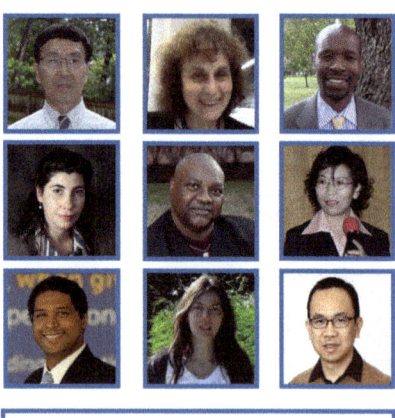
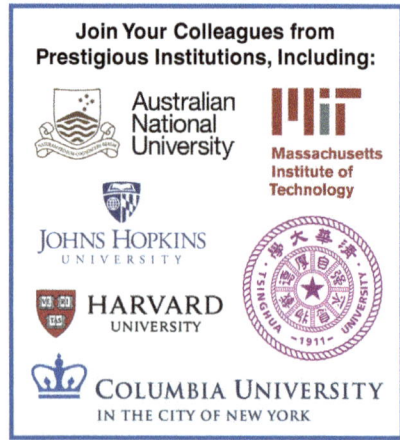

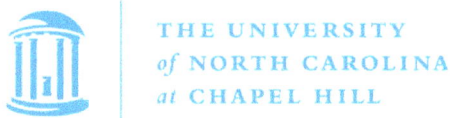
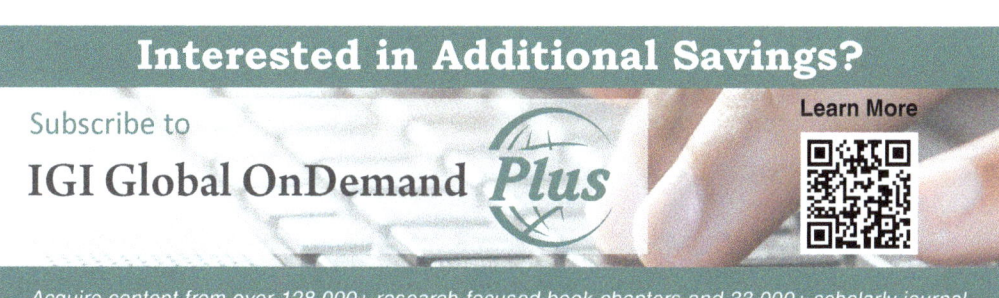

Ingram Content Group UK Ltd.
Milton Keynes UK
UKHW020643100423
419910UK00003B/26